# The Clinical Nurse Specialist in Theory and Practice

## Second Edition

*Edited by*

**Ann B. Hamric, M.S., R.N.**

*Associate Director of Nursing for*
*Research and Development*
*Medical College of Virginia Hospitals*
*Richmond, Virginia*

**Judith A. Spross, M.S., R.N., C.S., O.C.N.**

*Assistant Professor*
*MGH Institute of Health Professions;*
*Clinical Nurse Specialist*
*Massachusetts General Hospital*
*Cancer Pain Center*
*Boston, Massachusetts*

**W.B. SAUNDERS COMPANY**
Harcourt Brace Jovanovich, Inc.
*Philadelphia/London/Toronto/Montreal/Sydney/Tokyo*

**W. B. SAUNDERS COMPANY**

Harcourt Brace Jovanovich, Inc.

The Curtis Center
Independence Square West
Philadelphia, PA 19106

**Library of Congress Cataloging-in-Publication Data**

The clinical nurse specialist in theory and practice.

Includes bibliographies and index.

1. Nurse practitioners.   I. Hamric, Ann B.   II. Spross,
   Judith A.   [DNLM: 1. Nurse Clinicians.   WY 128 C639]

RT82.8.C573 1989      610.73′6      88-30612

ISBN 0-7216-4486-4

*Editor:*   Thomas Eoyang

*Manuscript Editor:*   Keryn Lane

*Production Manager:*   Frank Polizzano

*Indexer:*   Linda VanPelt

# CONTRIBUTORS

JOANNE BAGGERLY, M.S., R.N., C.R.R.N., C.N.R.N.
Clinical Nurse Specialist in Neuroscience and Rehabilitation Nursing, Department of Nursing, Massachusetts General Hospital, Boston, Massachusetts
*Models of Advanced Nursing Practice*

SUSAN B. BAIRD, M.P.H., R.N.
Doctoral Candidate and Research Associate, University of Pennsylvania School of Nursing, Philadelphia, Pennsylvania; Editor, *Oncology Nursing Forum*
*Administratively Enhancing CNS Contributions*

ANNE-MARIE BARRON, M.S., R.N., C.S.
Lecturer, Curry College, Division of Nursing Studies, Milton, Massachusetts
*The CNS as Consultant*

SARAH JO BROWN, M.S., R.N.
Doctoral Candidate, University of Rhode Island, Kingston, Rhode Island
*Supportive Supervision of the CNS*

SUSAN E. DAVIS DOUGHTY, M.S.N., R.N., C.S.
Director, Critical Care Nursing, Maine Medical Center, Portland, Maine
*The CNS in a Nurse-Managed Center*

SHIRLEY A. GIROUARD, Ph.D., R.N., F.A.A.N.
Program Officer, The Robert Wood Johnson Foundation, Princeton, New Jersey
*Health Policy: Implications for the CNS*

JOYCE L. GOURNIC, M.S.N., R.N.
Director, Cardiopulmonary Rehabilitation, Alexandria Hospital, Alexandria, Virginia
*Clinical Leadership, Management, and the CNS*

LORRY GRESHAM KENTON, M.S., R.N.
Formerly Assistant Professor, Rush University College of Nursing; formerly Practitioner-Teacher, Department of Gerontological Nursing, Rush-Presbyterian-St. Luke's Medical Center, Chicago, Illinois
*The CNS in Collaborative Relationships Between Nursing Service and Nursing Education*

KERRY V. HARWOOD, M.S.N., R.N.

Clinical Nurse Specialist, The Johns Hopkins Oncology Center, Department of Nursing, Baltimore, Maryland

*The CNS as Researcher*

HARRIET J. KITZMAN, Ph.D., R.N.

Associate Professor of Nursing and Pediatrics, University of Rochester, Rochester, New York

*The CNS and the Nurse Practitioner*

THERESA L. KOETTERS, M.S., R.N.

Assistant Clinical Professor, Department of Physiological Nursing, School of Nursing, University of California at San Francisco; Oncology Clinical Nurse Specialist, Sequoia Hospital District, Redwood City, California

*Clinical Practice and Direct Patient Care*

BEVERLY L. MALONE, Ph.D., R.N., F.A.A.N.

Dean of Nursing, North Carolina Agricultural and Technical State University, Greensboro, North Carolina

*The CNS in a Consultation Department*

DEBORAH B. McGUIRE, Ph.D., M.S., R.N.

Assistant Professor, The Johns Hopkins University School of Nursing; Director of Nursing Research, The Johns Hopkins Oncology Center, Department of Nursing, Baltimore, Maryland

*The CNS as Researcher*

ANN-REID PRIEST, M.S.N., R.N

Clinical Nurse Specialist, Liver Transplant Program, Medical College of Virginia Hospitals, Richmond, Virginia

*The CNS as Educator*

MARILYN P. PROUTY, M.S., R.N.

(Retired) Senior Vice-President of Nursing, Mary Hitchcock Memorial Hospital, Dartmouth Hitchcock Medical Center, Hanover, New Hampshire

*Administratively Enhancing CNS Contributions*

SALLY A. SAMPLE, M.N., R.N.

Assistant Dean for Clinical Affairs, University of Michigan School of Nursing; Associate Hospital Director for Nursing, University of Michigan Hospitals, Ann Arbor, Michigan

*Justifying and Structuring the CNS Role Within a Nursing Organization*

MARIAH SNYDER, Ph.D., R.N., F.A.A.N.

Professor, School of Nursing, University of Minnesota, Minneapolis, Minnesota

*Educational Preparation of the CNS*

PATRICIA STEWART, M.S., R.N., C.R.R.N.

Clinical Nurse Specialist and Rehabilitation Nursing Consultant, Rehabilitation Nursing Resources, P.C., Albuquerque, New Mexico

*The CNS in Private Practice*

JOYCE WATERMAN TAYLOR, M.S.N., R.N., C.S., F.A.A.N.

Clinical Nurse Specialist in Neuroscience, Kaiser Permanente Hospital, Fontana, California

*Role Development of the CNS*

ANNE EDGERTON WINCH, M.S.N., R.N., C.P.N.P.

Instructor, University of Virginia School of Nursing; Clinical Nurse Specialist, Pediatrics, University of Virginia Hospitals—Children's Medical Center, Charlottesville, Virginia

*Peer Support and Peer Review*

# ACKNOWLEDGMENTS

We acknowledge and appreciate the hard work of our contributors, most of whom created entirely new chapters for this edition. We are grateful to the CNSs, graduate students, educators, and administrators who have talked with us about the issues they face; these conversations helped us realize the need to revise this book and helped shape the revision. Finally, we are indebted to Thomas Eoyang, Senior Nursing Editor at W. B. Saunders Company, for his strong and thoughtful support and advocacy.

# PREFACE TO THE SECOND EDITION

In the six years since the publication of the first edition of *The Clinical Nurse Specialist in Theory and Practice*, much has been learned about the role of the clinical nurse specialist (CNS), and much has changed in the health care system. Significant developments, such as DRG-based reimbursement mechanisms, increased acuity of hospitalized patients, high-tech home care, and the nursing shortage, have underscored and supported the need for the expertise of the CNS. At the same time, cost containment has placed severe constraints on health care institutions; as a result, CNS positions have been jeopardized in some areas of the country, while in others the role has flourished.

Despite regional variability in the development of the role, the CNS is certainly a more visible presence within nursing today than when the first edition appeared. There are more publications by and about CNSs, including a journal, *The Clinical Nurse Specialist*, devoted exclusively to CNS role issues. The nature of expert practice has been better defined, and literature in specialty journals also addresses CNS practice more frequently.

Taking advantage of this burgeoning knowledge base, the second edition of *The Clinical Nurse Specialist in Theory and Practice* is theoretically as well as experientially grounded. In addition to referring broadly to the current literature, the contributing authors share wisdom and strategies gained from experience in CNS practice or from teaching and supervising student and practicing CNSs. This revision is essentially a new work, with over 70% of the material original to the second edition. Although it rests on the shoulders of the first edition, this book is considerably different in scope and content from our first effort. The thorough nature of this revision reflects the growth in our understanding about the realities of CNS practice as well as changes in the health care system that have had a decided impact on the CNS role.

The first section, "Theoretical Aspects of the CNS Role," explores the historical, theoretical, and conceptual bases of role development, advanced practice, and evaluation. These concepts and models are followed throughout the book, which we believe gives the second edition considerably more conceptual clarity and consistency than we were able to effect with the first edition. New research-based data is the basis for discussion of developmental phases and practical strategies to enhance CNS role development.

The second section, "Subroles and Competencies," has been expanded to address all subroles. In addition to a more complete description of the direct care role and its importance, new chapters on the education subrole, collaboration, and leadership competencies have been added. Readers will appreciate the clear description of the research subrole.

The third section, "Nursing Administration and the CNS," examines the CNS role from an administrative perspective, with a focus on utilization, placement, and support of those in CNS positions. The fourth section addresses several contemporary concerns: CNS education, collaborative relations between service and education, the CNS and health policy, and CNS and nurse practitioner roles. Rather than speculate on the future as we did in the first edition, the final section describes innovative models that promote and support advanced practice and also offers practical advice for initiating them.

As with the first edition, this book is intended for practicing CNSs, graduate students, educators, and administrators. For practicing CNSs and students, the book contains both theoretical and practical content to guide role implementation. Educators can use the text in graduate classes for anticipatory guidance of student CNSs. Administrators can use the text to help make decisions about utilization and evaluation of CNSs and to assist in analyzing problem situations.

The editors remain committed to the worth and necessity of the CNS role to advance the practice of nursing. We hope that this edition of *The Clinical Nurse Specialist in Theory and Practice* provides an authoritative and accessible resource for understanding the versatile and complex CNS role. In addition, we offer the second edition as a practical guide for promoting, strengthening, and evaluating CNS practice.

# CONTENTS

# PART V  INNOVATIVE PRACTICE MODELS

# PART I

# THEORETICAL ASPECTS OF THE CNS ROLE

# History and Overview of the CNS Role

*Ann B. Hamric*

## HISTORICAL DEVELOPMENT OF THE CNS ROLE

The idea of specialists in nursing is not new to the profession. The first issue of the *American Journal of Nursing* contains an article entitled "Specialties in Nursing" (DeWitt, 1900), and as early as 1910, nurses were designated as specialists. For the first half of the twentieth century, however, the term "specialist" denoted a nurse with extensive experience in a particular area of nursing, a nurse who completed a hospital-based "postgraduate" course, or a nurse who performed with technical expertise. Private duty nurses are prime examples of these early specialists. Nurses with extensive experience in one clinical area have continued to consider themselves specialized.

The idea of a specialist in clinical nursing prepared at the master's level represented a significant variation from traditional practitioners. Originated for the purpose of improving the quality of nursing care provided to patients, the clinical nurse specialist (CNS) role is a relatively recent development within the profession. Various authors have assigned the origin of the CNS concept to different groups at different times. Peplau stated that the title dates from 1938 (Peplau, 1965). Reiter first used the title "nurse clinician" in 1943 to describe a nurse with advanced knowledge and clinical competence committed to providing the highest quality of nursing care (Reiter, 1966). Although Reiter did not believe that a master's degree alone qualified one to be a nurse clinician, she noted that organized graduate education programs represented the most efficient means of quickly preparing such practition-

3

ers. Norris stated that the CNS concept was first advanced in 1944 with the Committee to Study Postgraduate Clinical Nursing Courses of the National League for Nursing Education (Norris, 1977). Smoyak credited a national conference of directors of graduate programs, held in 1949 and sponsored by the University of Minnesota, with advancing the concept in a formal setting (Smoyak, 1976). A major impediment to the realization of the CNS concept during this period was the existing assumption that education for nursing practice ended at the diploma level. "Postgraduate" courses were offered in specialty hospitals as supervised on-the-job training experiences (Norris, 1977). Even into the 1950s, nurses in both baccalaureate and master's level courses were in the same classroom, receiving the same instruction (Smoyak, 1976).

For the first half of the twentieth century, specialization in graduate education in nursing consisted of functional rather than clinical preparation. Nurses who wished to become specialized took courses in administration, teaching, or supervision (Smoyak, 1976). Sills noted the following reasons for this direction in nursing: the preparation of nursing's early graduate leaders at Teachers College, Columbia University; the post–World War II increase in hospital care demands and nursing's subsequent shift from a private duty model to a supervisory model within a hospital's bureaucratic structure; and the attendant issues associated with nursing being predominantly a woman's profession. All these factors "created situations which were inimical to the growth of clinical practice in nursing" (Sills, 1983, p. 565).

The specialty of psychiatric nursing is credited with being the first to develop graduate level clinical experiences. Critchley noted the dramatic effect of nurses returning from service during World War II eligible for advanced education under the GI Bill. "The existing programs were unable to meet the demand. In 1946, with the passage of the National Mental Health Act research and training funds were provided for the core mental health disciplines. Psychiatric nursing was designated a core discipline and thus received federal funds for both undergraduate and graduate nurse education. The National Mental Health Act provided funding and influenced the scope and direction of nursing and psychiatric nursing education" (Critchley, 1985, p. 12). In 1954, Peplau developed the first master's program focused exclusively on the development of an advanced practitioner in psychiatric nursing at Rutgers University. Sills considered Peplau's work to be "the major driving force for the preparation of clinical specialists at the graduate (master's) level" (Sills, 1983, p. 566).

Oncology nursing is another area that developed graduate education for specialization early in its evolution. In 1947, Nelson initiated a graduate course in cancer nursing. Early efforts were spearheaded by the American Cancer Society and the National Cancer Institute (Craytor, 1982). The American Cancer Society continues to take a keen interest in the development of CNSs in oncology, as exemplified by its curriculum guide and role definition, "The Master's Degree with a Specialty in Cancer Nursing" (American Cancer Society, 1979). The Oncology Nursing Society has also been credited with establishing cancer nursing as a specialty and contributing to the development of the oncology CNS role (Spross, 1983).

In 1963, expansion of the Professional Nurse Traineeship Program to include CNS education provided a major impetus to develop graduate program content in advanced clinical nursing. This expansion, together with a growth in the number of baccalaureate-prepared nurses and the profession's increasing interest in graduate education, led to the firm establishment of education for clinical specialization within graduate programs. By 1984, there were 129 accredited programs preparing clinical nurse specialists (National League for Nursing, 1984).*

Evidence of the growing acceptance of the CNS role can be seen from the report of the Task Force on Nursing Practice in Hospitals: "Apparently many of the hospitals employ clinical specialists, who add a dimension of nursing care that would otherwise not be available to patients and their families. The participants in the study consider these individuals, because of their advanced knowledge and skills, to be valuable resources to the staff as well as enriching the practice environment" (McClure, et al., 1983, p. 90). And, in the final report of the National Commission on Nursing, the continuing need for specialists was recognized. "The complexity of patient care continues to require more sophisticated nursing roles and functions, and the educational requirements for quality nursing care have increased. . . . Effective leadership by clinical nurse specialists, managers of nursing divisions, and head nurses in patient care units is viewed by nurses as critical to developing an appropriate environment for clinical nursing practice" (1983, p. 5). The American Nurses Association (ANA) stated, "Specialization in nursing is now clearly established" (ANA, 1980, p. 22). Yet concerns continue to be expressed regarding the future of the CNS

---

*Development of the CNS role in England is relatively recent in comparison with the U.S., although it appears to be occurring along similar lines. In a series of articles in *Nursing Mirror*, Castledine noted that nurses who perform a particular technical skill very well consider themselves specialists. In a study on the role and function of CNSs in England and Wales, Castledine found that of 300 respondents, only 2 had master's degrees in nursing. At the time of these articles, there was only one university in England where a master's degree with a clinical option was available. Castledine echoes U.S. nursing's past optimism about the potential of the CNS in stating, "I believe that the creation and development of the CNS holds the key to the future." (Castledine, 1983, p. 52).

role and its viability in the face of mounting pressures within the health care system to decrease costs.

## SPECIALIZATION AND THE CNS ROLE

Before describing the CNS role in detail, it is important to distinguish between specialization in nursing and the clinical nurse specialist role. As the ANA noted, "Specialization is a mark of the advancement of the nursing profession" (ANA, 1980). Specialization involves concentration on selected phenomena within the domain of nursing. Both societal and professional forces continue to shape the direction of nursing specialization. Societal forces that have contributed to the increase in specialization include growth in the amount and complexity of knowledge and technology, the focus of public attention on the need for specialization and funds available for a specific area of practice (ANA, 1980, p. 21), and rapid change with the concomitant need for institutions and individuals to adapt and respond to this change (Naisbitt, 1982). Professional forces include the presence within nursing of pioneers who test out new practices and obtain greater depth of understanding of a segment of nursing, response to expansion in a part of a professional field, increase in complexity of services (ANA, 1980), and nursing's desire to advance in a more clinical direction (Christman, 1965). The nursing profession has responded in various ways to these driving forces for specialization. The implementation of training programs for nurse midwives, nurse anesthetists, and nurse practitioners has been one response; the development of specialized faculty and researchers has been another; and the creation of specialty organizations can be considered a third.

The development of the CNS has been yet another response to these forces. It is important to distinguish between nurses who have specialized in an area of nursing and those who are clinical nurse specialists. As can be seen above, nurse anesthetists, nurse practitioners, nurse faculty, and nurse researchers can all be considered specialists in an area of nursing; some of them may have advanced education in a clinical specialty as well. They are not necessarily clinical nurse specialists, however. How then can one distinguish between clinical nurse specialists and those who have specialized within nursing? And why is this distinction important for understanding and strengthening the CNS role?

The CNS role has been broadly conceived in nursing literature. Early writers emphasized the CNS as an expert direct care provider, "who serves as a model of expertness representing advanced or newly developing practices to the general staff nurse . . . who gives direct care to a selected case load of patients, who studies and reports her practices through publications" (Peplau, 1965, pp. 276–284). Christman outlined other roles for the CNS: experiential teaching to help less trained personnel, serving as a resource to other personnel, assisting in establishing standards, and possessing "some beginning investigatory competency" (Christman, 1965, pp. 450–451). These indirect functions of education, consultation, and research have received a great deal of attention in the literature (Baker & Kramer, 1970; Georgopoulos & Christman, 1970; Riehl & McVay, 1970; Padilla & Padilla, 1979), with writers emphasizing the CNS role in facilitating the clinical competence of nursing staff (Blount, et al., 1981), as well as the CNS role as consultant and liaison in developing staff (Everson, 1981). Everson went so far as to deny a direct practice role for the CNS in writing, "If both the system and the specialist agree that she should be a resource for broad system changes, then diluting her efforts toward this goal with administrative or direct patient care responsibilities confuses and weakens her role" (Everson, 1981, p. 17).

This versatility of role definition has been both a bane and a blessing. In spite of the efforts of professional organizations and selected individuals to define the CNS, as recently as 1983, Sills felt safe in assuming that there is "a low level of consensus about what should be the normative dimensions of the position" (Sills, 1983, p. 567). Within the profession, nurses who function solely as staff educators call themselves CNSs, nurses in administrative positions call themselves CNSs, and nurses with extensive experience but no master's degree call themselves CNSs. Unfortunately, the title has been seen by some nurses as a professional attribute, a mark of their achievement of a graduate clinical education or clinical expertise, rather than as a discrete work role with describable functions. In its enthusiasm over the potential of the role, the profession has tended to make the CNS "all things to all people." As a result, "individual specialists are often left to define and develop their own positions within institutions. These efforts have produced widely differing practice modes, role confusion as well as role diversity, and varying degrees of success in achieving the original goal of improved nursing practice" (Hamric, 1983, p. xi).

While it seems desirable for the profession to view specialization in nursing broadly so that innovative strategies continue to be developed to meet changing needs, at a professional and institutional level, the role of the CNS must be clarified in order to reduce confusion. Consensus regarding the defining characteristics of the CNS role and restriction of the title of CNS to those nurses who meet the defining characteristics will strengthen the role in a number of ways. Such consensus will allow for more consistency in graduate curricula and in the competencies of graduates. Role clarity is especially critical in explaining the CNS to consumers, administrators, and third party payors. Agreement on the role parameters of the CNS can improve the understanding of other health care disciplines and consequent collaborative efforts with these disciplines. Building advocacy for the role within the nursing profession, especially among staff nurses and administrators, will be enhanced by such consensus. It is difficult, if not impossible, to justify CNS positions in an institution when ambiguity in CNS definition and resultant lack of performance criteria abound. Different institutions will have different emphases, and emphases will shift over time as institutional needs change and as the individual CNS evolves the role. But the framework must be stable and the expectations clear and realistic.

## DEFINING CHARACTERISTICS OF THE CNS ROLE

The ANA defined the CNS as a registered nurse "who, through study and supervised practice at the graduate level (master's or doctorate), has become expert in a defined area of knowledge and practice in

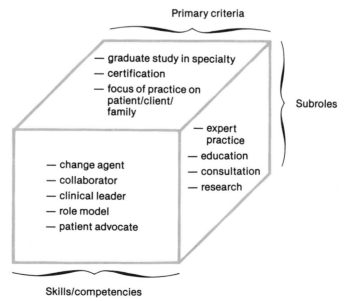

**Figure 1–1.** Defining characteristics of the CNS role.

a selected clinical area of nursing" (ANA, 1980, p. 23). The CNS role is multifaceted, with many components and defining characteristics. Any attempt to fully describe the CNS must be multifaceted as well. This discussion will examine the role from four perspectives. First, certain baseline or primary criteria must be met before one can be considered a CNS. Second, the four major subroles of the CNS must be practiced. Third, there is a set of skills or competencies the CNS uses in implementing the subroles. These three sets of characteristics form the core definition of the CNS. Relationships between these defining characteristics are shown in Figure 1–1.

There is a fourth set of characteristics that, while not an inherent part of the definition, influence CNS role expression. These variables are diagrammed in Figure 1–2. Each of these areas will be discussed in depth in subsequent chapters, so this will be an overview discussion. The goal is to identify the multiple responsibilities and competencies of the CNS and to demonstrate the complex interplay between elements that combine to form this advanced practice role.

## Primary Criteria for CNS Practice

The ANA has identified two primary criteria for specialists in nursing practice: "(1) an earned graduate degree (master's degree or doctorate) that represents study of scientific knowledge and supervised

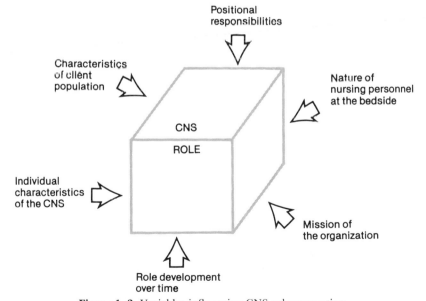

**Figure 1–2.** Variables influencing CNS role expression.

advanced clinical practice related to a particular area within the scope of nursing; (2) eligibility requirements for certification through the professional society or completion of the certification process" (ANA, 1980, p. 24). Graduate study prepares the CNS for expert practice, including the abilities to analyze complex clinical problems, to consider a wide range of theory, to selectively apply theories appropriately, and to foresee short- and long-range consequences of nursing actions (ANA, 1980). Certification is a judgment made by the profession that the specialist meets criteria of expert competence. "Through credentialing of those nurses who claim competence at an expert level, the nursing profession assures the public that these claims of a higher standard of nursing competence are not false" (ANA, 1980, p. 24).

The third primary element essential to the definition of the CNS is the focus of practice on the patient/client/family. Regardless of setting, the CNS's practice is directed toward improving patient care and nursing practice. The ANA Council of Clinical Nurse Specialists has clearly articulated the primary nature of this criterion: "To fulfill the clinical nurse specialist's role, the nurse must have a client-based practice" (ANA, 1986, p. 2). It is clear from this statement that if the focus of the practice shifts to education, the CNS becomes a nurse educator; if the shift is to research, the CNS becomes a nurse researcher. If the CNS does not maintain a clinical practice and a focus on the patient/client/family, that individual ceases to be a CNS and should not use the title.

### Subroles of CNS Practice

While these characteristics are necessary to define the CNS role, they are not sufficient. There is a complex interplay of subroles and competencies that further define the CNS and differentiate this nurse from other advanced practitioners. The four generally accepted subroles that the CNS uses are: expert practice, consultation, education, and research. The CNS role was created to bring the expertise of advanced practitioners directly to the patient/client, so the expert practitioner component is really the sine qua non of the CNS role. As Norris stated, ". . . specialization is synonymous with practice, i.e., one simply cannot remain a specialist and function only as a teacher or coordinator or administrator" (Norris, 1977, p. 23). CNSs give highly expert nursing care to patients with complex health problems by virtue of their advanced education and expanded practice base.

The remaining subroles have been characterized as indirect practice roles in contrast to the direct practice role discussed above (Hamric, 1983; Sills, 1983). The consultation subrole involves both intra- and inter-professional consultation (ANA, 1980, p. 26). The importance of this subrole has been identified by Fenton in an ethnographic study of the CNS role (1985). The education subrole includes formal and informal teaching of staff nurses, graduate, and undergraduate students in nursing and other disciplines. (Patient education is commonly considered to be an element of expert practice [Benner, 1984], rather than part of this sub-role.) The fourth subrole is that of research. "The CNS is expected to initiate relevant clinical studies, as well as translate research findings into routine clinical practice" (Hamric, 1983, p. 42). It is difficult to prescribe a level of activity in each subrole, although different time percentages in each category have been identified (Wright, 1984; Walker, 1986; Topham, 1987), as the focus of practice changes over time and is highly sensitive to the variables influencing role expression. However, each subrole should be enacted in some degree for the nurse to be considered a CNS.

## Skills/Competencies of the CNS

The next group of defining characteristics reflects the skills or competencies the CNS uses in practicing the role components. These are not subroles because the CNS utilizes these skills in all the subroles. The first and perhaps the most classic competency is that of change agent. "Indeed, central to the position of the C.N.S. is a set of ideas about change. Inherent in all that the C.N.S. does is the fundamental notion of attempting to alter or change the course of some human experience. . ." (Sills, 1983, p. 571). Fenton's study documented that "the CNS is most creative in developing ways to institute change in an organization that resists change" (Fenton, 1985, p. 33). This competency involves innovation as well. CNSs bring bold new ideas to nursing practice. They are not afraid to try new approaches to "shake up" the system for the sake of improved patient care (Hamric, 1983, p. 42).

The competency of collaboration, i.e., working together with colleagues in different disciplines as well as within nursing, includes liaison activities as well. Collaboration requires skill in communication and in maintaining effective interpersonal relationships. The CNS continually interacts with other caregivers and organizational units to achieve patient care goals (Holt, 1984). The CNS serves as a link of communication, a bridge of continuity between disparate parts of the health care system. "Building and maintaining a therapeutic team in order to provide optimum therapy," one of Benner's expert nurse competencies, was found by Fenton to be very significant in CNS practice in providing effective patient care and in maintaining morale among treatment team members (Fenton, 1985).

Clinical leadership is another important skill needed by CNSs. "Clinical and professional leadership is inherent in the CNS role—it is not optional" (Spross and Donoghue, 1984, p. 78). The importance of this competency is being increasingly recognized (Paulen, 1985). Hodges, Poteet, and Edlund asserted, "Clinical nurse specialists need sharply-honed leadership and management skills to work effectively in today's complex hospital organizations. Below par skills are threatening the demise of this nursing role" (1985, p. 193). Leadership involves many activities, such as problem-solving, setting priorities, exercising authority by virtue of one's expert power base, and providing emotional and situational support. Fenton noted, "The finding that the CNS has the emotional support of the nursing staff as a primary activity was a surprise, as it is not usually included in job descriptions. . . .The CNS may work only with the nurse to resolve the problem or she may use her skills and contacts to get the system to respond to the problem" (Fenton, 1985, p. 33).

A competency long recognized as inherent in CNS practice is that of professional role model for staff nurses. The CNS demonstrates desirable practice behaviors for others to emulate. Indeed, whether consulting, teaching, or conducting research, the CNS models professional behaviors for professional staff.

The CNS also demonstrates skill as a patient advocate. Although all nurses should be patient advocates, this competency requires self-confidence, assertiveness, and a sense of assurance that comes from expertise. These requirements make patient advocacy a difficult competency for staff nurses to actualize. The CNS's primary commitment is to help the patient, rather than the institution, physicians, or staff members. Patient advocacy was identified in Fenton's study as a major function of the expert nurse in working with nursing staff, other professionals, and the bureaucratic system. "The CNS serves as a path finder for those patients whose needs get lost in the system" (Fenton, 1985, p. 34). Fenton identified "massaging the system" to make the bureaucracy respond to patients and family needs as an organizational competency; to this author, massaging the system is an integral aspect of patient advocacy. Although Fenton identified patient advocacy as part of the consultant subrole, this author believes it transcends that role component and is a skill used by the CNS in each subrole.

## VARIABLES INFLUENCING CNS ROLE EXPRESSION

The criteria, subroles, and skills/competencies described above comprise the core definition of the CNS role. There are, however, other variables that influence role implementation, as represented in Figure 1–2. Although not inherent in the role's definition, they significantly affect how the role will be expressed. These variables are: responsibilities related to the type of position the CNS has within the organization (whether line, staff, or joint appointment; whether unit-based or population-based); characteristics of the client population (whether primarily inpatient or outpatient, type of illness, age); the mission of the organization in which the CNS practices (a small community hospital, a large tertiary teaching center, a community center, or a private practice may each have very different missions, as well as missions that change over time); individual characteristics of the CNS; and role development over time.

All CNSs have certain organizational responsibilities such as committee activities, but the type and amount of responsibility vary greatly according to the expectations of the position and type of organization in which the CNS practices. Administrative or managerial responsibilities assume increased importance for the CNS in a line position. Staff supervision, budget preparation, participation in strategic planning, and organizational goal-setting are examples of activities that CNSs may be involved in depending upon their position. Some authors maintain that supervisory functions are an inherent part of the CNS's function (Sills, 1983, p. 571). This author disagrees, although the competencies possessed by the CNS, especially leadership skills, can make the CNS an ideal candidate for supervisory positions. It is possible to integrate administrative responsibilities successfully into the CNS role while maintaining the focus of practice on the patient/client/family. However, administration is not an inherent part of the role, and care must be taken to allow the CNS in a line position to practice the other role components. In joint appointment positions with schools of nursing, the educational component of the role receives increased importance. While positional responsibilities may result in emphasis upon one role component or competency, especially in complex organizations, some balance between subroles must be maintained for the CNS to continue to be considered a CNS.

Characteristics of the CNS's client population may also shape the practice. As more chronically ill patients are cared for in outpatient settings or at home, the CNS may move outside the primary institution as well.

The type of organization in which the CNS practices and the mission identified by the organization can affect the CNS role expression. Small community hospitals may have CNSs involved in community activities and patient education in the community, while teaching centers may wish the CNS focused entirely on the inpatient population. An institution may also redefine its mission over time and in response to community needs or marketplace forces. Such redefinition can subsequently spur a reconfiguration of the CNS role within the setting.

The nature of nursing personnel at the bedside can influence the CNS's role. In institutions with primary nursing as the model of practice, the CNS may emphasize consultation to staff and working through staff. In situations in which the primary caregivers are nonprofessional staff, the CNS may need to be more directly involved with patient care and teaching the staff. Joel felt that this was the determining factor in deciding whether the CNS should be in a line or staff position, with line authority necessary when dealing with nonprofessional nursing personnel (Joel, 1985).

Individual characteristics of the CNS influence role expression. Individuals may emphasize certain role components or feel more comfortable with certain skills and tend to emphasize them in developing their practice. The individual's philosophy of care also guides role expression. The importance of this variable was discussed by Sills: "First and foremost, the C.N.S. must have a personal philosophy of care. In this philosophical matrix are located the essences of the practice—the rationale for the practice, the belief in the theoretical and conceptual frameworks which guide the practice, the commitment to inquiry which governs the practice, the ethical and moral values which metagovern the practice. . ." (1983, p. 567).

Role development over time is a potent factor in shifting role emphases. As the CNS becomes more experienced, certain subroles may assume more importance. Different developmental phases may lead to changes in role expression. Detail on this important variable will be given in Chapter 3.

## IMPLICATIONS OF THIS DEFINITION OF THE CNS ROLE

The CNS role involves many components and competencies. As Sills noted, "Obviously, ability to give such a high quality of care does not emerge full-bloom from a master's program, but requires nourishment to grow and flourish" (1983, p. 569). The individual CNS requires a considerable period of role development to fully implement the varied aspects of this practice. Numerous authors have identified use of mentors, peer support, networking between CNSs, supervision of an expert in one's specialty, and anticipatory socialization in graduate school as facilitators of this development (Sills, 1983; ANA, 1980; Hamric, 1983). It is important that graduate programs include clinical practice in the various role components as well as a sound theoretical base. Even with the most excellent graduate education, however, no CNS new to the role can be expected to perform all the role components and competencies with equal skill.

Another implication of the definition is that if an individual nurse does not possess the primary criteria, does not perform all the role components, and does not demonstrate the competencies, then that individual is not a CNS and should not use the title. Consistent application of these criteria will clarify the role of this practitioner. There will continue to be considerable variation in individual role enactment; this flexibility is inherent in and essential to CNS function, as explained by the multiple variables that influence role expression. The CNS can change priorities and attendant activities on the basis of identified needs and develop different strategies that will meet those needs.

One further implication of the definition is that the CNS is clinically expert. Expertise requires experience in addition to education. The author has previously noted problems with role enactment which occur when the CNS is not clinically expert (Hamric, 1983). In the last few years, programs preparing non-nurse baccalaureate graduates for CNS roles have been created. Such programs can be successful, if they admit students who have prior relevant experience in the area in which they wish to specialize, and if they emphasize clinical practice experiences. Graduates of such programs should develop clinical expertise as their first priority upon assuming a CNS position.

## PROBLEMS WITH ROLE ENACTMENT

Problems experienced by CNSs have been described by Holt and include: inadequate academic preparation, lack of clarity or agreement regarding goals, pressure for quick results, overextending oneself in an effort to practice all components simultaneously, moving into staff development or consultation exclusively, and finding the most effective organizational placement (Holt, 1984). These difficulties, as well as problems with applying the theory of the CNS role to its practice, continue to be experienced by CNSs. These latter problems include the numerous blocks to the effectiveness of role modeling as a change strategy, maintaining patient advocacy while trying to prove one's worth, pressuring the individual CNS to "sell" the role, and attempting to make change without a strong, legitimate power base (Hamric, 1983). Other writers have noted the isolation and rejection encountered by CNSs (Woodrow and Bell, 1971; Everson, 1981). The CNS is a nontraditional nurse whose presence "indicates that something needs changing" (Smoyak, 1976, p. 681). This feature can cause those in traditional nursing roles to view the CNS with suspicion and hostility (Hamric, 1983, p. 44) and can create a powerful sense of "not belonging" within the CNS. Strategies for dealing with this phenomenon will be addressed in Chapter 3.

One final issue to be examined in this discussion of problems with role definition is writing one's own job description. The ANA asserted, "When nurse specialists are employed in health care settings, descriptions of their position and functions ought not to be standardized. The work rules for the specialist must be jointly determined and negotiated by the applicant and the employing institution. The emphasis should be on developing negotiated positions and organizational arrangements that are most likely to result in freedom and responsibility for maximum use of the abilities of the particular specialist in the particular health care setting" (ANA, 1980, p. 26–27). Other authors have contended that CNSs should view with suspicion the "opportunity" to write their own job description, as it may indicate a lack of clear employer expectations (Kwong, Manning, Koetters, 1982). Colerick, Mason and Proulx advocated "a balance between role ambiguity and the rigid job descriptions used traditionally in nursing" (1980, p. 29). The core definition of the CNS role presented here and the positional responsibilities identified by the employing agency should form the basis of a new CNS's job description. Within this framework, the individual CNS and supervisor should then negotiate a balance of role components and expectations which matches the institution's goals for the position with the particular skills of the CNS. Subsequent renegotiation will need to occur on a regular basis. Totally open-ended job descriptions make one question whether the institution has carefully identified its clinical needs and the appropriateness of the CNS role in meeting those needs. A strict, predeveloped job description denies the flexible and self-directed nature of CNS practice.

## SUMMARY

"Specialization is the inevitable result of new knowledge within fields and demands from the public for new service" (Smoyak, 1976, p. 678). Specialization in nursing has been distinguished from the CNS role, which is one response to increasing specialization within the profession. Characteristics of the CNS have been proposed to clarify CNS role definition and practice. Continued refinement of role definition and expression will lead to improved specialist practice and advancement of the profession.

## References

American Cancer Society: The Master's Degree with a specialty in cancer nursing: Curriculum guide and role definition. New York, American Cancer Society, Inc., 1979.

American Nurses Association: Nursing: A Social Policy Statement. Kansas City, ANA, 1980.

Baker, C., & Kramer, M.: To define or not to define: The role of the clinical nurse specialist. Nurs Forum 9(1):45–55, 1970.

Benner, P.: From Novice to Expert. Menlo Park, CA, Addison-Wesley, 1984.

Blount, M., Burge, S., Crigler, L., et al.: Extending the influence of the clinical nurse specialist. Nurs Admin Q 6(1):53–63, 1981.

Castledine, G.: Clinical nurse specialist. Nurs Mirror 156(19):52, 1983.

Christman, L.: The influence of specialization on the nursing profession. Nurs Sci 3:446–453, 1965.

Colerick, E., Mason, P., and Proulx, J.: Evaluation of the clinical nurse specialist role: Development and implementation of a dual purpose framework. Nurs Leadership 3(3):26–33, 1980.

Council of Clinical Nurse Specialists: The Role of the Clinical Nurse Specialist. Kansas City, ANA, 1986.

Craytor, J.: Highlights in education for cancer nursing. Oncol Nurs Forum 9(4):51–59, 1982.

Critchley, D.L.: Evolution of the role. In Critchley, D.L., and Maurin, J.T. (eds): The Clinical Specialist in Psychiatric Mental Health Nursing. New York, John Wiley & Sons, 1985, pp. 5–22.

DeWitt, K.: Specialties in nursing. Am J Nurs 1:14–17, 1900.

Everson, S.A.: Integration of the role of clinical nurse specialist. J Cont Ed Nurs 12(2):16–19, 1981.

Fenton, M.V.: Identifying competencies of clinical nurse specialists. J Nurs Admin 15(12):31–37, 1985.

Georgopoulos, B.S., & Christman, L.: The clinical nurse specialist: A role model. Am J Nurs 70(5):1030–1039, 1970.

Hamric, A.B.: Role development and functions. In Hamric, A.B., and Spross, J. (eds): The Clinical Nurse Specialist in Theory and Practice. New York, Grune and Stratton, 1983, pp. 39–56.

Hodges, L.C., Poteet, G.W., and Edlund, B.J.: Teaching clinical nurse specialists to lead . . . and to succeed." Nurs Health Care 6(4):193–196, 1985.

Holt, F.M.: A theoretical model for clinical specialist practice. Nurs Health Care 5(8):445–449, 1984.

Joel, L.A.: Preparing clinical specialists for prospective payment. In: Patterns in Education. The Unfolding of Nursing. New York, National League for Nursing, 1985, pp. 171–178.

Kwong, M., Manning, M.P., and Koetters, T.L.: The role of the oncology clinical nurse specialist: Three personal views. Cancer Nurs 5(6):427–434, 1982.

Lewis, E.P. (ed): The Clinical Nurse Specialist. New York, American Journal of Nursing, Educational Services Division, 1970.

McClure, M.L., Poulin, M.A., Sovie, M.D., and Wandelt, M.A.: Magnet Hospitals. Kansas City, ANA, 1983.

Naisbitt, J.: Megatrends. New York, Warner Books, 1982.

National Commission on Nursing: Summary Report and Recommendations. Chicago, The Hospital Research and Educational Trust, 1983.

National League for Nursing: Master's Education in Nursing: Route to Opportunities in Contemporary Nursing, 1984–1985. New York, National League for Nursing, 1984.

Niessner, R.: The clinical specialist's contribution to quality nursing care. Nurs Leadership 2(1):21–30, 1979.

Norris, C.M.: One perspective on the nurse practitioner movement. *In* Jacox, A., and Norris, C. (eds): Organizing for Independent Nursing Practice. New York, Appleton-Century-Crofts, 1977, pp. 21–33.

Padilla, G.V., and Padilla, G.J.: Nursing roles to improve patient care. *In* Padilla, G.V. (ed): The Clinical Nurse Specialist and Improvement of Nursing Practice. Wakefield, MA, Nursing Resources, 1979, pp. 1–13.

Paulen, A.: Practice issues for the oncology clinical nurse specialist. Oncol Nurs Forum 12(2):37–39, 1985.

Peplau, H.E.: Specialization in professional nursing. Nurs Sci 3(8):268–287, 1965.

Reiter, F.: The nurse-clinician. Am J Nurs 66(2):274–280, 1966.

Riehl, J.P., and McVay, J.W. (eds): The Clinical Nurse Specialist: Interpretations. New York, Appleton-Century-Crofts, 1970.

Sills, G.M.: The role and function of the clinical nurse specialist. *In* Chaska, N.L. (ed): The Nursing Profession: A Time to Speak. New York, McGraw-Hill, 1983, pp. 563–579.

Smoyak, S.A.: Specialization in nursing: From then to now. Nursing Outlook 24(11):676–681, 1976.

Spross, J.A.: An overview of the oncology CNS role. Oncol Nurs Forum 10(3):54–58, 1983.

Spross, J.A., and Donoghue, M.: The future of the oncology clinical nurse specialist. Oncol Nurs Forum 11(1):74–78, 1984.

Topham, D.L.: Role theory in relation to roles of the clinical nurse specialist. Clinical Nurse Specialist 1(2):81–84, 1987.

Walker, M.L.: How nursing service administrators view clinical nurse specialists. Nurs Management 17(3):52–54, 1986.

Woodrow, M., and Bell, J.: Clinical specialization: Conflict between reality and theory. J Nurs Admin 1(6):23–27, 1971.

Wright, L.K., Owen, J., Murphy, K., et al.: Work activities of clinical nurse specialists. J Nurs Admin 14(3):9–36, 1984.

# Models of Advanced Nursing Practice

*Judith A. Spross*
*Joanne Baggerly*

## INTRODUCTION

Nurses, physicians, and other health care providers often ask how the CNS is different from the non-master's–prepared experienced nurse clinician. Nurses may find it difficult to articulate the differences. Too often nurses have sensed differences but have been unable to explain them. It is important that nurses, particularly CNSs and administrators, be prepared to answer this important question. For CNSs, this question may not be directly asked, but certainly staff nurses and other health care providers with whom CNSs work look for what is different, what CNSs have to offer that is unique. For neophyte CNSs, experienced clinicians often challenge their suggestions for improved care. For CNSs who are in staff positions that are vulnerable to cost containment pressures, it is vital to clearly articulate what it is that makes CNSs different from clinicians and equally valuable to the care of clients. Some of the differences between CNSs and experienced clinicians are apparent in the range and depth of the CNSs' clinical knowledge; in their ability to anticipate patient responses to health, illness, and nursing interventions; in their ability to analyze clinical situations, to be explicit about their clinical judgments, and to explain why a phenomenon has occurred or why a particular intervention has been chosen; and in their skill in assessing and addressing nonclinical variables that influence patient care. In addition, CNSs are expected to perform well in a range of subroles and also to function with more autonomy than do most nurse clinicians. The authors believe it is important for CNSs, CNS educators, and administrators to examine models of advanced practice which may help to explain, justify, and support different levels of

**19**

practice, including the advanced clinical practice of master's-prepared nurses. For the purposes of this chapter, advanced practice refers only to the practice of master's-prepared nurses. Although the authors refer specifically to the CNS, these models are also applicable to the master's-prepared nurse practitioner (NP).

A model can be defined as a symbolic depiction in logical terms of an idealized, relatively simple situation representing the structure of the original system (Hazzard, 1971). Therefore, a model can be thought of as a conceptual representation of reality. A model includes the concepts and assumptions that integrate them into a meaningful configuration (Nye & Berardo, 1966). The authors have identified models in the literature which can be regarded as models for advanced practice. It is important for the reader to realize that this chapter is not examining conceptual models of nursing (i.e., models that include the four phenomena of concern to nurses—person, environment, health, and nursing). Rather, the authors have tried to describe and critique models in order to clarify the nature of advanced CNS practice.

## COMPONENTS OF A MODEL FOR ADVANCED PRACTICE

The concepts the authors believe to be essential to a model of advanced practice are *clinical judgment* and *leadership*. Although clinical judgment is exercised by all nurses when they make decisions about patient care, CNSs are expected to demonstrate an advanced level of clinical judgment. The authors believe this advanced level of judgment becomes particularly apparent when CNSs care for clients with complex physiologic and psychosocial problems. Because of the interaction and integration of graduate education in nursing practice and years of clinical experience, the CNS is able to exercise a level of discrimination that is unavailable to other experienced clinicians.

Statements about CNS education and practice promulgated by the National League for Nursing (1983), the American Nurses Association (1986), specialty nursing journals, and nursing organizations clearly indicate that CNSs are expected to demonstrate leadership behaviors. In the most recent (ANA) publication on CNSs (1986), particular areas in which CNSs contribute to activities of the nursing profession were identified. The term leadership was specifically used: "The [CNS] will continue to be a source of leadership in the expansion of nursing services" (p. 7); "[CNSs] can assist the profession in [providing] leadership in exploring and molding career options for the [CNS]" (p. 7); and "economic constraints require the [CNS] to take leadership in securing a financial base for research, program development, educational advancement, patient care and patient education" (p. 8). The authors agree that "leadership is not an option" (Spross & Donoghue, 1984, p. 78). Success as a CNS depends upon exquisite clinical judgment and effective leadership.

Clinical judgment is a complex intellectual process of decision-making which typically includes: (1) decisions regarding what to observe in a patient situation; (2) inferential decisions, deriving meaning from data observed (diagnosis); and (3) decisions regarding actions that should be taken which will be of optimal benefit to the patient (Tanner, 1983). Leadership uses communication processes to influence the activities of an individual or group toward the attainment of a goal or goals in a given situation (LaMonica, 1983). For the CNS this includes guiding staff nurses in the acquisition of clinical skills and knowledge, interpreting nursing practice to nurses and non-nurses, developing innovative approaches to clinical practice, promoting interdisciplinary collaboration, and advancing the practice and profession of nursing (for further discussion of leadership see Chapter 6). A model that includes these two elements can help CNSs analyze their advanced practices.

## BENNER'S MODEL OF EXPERT PRACTICE

### Description of the Model

Benner's landmark research on clinical expertise has important implications for CNSs (Benner, 1984; 1985). Through this research, Benner identified seven domains of nursing practice which describe the process of clinical judgment. These domains include:

* the helping role
* administering and monitoring therapeutic interventions and regimens
* effective management of rapidly changing situations
* the diagnostic and monitoring functions
* the teaching-coaching function
* monitoring and ensuring the quality of health care practices
* organizational and work role competencies

Specific competencies found within each domain are listed in Table 2–1. Benner's initial research focused on expert clinicians, the majority of whom were not master's-prepared CNSs.

Later, Benner described the expertise of the CNS as a hybrid of practical knowledge gained in front line practice and of the most

## TABLE 2–1. Domains of Nursing Practice

**DOMAIN: THE HELPING ROLE**

The healing relationship: Creating a climate for and establishing a commitment to healing

Providing comfort measures and preserving personhood in the face of pain and extreme breakdown

Presencing: being with a patient

Maximizing the patient's participation and control in his or her own recovery

Interpreting kinds of pain and selecting appropriate strategies for pain management and control

Providing comfort and communication through touch

Providing emotional and informational support to patients' families

Guiding a patient through emotional and developmental change; providing new options, closing off old ones

Channeling, teaching, mediating

Acting as a psychological and cultural mediator

Using goals therapeutically

Working to build and maintain a therapeutic community

**DOMAIN: ADMINISTERING AND MONITORING THERAPEUTIC INTERVENTIONS AND REGIMENS**

Starting and maintaining intravenous therapy with minimal risks and complications

Administering medications accurately and safely: monitoring untoward effects, reactions, therapeutic responses, toxicity, and incompatibilities

Combating the hazards of immobility; preventing and intervening with skin breakdown, ambulating and exercising patients to maximize mobility and rehabilitation, preventing respiratory complications

Creating a wound management strategy that fosters healing, comfort, and appropriate drainage

**DOMAIN: EFFECTIVE MANAGEMENT OF RAPIDLY CHANGING SITUATIONS**

Skilled performance in extreme life-threatening emergencies: rapid grasp of a problem

Contingency management: rapid matching of demands and resources in emergency situations

Identifying and managing a patient crisis until physician assistance is available

**DOMAIN: THE DIAGNOSTIC AND MONITORING FUNCTION**

Detection and documentation of significant changes in a patient's condition

Providing an early warning signal: anticipating breakdown and deterioration prior to explicit confirming diagnostic signs

Anticipating problems: future thinking

Understanding the particular demands and experiences of an illness: anticipating patient care needs

Assessing the patient's potential for wellness and for responding to various treatment strategies

**DOMAIN: THE TEACHING-COACHING FUNCTION**

Timing: capturing a patient's readiness to learn

Assisting patients to integrate the implications of illness and recovery into their lifestyles

Eliciting and understanding the patient's interpretation of his or her illness

Providing an interpretation of the patient's condition and giving a rationale for procedures

The coaching function: making culturally avoided aspects of an illness approachable and understandable

**DOMAIN: MONITORING AND ENSURING THE QUALITY OF HEALTH CARE PRACTICES**

Providing a backup system to ensure safe medical and nursing care

Assessing what can be safely omitted from or added to medical orders

Getting appropriate and timely responses from physicians

**DOMAIN: ORGANIZATIONAL AND WORK-ROLE COMPETENCIES**

Coordinating, ordering, and meeting multiple patient needs and requests; setting priorities

Building and maintaining a therapeutic team to provide optimum therapy

Coping with staff shortages and high turnover: Contingency planning

Anticipating and preventing periods of extreme work overload within a shift

Using and maintaining team spirit; gaining social support from other nurses

Maintaining a caring attitude toward patients even in absence of close and frequent contact

Maintaining a flexible stance toward patients, technology, and bureaucracy

(Excerpted from Benner, P.: From Novice to Expert: Excellence and Power in Clinical Nursing Practice. Menlo Park, CA, Addison-Wesley Publishing Company, 1984; as it appeared in Fenton M.V.: Identifying competencies of clinical nurse specialists. J Nurs Admin *15*(12):31–37, 1985.)

sophisticated skills of knowledge utilization (1985). Benner described the CNS as having in-depth knowledge of a particular clinical population and as grasping in theory and practice the illness and disease trajectory of the particular patient population. The clinical judgment of the expert CNS allows the CNS to recognize subtle changes in patient condition, the meanings the illness might have for the patient based on the patient's interpretation of the experience, and common cultural meanings of illness and therapy. "The hallmarks of clinical expertise are an in-depth knowledge of a particular clinical population; advanced recognitional abilities; and increased use of past whole situations or situation specific referents for understanding the clinical situation" (Benner, 1985, p. 41). To describe and refine expert knowledge, she suggested that nurses must share their experiences—through rounds, small group discussions, and documenting clinical experiences. She also cited the importance of clinical ethnographies as a way of documenting many clinical experiences. The documentation of a series of exemplars can foster understanding of relationships between the disease process and the patient's experience of illness (Benner, 1984; 1985).

Further application of Benner's model to CNSs was done by Fenton (1985). Fenton verified that CNSs practice as experts and identified some CNS behaviors that had not been noted by Benner in her original work on developing nursing expertise. These additional CNS behaviors are listed in Table 2–2.

**TABLE 2–2. New Areas of Skilled Performance and Competencies of CNSs**

| Domain: Monitoring and Ensuring the Quality of Health Care Practices | Domain: Organizational and Work-Role Competencies |
|---|---|
| Recognition of a generic recurring event or problem that requires a policy change | Building and maintaining a therapeutic team to provide optimum therapy<br>Providing emotional and situational support for nursing staff<br>Competencies developed to cope with staff and organizational resistance to change<br>Showing acceptance of staff persons to resist system change<br>Using formal research findings to initiate and facilitate system change<br>Using concurrent or mandated change to facilitate other system changes<br>Making the bureaucracy respond to patient's and families' needs (massaging the system) |
| **Domain: The Consulting Role** | |
| Providing patient care consultation to the nursing staff through direct patient intervention and follow-up<br>Interpreting the role of nursing in specific clinical patient care situations to nursing and other professional staff<br>Providing patient advocacy by sensitizing staff to the dilemmas faced by patients and families seeking health care | |

(Reprinted with permission from Fenton, M.V.: Identifying competencies of clinical nurse specialists. J Nurs Admin *15*(12):31–37, 1985.)

Of the CNS competencies described by Fenton, two deserve particular mention because they are not cited in other CNS literature (even though practicing CNSs certainly recognize the behaviors as ones they use often). Fenton found that a very important role for CNSs is the support of staff nurses and that this leadership function often goes unstated and/or unrecognized by administrators and in job descriptions (1985). Fenton also found that CNSs often "massaged the system" to improve situations for patients and staff.

## Critique

Benner's and Fenton's research are clear attempts to describe the skills involved in clinical judgment. The domains and competencies identified by Benner describe the clinical judgment exercised by experienced clinicians. Leadership is not specifically addressed by Benner. However, it could be argued that some competencies within the "Monitoring and Ensuring Quality" and the "Organizational and Work Role" domains describe leadership behaviors. The scope of leadership described in Benner's initial research is limited to care of specific patients (e.g., the work of a primary nurse) or to managing workload/co-workers within a specific shift (e.g., the leadership one expects of a charge nurse).

The additional CNS competencies identified by Fenton (Table 2–2) describe leadership skills rather than ones of clinical judgment. It would seem that CNSs use clinical judgment competencies similar to those of the experienced clinician (Fenton, 1985). The authors of this chapter believe that CNSs are able to be more explicit about clinical judgment processes and that their clinical knowledge is less likely to be embedded or buried in their practices. The new domain described by Fenton, i.e., the "Consulting Role," and the competencies within this domain are clearly focused on influencing others (i.e., exercising leadership). Within the "Organizational and Work Role" domain, supporting staff nurses, dealing with change, and "massaging the system" are CNS behaviors that demonstrate leadership. The importance of these findings is that they begin to differentiate the practice of experienced clinicians from that of CNSs. The integration of Benner's and Fenton's research provides a model of advanced practice which includes the essential concepts of clinical judgment and leadership that can be useful to CNSs.

The model's usefulness can be examined by applying it to the subroles of the CNS. As a practitioner, the CNS can use the seven domains of nursing practice as a means of self-assessment, as a framework for analyzing practice, and as a basis for documenting paradigm cases. CNSs can build on Benner's and Fenton's work by identifying new domains and competencies or by refining those that seem to have particular usefulness.

With regard to the educator subrole, the authors believe that the teaching/coaching function that Benner identified in relation to patients can also be applied to the coaching of staff nurses. Table 2–3 illustrates possible CNS roles in coaching other nurses. For example, a staff nurse who has consulted an oncology CNS to help assess and plan the care of a patient with chronic pain indicates an interest in improving her assessment skills and using relaxation to treat pain. The CNS uses the next few consultations on the unit to bring the nurse to the bedside to observe the CNS's assessment process and how the CNS coaches a patient through relaxation. The CNS observes the staff nurse perform a pain assessment on one of her patients. The patient is a candidate for relaxation techniques. Initially, the CNS coaches the patient. The staff nurse practices the relaxation sequence with a tape recorder. The staff nurse indicates that she is ready to coach the patient, and at the next session, she guides the patient's relaxation exercise while the CNS observes. The CNS gives the nurse feedback on both activities—assessment and relaxation coaching—and concludes that the nurse has become competent in assessing pain and using relaxation as an intervention.

The consultant subrole of the CNS role is well-documented (Barron, 1983; Simmons, 1985). The consulting role competencies described by Fenton are consistent with descriptions of the consultant subrole found in the literature and in CNS position descriptions. While the consulting role competencies do not add anything new to characterizations of the CNS as consultant, they are important because they help to discriminate two levels of practice.

CNSs sometimes experience frustration in implementing the research subrole. A variety of personal, clinical, and organizational variables may account for this. For CNSs who believe that clinical needs interfere with their research efforts, Benner's suggestions for capturing the knowledge embedded in practice offer a means of transforming clinical experiences into descriptive research. Clinical record-keeping

**TABLE 2–3.  Competencies of CNSs for Teaching and Coaching Staff Nurses**

- Timing: capturing nurse's readiness to learn
- Assisting staff nurse to integrate implications of a clinical situation into practice
- Eliciting and understanding nurse's interpretation of a clinical situation
- Providing an interpretation of a clinical situation
- Coaching: making culturally avoided aspects of a clinical situation approachable and understandable

in the form of ethnographies can advance the practice of nursing. Ethnographies will uncover practical knowledge that can be used to develop expert nurses and refine their skills. CNSs are the logical choice for providing this kind of clinical leadership and scholarship. CNSs can use not only their own practice but also the practices of the staff with whom they work to generate both exemplars of expert practice and clinical ethnographies. The model offers CNSs a practical way to implement the research subrole.

The Benner model of clinical expertise, together with the refinements provided by Fenton, make this approach very useful to CNSs. Areas that need further development include:

- further application of the model to CNS practice
- extension of the teaching/coaching domain to teaching nurses
- comparison of clinician and CNS competencies to further elucidate components of expert practice
- incorporation of knowledge of and practice with ethnographic methods in graduate programs so CNSs can provide clinical leadership to address Benner's challenge to uncover knowledge embedded in practice.

## ROY AND MARTINEZ' CONCEPTUAL FRAMEWORK FOR CNS PRACTICE

### Description of the Model

Roy's adaptation model has been well-documented. A deliberate effort was made to look at a systems model for CNS practice (Roy & Martinez, 1983). This framework is based on systems theory and humanistic values. Systems theory helps one see how a person or group functions as a whole within a dynamic environment. Systems arc characterized by inputs, outputs, and control and feedback processes (Roy & Martinez, 1983). The systems framework for CNS practice is found in Figure 2–1. Roy and Martinez also described systems frameworks that CNSs can use for viewing individuals and groups (Figures 2–2 and 2–3). Roy and Martinez described clinical applications of both the individual and group frameworks in their publication.

The systems framework clearly specified judgment as an integral part of the model. Internal inputs, particularly education and experience, are important and, in fact, prescribed. As in the Roy adaptation model, this model for CNS practice discriminated two types of processes—regulator and cognator. In addition to elementary neural re-

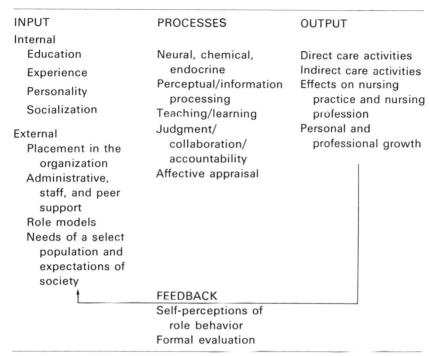

| INPUT | PROCESSES | OUTPUT |
|---|---|---|
| Internal | | |
| Education | Neural, chemical, endocrine | Direct care activities |
| Experience | | Indirect care activities |
| Personality | Perceptual/information processing | Effects on nursing practice and nursing profession |
| Socialization | Teaching/learning | |
| | Judgment/ collaboration/ accountability | Personal and professional growth |
| External | | |
| Placement in the organization | Affective appraisal | |
| Administrative, staff, and peer support | | |
| Role models | | |
| Needs of a select population and expectations of society | | |
| | FEEDBACK | |
| | Self-perceptions of role behavior | |
| | Formal evaluation | |

**Figure 2–1.** A systems framework for clinical specialist practice. (Reprinted with permission from Roy, C., & Martinez, C.: A conceptual framework for CNS practice. *In* Hamric, A.B., and Spross, J. (eds): The Clinical Nurse Specialist in Theory and Practice. New York, Grune and Stratton, 1983.)

sponses, the CNS was seen as having highly developed cognator responses. The CNS's ability to perceive and process both covert and overt information within the environment is well-developed. Roy and Martinez believed that the cognitive processes of judgment, collaboration, and accountability most definitively distinguish CNS practice. These abilities are reflected in mature clinical and professional judgment.

Leadership is an expectation of the systems model. One goal of developing an expert practice role is improving patient care. The systems model assumed that direct and indirect care activities affect both nursing practice and the profession. Roy and Martinez stated that "the achievement of this goal (improvement of patient care) can obviously affect the image, authority and autonomy of the nursing profession" (1983, p. 6). Two case studies presented by Roy and Martinez illustrate the application of their model of CNS practice to an individual patient and a group of patients.

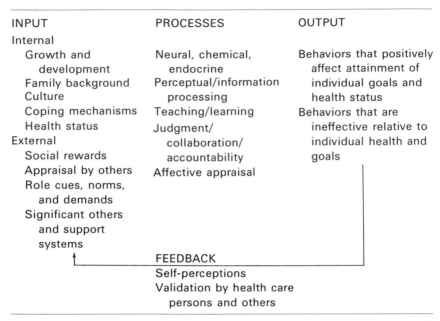

| INPUT | PROCESSES | OUTPUT |
|---|---|---|
| Internal | | |
| Growth and | Neural, chemical, | Behaviors that positively |
| development | endocrine | affect attainment of |
| Family background | Perceptual/information | individual goals and |
| Culture | processing | health status |
| Coping mechanisms | Teaching/learning | Behaviors that are |
| Health status | Judgment/ | ineffective relative to |
| External | collaboration/ | individual health and |
| Social rewards | accountability | goals |
| Appraisal by others | Affective appraisal | |
| Role cues, norms, | | |
| and demands | | |
| Significant others | | |
| and support | | |
| systems | | |
| | FEEDBACK | |
| | Self-perceptions | |
| | Validation by health care | |
| | persons and others | |

**Figure 2–2.** A systems framework to use in viewing an individual. (Reprinted with permission from Roy, C., & Martinez, C.: A conceptual framework for CNS practice. *In* Hamric, A.B., and Spross, J. (eds): The Clinical Nurse Specialist in Theory and Practice. New York, Grune and Stratton, 1983.)

## Critique

The systems framework addresses both clinical judgment and leadership and is specific to the CNS. The frameworks proposed for viewing CNS practice, individual clients, and groups enable the CNS to analyze and integrate role components, clinical judgment, and leadership. The strength of the systems model lies in the framework offered by Roy and Martinez. They provide a structure for CNSs to analyze their subroles as well as leadership and change agent activities. The framework for CNS practice (see Figure 2–1) enables CNSs to assess their own knowledge and skills as well as organizational and other variables that may influence role implementation.

The systems framework for viewing an individual can be used by CNSs to understand a particular patient or staff member. For the individual patient, CNSs might find it useful to modify this framework to reflect specialty content, issues, and processes. The framework for viewing a group appears to focus on organizational groups, although

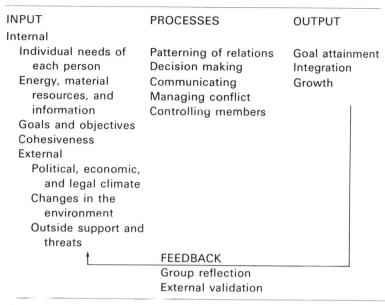

| INPUT | PROCESSES | OUTPUT |
|---|---|---|
| Internal | | |
|   Individual needs of | Patterning of relations | Goal attainment |
|     each person | Decision making | Integration |
|   Energy, material | Communicating | Growth |
|     resources, and | Managing conflict | |
|     information | Controlling members | |
|   Goals and objectives | | |
|   Cohesiveness | | |
| External | | |
|   Political, economic, | | |
|     and legal climate | | |
|   Changes in the | | |
|     environment | | |
|   Outside support and | | |
|     threats | | |
| | FEEDBACK | |
| | Group reflection | |
| | External validation | |

**Figure 2–3.** A systems framework to use in viewing a group. (Reprinted with permission from Roy, C., & Martinez, C.: A conceptual framework for CNS practice. *In* Hamric, A.B., and Spross, J. (eds): The Clinical Nurse Specialist in Theory and Practice. New York, Grune and Stratton, 1983.)

Roy and Martinez applied the framework to a group of clients in the aftermath of an air disaster.

It is difficult to apply the systems model to each subrole, since the emphasis of the model is on systems and integration of roles and leadership. The authors believe the model is most useful for applying leadership aspects of the CNS role rather than for analyzing clinical judgment. For example, CNSs could use the model to plan entry into a new setting or to plan, implement, and evaluate change.

Areas for further development and testing of this framework for CNS practice include:

- development and testing of specialty-specific systems frameworks
- evaluation of the model's efficacy in discriminating between CNS and experienced clinician practices
- evaluation of the individual and group impact of CNSs on patients, staff, and organizations
- identification of other key components of input, output, and feedback processes that are relevant to CNS practice.

# HOLT'S THEORETICAL MODEL FOR CLINICAL SPECIALIST PRACTICE

## Description of the Model

Holt offered a practical model encompassing concepts relevant to definition, goals, and growth and development of the CNS role (1984). She considered relationships and effective communication skills to be as important as clinical acumen in actualizing the role. Holt emphasized that maintaining and refining the art of nursing requires regular practice. The skills required for leadership aspects of the role were clearly articulated. The model stressed that specialty expertise, with continued expansion of clinical knowledge, form the cornerstone and remain the focus of the CNS role. The goal of the CNS role is to improve patient care; expert direct care and effective indirect care activities are the vehicles by which this is achieved.

Clinical judgment was not explicitly described. However, Holt alluded to it when she discussed the CNS's abilities to connect concepts, both clinical and process-oriented, to determine interventions, and to predict outcomes. Elements of clinical judgment are contained in her discussion of leadership, and, in fact, the two concepts seem inextricably linked in this model.

Leadership was described mainly in the context of indirect roles, such as the ability to influence others. Effective implementation of indirect care roles, such as teacher, researcher, change agent, and role model, was viewed by Holt as essential if CNSs are to influence the quality of care in general rather than only for those for whom they provide direct care.

As stated by Holt, implementing direct and indirect role components requires adroit interpersonal relationships, communication, and problem-solving ability. Developing effective relationships with the myriad of individuals with whom CNSs interact (including patients, families, staff, peers from other disciplines, and administrators) facilitates information sharing, learning, and achievement of patient care outcomes. Frequently, CNSs collaborate with others to accomplish patient care goals; effective collaboration is often contingent upon their interpersonal skills. Collegial relationships allow for mutual insights relative to management of specific patient problems and identification of the health care provider best able to provide interventions.

A major leadership objective for the CNS is to improve care for all patients in the specialty area. Success, in Holt's model, is contingent upon maturation in CNS role components, leadership, and proficiency in the use of change theory. Once credibility is established at the unit or specialty level within the institution, CNSs can widen their spheres of influence. This process begins with the initiation of surveys and projects to promote a change in practice by capitalizing on facts, rather than on preconceived ideas. The data obtained, adeptly presented to and shared with staff, serve as a catalyst for change. Built upon such a foundation, established over time, the change agent role allows the CNS to have an impact on the health care system.

According to Holt, engagement in research projects and subsequent publication of findings were identified as mechanisms for extending influence and affecting care for all patients. Access to patients through the direct care role yields a rich source for identifying clinical research problems and subsequent development of new or validated approaches to care. Holt also presented her views on CNS role development and described potential obstacles.

### Critique

The value of this model for CNSs is its emphasis on leadership skills based on the premise that "a clinical nurse specialist must influence the quality of nursing care in a larger group of patients than she can personally attend" (Holt, 1984, p. 446). The discussion of change agency and ways of influencing care is useful. Holt cautioned that major changes require years of experience in the role (p. 448). The authors believe that such caution may not be well-advised and do not agree that it may take years to establish credibility and realize change. If it takes years for CNSs to establish credibility, an administrator might have reason to question whether there is a good match between the institution and the CNS. In addition, since health care organizations are so dynamic, the authors suggest that change is normal. Fenton found that CNSs use mandated change to implement other changes simultaneously. It is important for CNSs to have a thorough grasp of change theories and strategies, an ability to analyze organizations, and a good sense of timing. The model's strength is also its weakness in that it primarily focuses on leadership with a particular emphasis on change agent skills. While the change agent function of the CNS is important, it is not the only way a CNS can exercise leadership (see Chapter 6). However, the CNS who has been hired with a primary mission of effecting change should find this model useful.

There is not a systematic discussion of subroles. Holt valued the direct care role but did not offer strategies for implementing it. The educator subrole is alluded to in a brief discussion of role modeling. Consultation is not addressed directly, although one assumes it is included in the indirect role activities. Holt reaffirmed the importance of the research subrole and believed that CNSs must be responsible for increasing the knowledge base of nursing care in their specialties. Like Benner, Holt suggested that patient care or case studies can build such a knowledge base.

Holt's description of role development and potential obstacles offers practical anticipatory guidance for CNSs. The weakness of this aspect of the model is that these observations have not been tested; Holt also did not identify the source of her observations. An explanation of the source of these observations (e.g., personal experience, experience with students and graduates, and so forth) would enable readers to better determine her model's applicability. Aspects of Holt's model which merit further testing include:

- evaluation of the description of role development
- clarification of the art of nursing as it reflects clinical judgment and how the CNS's art differs from that of the experienced clinician
- demonstration of a relationship between indirect care activities of the CNS and improvement in quality of care.

## CALKIN'S MODEL OF ADVANCED NURSING PRACTICE

### Description of the Model

Calkin's model of advanced nursing practice was developed from a management perspective. Calkin used the term advanced nurse practitioner (ANP) to refer to master's-prepared nurse practitioners and CNSs. CNS will be used in this discussion. Calkin provided a clear definition of advanced practice. From an administrator's viewpoint, she described the advantages of employing a CNS. She delineated specific functions and expectations of the CNS with an emphasis on analytical skills and the ability to articulate practice needs, rather than on a task focus of the role. Guidelines were offered to assist nurse administrators in determining the need for a CNS and with decisions regarding whether the CNS should be in a line, staff, or consultative capacity.

Calkin defined the clinical judgment abilities of three professional nursing practice levels—novice, expert by experience, and the master's-prepared practitioner. Utilizing the definition of nursing as the "diagnosis and treatment of human responses to actual or potential health problems" (ANA, 1984), Calkin postulated that nurses deal with responses that exist in a normal distribution. The novice is prepared to manage a circumscribed group of responses. Experts by experience demonstrate skills superior to novices when faced with similar situations and are capable of identifying and intervening for a more extensive range of human responses. Calkin stated that, in general, interventions employed by such experts tend to be more intuitive, while CNS actions are based on deliberate reasoning and analytical skills. Not only are the CNS's actions deliberative, but also the range of responses to which the CNS can respond is broader. The CNS is academically and clinically prepared to "diagnose and treat a *full range* [emphasis added] of human responses to actual or potential problems" (Calkin, 1984). Calkin's conceptualization of these three levels of practice is graphed in Figure 2–4.

The essence of the CNS's direct care role lies in the ability to recognize and capitalize on positive human responses with a focus on responses that occur in the distribution's extremes. The identification of positive responses expedites the achievement of outcomes, resulting in improvements in the quality of care for individuals and groups of patients. An extensive repertoire of strategies developed by the CNS also facilitates CNS efforts to effect change when negative or nonhelpful responses are demonstrated. In addition to these practice benefits, Calkin noted other implications for the CNS role in the treatment of extremes in human responses. In terms of research, the CNS is in the ideal position to examine conditions or requisites that lead to positive responses or predict negative ones. By virtue of their knowledge of the patient population, CNSs can offer input regarding the range of responses for which new graduates need to be prepared.

Calkin elucidated concomitant activities required by this focus on extremes, including a continuing expansion of clinical knowledge through utilization of resources, such as colleagues, literature, and professional organizations, and development of skills in others through teaching-learning activities.

Leadership aspects of the CNS role described in this model include the abilities "to be articulate about the nature of nursing practice, to use reasoning to deal with practice innovations and to develop or contribute to newer forms of practice" (Calkin, 1984, p. 30). Research efforts directed at exploring conditions that enhance and elicit positive human responses are identified as appropriate CNS endeavors. All of these represent leadership behaviors. Calkin described conditions in the practice setting which direct the expression of leadership activities. Conventional use of the CNS has been in teaching or tertiary care institutions where rapid scientific and technological advances, complex care needs, and divergent patient populations combine to increase the likelihood of unusual or aberrant human responses. The ability to diagnose and treat responses at extremes of the normal distribution is essential in these settings. The CNS possesses these skills and assists

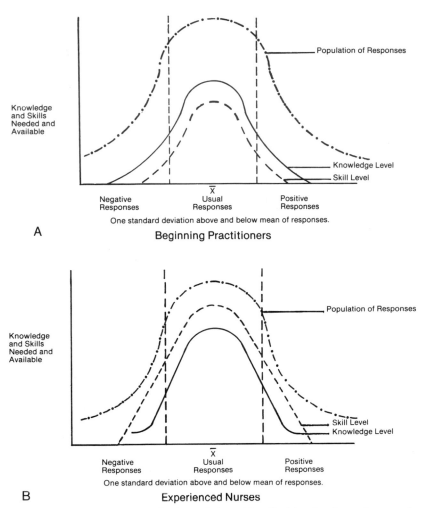

**Figure 2–4.** Calkin's conceptualization of three identified levels of practice correlated with population of responses and knowledge and skills needed to respond. (From Calkin, J.D.: A model for advanced nursing practice. J Nurs Admin *14*(1):25–27, 1984.)

*Illustration continued on opposite page*

staff and students in acquiring the skills needed to care for patients. CNSs also anticipate factors that might cause unfamiliar responses and prepare staff to meet these needs. The CNS can provide anticipatory guidance to administrators by describing the needs identified in the clinical setting. As Calkin indicated, a distinguishing component of advanced practice is the ability to analyze situations and to articulate information that will effect change. Thus, the CNS may be expected to develop and implement programs or adapt them from other settings.

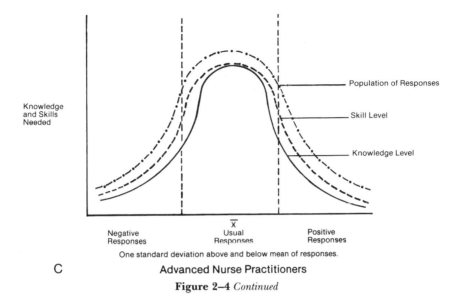

Negative Responses · Usual Responses $\overline{X}$ · Positive Responses

One standard deviation above and below mean of responses.

C                              **Advanced Nurse Practitioners**

**Figure 2–4** *Continued*

## Critique

Of all the models described in this chapter, Calkin provides the most explicit answer to the question posed at the beginning of the chapter—by clearly articulating the differences between an experienced clinician and a CNS. It is significant that this model has been proposed by an administrator and, in the authors' view, is a good explanation of the differences among three practice levels.

A major strength of this model lies in its pragmatic applicability in the practice setting. Calkin's description of advanced practice and circumstances in the setting which would support the need for a CNS helps to define role parameters and expectations for both the nurse administrator and the CNS. Administrators can use the model as a guide to ascertain information about the mix of novices, experts by experience, and CNSs which will be required to meet the needs of specific patient populations. For the CNS focusing on extremes in human responses, the model provides a way to determine the most appropriate caseload and a way to establish practice development priorities.

Since the focus of the article is on advanced practice, leadership, and administrative utilization of advanced practice nurses, there is little specific discussion of subroles other than practice. For the practice subrole, the CNS is offered a way to analyze practice from the perspective of nursing diagnoses and human responses. CNS practice is viewed as a vital component of the role, and the communication of practice issues by CNSs to administrators is valued. This assertion by Calkin is an important addition to the few articles that address administrator/ CNS communication and relationships (Brown, 1983; Baird, 1985; see Chapters 12 and 13). Calkin reaffirms the educator and consultant subroles when she describes how CNSs prepare staff nurses to respond to extremes of human responses and how CNSs intervene when such responses occur. Like Holt and Benner, Calkin believes CNSs must use their clinical experiences to add to the research and clinical knowledge base of nursing practice.

The following clinical example illustrates the Calkin model. One of the authors was consulted by an experienced staff nurse about a competent, ambulatory client (Mr. C.) who refused to do his Hickman catheter dressing after being taught and performing a satisfactory return demonstration. Mr. C. would accuse the nurse of being lazy and wanting him to do her work. The CNS asked the primary nurse questions about the patient's return demonstration and about the man's interaction with his wife when she visited. The nurse admitted that when she pressed Mr. C. about the need to be able to do the dressing at home, he said his wife would do it. (She had been taught and had dressed the catheter successfully.) He had also commented from time to time that if the nurse did not do the dressing, he would have his wife do it when she came in. The CNS knew the patient. Based on the information the staff nurse had provided and the CNS's own experience with the patient, the CNS suggested that the patient's behavior toward the nurse was similar to his behavior toward his wife, and probably toward women in general—i.e., he expected that women would indulge his wishes and wait on him. The nurse was advised that since Mr. C.'s socialization had been acquired over a lifetime, it was unreasonable to expect that he would change. Therefore, since the goal of patient education had been met—he had done a meticulous return demonstration of the dressing and could consistently describe the steps of the procedure and the principles of asepsis—the struggle should be abandoned. The nurse continued to do the dressing until discharge and reduced both her stress and that of the patient. The CNS brought an understanding of behavior and sociology to interpret and resolve a clinical problem—perspectives often unavailable to the expert by experience.

Several aspects of the Calkin model should be developed and tested. While it would seem plausible to accept the premise that human responses occur in a normal distribution and that the CNS is prepared to diagnose and treat these responses, both concepts require further scrutiny. Consensus among practitioners regarding responses designated as falling within distribution extremes needs to be determined.

The use of ethnographies, as suggested by Benner, would seem to be a reasonable approach to clarify what responses represent extremes on a normal curve and how CNS interventions influence patient outcomes. What discriminates these interventions and outcomes from those of the novice and the expert by experience needs further study. In addition to efforts undertaken by CNSs to evaluate this model, administrators and managers could contribute by documenting (through "administrative ethnographies") their interactions with and evaluations of individual nurses and groups of nurses who represent the three levels of practice described by Calkin. Such administrative ethnographies could also be used to document the impact of CNSs on organizations.

## BROWN'S MODEL: THE CNS IN A MULTIDISCIPLINARY PARTNERSHIP

### Description of the Model

In 1983 Brown described a model she called a multidisciplinary partnership. Brown proposed her model as one that would keep nursing's best prepared practitioners in direct care roles. She voiced a concern that indirect care functions remove many CNSs from interacting with patients. Brown asserted that clinical experience and graduate education enable CNSs to assume responsibility for the nursing care patients receive. Graduate education develops the knowledge base, cognitive processes, and assertiveness that enable CNSs to work with physicians as colleagues. In a joint practice partnership, CNSs and physicians would manage the care of a specific patient population regardless of setting. The CNS would become the attending nurse in relation to staff nurses similar to the way attending physicians relate to residents and interns. Brown proposed an organizational structure to accommodate such an arrangement, which is very different from current institutional arrangements for nursing practice. The nursing department would employ mentors (experienced, non-master's-prepared clinicians), staff nurses (more than one year of experience), and tyros (neophyte nurses). Brown did not describe the nature of clinical judgment exercised by the CNS but suggested that the exercise of clinical judgment and the coaching of others in developing clinical judgment would constitute a large component of the CNS role.

Brown addressed the leadership aspects of the CNS role when she described the qualities necessary to make partnerships viable. CNSs should "be able to define nursing practice creatively and soundly. They are on the frontier of interprofessional relationships, thus they require courage and skill" (Brown, 1983, p. 39). CNSs can enhance the image of nursing in the eyes of clients and other health care providers and can define the scope of nursing practice. These last two qualities are also leadership skills.

## Critique

On the face of it, the model seems more structural than conceptual. However, the authors believe it has the elements of a model for advanced practice and deserves scrutiny so that others might further develop Brown's ideas. The focus of this model is on the practitioner and educator subroles and on collaboration as a leadership skill. Consultant and research subroles are not addressed. The strength of the model is the blueprint Brown offers for advancing hospital nursing practice and nurse–physician collaboration. The CNS interested in implementing a joint practice, particularly in the hospital setting, would find Brown's vision instructive.

The direct care subrole of the CNS, which Brown advocates (and the authors support), provides an interesting view quite different from one proposed by Joel, who argues that CNSs are too expensive to provide direct care as a major function of their jobs (1985). The most clearly articulated aspects of leadership are the collaborative relationships among CNSs and physicians and the CNS as clinical leader and role model for staff nurses. Brown proposes an organizational structure that would support the multidisciplinary partnerships she envisions. Brown's model is somewhat similar to Calkin's model. Both authors propose levels of nursing practice. Brown adds a level between the tyro (novice) and the mentor (expert by experience): that of staff nurse with one year of experience.

Although there are descriptions of joint practices in the literature, most are between nurse practitioners and physicians, some are between CNSs and physicians, and most are in the context of office/private practice settings. Existing joint practices in which the CNS has hospital privileges are not structured so that CNSs are held accountable for the care delivered by other nurses. Brown's model contains some creative, innovative ideas, the implementation of which would require significant social change. However, elements of the model could be applied and evaluated. The authors believe many of the elements of joint partnerships can be implemented even without the organizational structure proposed by Brown.

## SUMMARY

There are a variety of models that may be useful for analyzing the advanced practice role of the CNS. From this review of models, it is clear that none are fully developed in terms of advanced practice and the CNS. Conceptualizing advanced practice and being able to discriminate it from the practice of a neophyte or an expert by experience is vital. In any system of health care, both consumers and employers want to know what the CNS has to offer, how CNS services differ from care given by novices and clinicians, why CNS services should be chosen, and whether CNS care is worth the expense. There are some who believe that direct care by a CNS is too expensive and that the role of the CNS should be to influence those direct caregivers who are less expensive (Joel, 1985). As CNSs themselves, the authors know there are clients who cannot afford *not* to be cared for by CNSs. Selecting and developing a model of advanced practice will enable CNSs to articulate and demonstrate the knowledge and skills they have that consumers and employers need. Such a model can help administrators justify hiring CNSs. The viability of the practice component of the CNS role will depend upon the CNS's ability to describe and demonstrate that advanced practice makes a difference.

### *References*

American Nurses Association: Nursing: A social policy statement (Publ. No. NP 63 35M). Kansas City, MO, ANA, 1983.
American Nurses Association: The role of the clinical nurse specialist. Kansas City, MO, ANA, 1986.
Baird, S.B.: Administrative support issues and the oncology clinical nurse specialist. Oncol Nurs Forum *12*(2):51–54, 1985.
Barron, A.: The CNS as consultant. *In* Hamric, A.B., and Spross, J. (eds): The Clinical Nurse Specialist in Theory and Practice. New York, Grune and Stratton, 1983.
Benner, P.: From Novice to Expert: Excellence and Power in Clinical Nursing Practice. Menlo Park, CA, Addison Wesley, 1984.
Benner, P.: The oncology clinical nurse specialist as expert coach. Oncol Nurs Forum *12*(2):40–44, 1985.
Benner, P., & Tanner, C.: How expert nurses use intuition. Am J Nurs *87*(1):23–31, 1987.
Brown, S.J.: The clinical nurse specialist in a multidisciplinary partnership. Nurs Admin Q *8*(1):36–46, 1983.
Brown, S.J.: Administrative support. *In* Hamric, A.B., and Spross, J. (eds): The Clinical Nurse Specialist in Theory and Practice. New York, Grune and Stratton, 1983.
Calkin, J.D.: A model for advanced nursing practice. J Nurs Admin *14*(1):24–30, 1984.
Donoghue, M., & Spross, J.: Proceedings from the first invitational conference on the oncology clinical nurse specialist. Oncol Nurs Forum *12*(2):35–37, 66–73, 1985.
Fenton, M.V.: Identifying competencies of clinical nurse specialists. J Nurs Admin *15*(12):31–37, 1985.
Hazzard, M.E.: An overview of system theory. Nurs Clin North Am *6*(3):385–393, 1971.
Holt, F.M.: A theoretical model for clinical specialist practice. Nurs Health Care *5*(8):445–449, 1984.

Joel, L.A.: Master's prepared caregivers in line positions: A case study. *In* National League for Nursing (ed): Patterns in Specialization: Challenge to the Curriculum. (NLN publ. #15–2154). New York, NLN, 1985.

LaMonica, E.: Nursing Leadership and Management: An Experiential Approach. Monterey, CA, Wadsworth Health Sciences Division, 1983.

National League for Nursing. Criteria for the evaluation of baccalaureate and higher degree programs in nursing (Publ. No. 15–1251). New York, NLN, 1983.

Nye, F.I., & Berardo, F.M.: Emerging Conceptual Frameworks in Family Analysis. New York, Macmillan, 1966.

Roy, C., & Martinez, C: A conceptual framework for CNS practice. *In* Hamric, A.B., and Spross, J. (eds): The Clinical Nurse Specialist in Theory and Practice. New York, Grune and Stratton, 1983, pp. 3–20.

Simmons, M.K.: Psychiatric consultation and liaison. *In* Critchley, D., and Maurin, J. (eds): The Clinical Specialist in Psychiatric-Mental Health Nursing. New York, John Wiley & Sons, 1985.

Spross, J.A., & Donoghue, M.: The future of the oncology clinical nurse specialist. Oncol Nurs Forum *11*(1):74–78, 1984.

Tanner, C.A.: Research on clinical judgment. *In* Holzemer, W.L. (ed): Review of Research in Nursing Education. Thorofare, NJ, Charles B. Slack, 1983, pp. 2–32.

# Role Development of the CNS

*Ann B. Hamric*
*Joyce Waterman Taylor*

> Socialization, the process by which one learns to perform his various roles adequately, is continuous throughout life. . . . Chief among the roles for which adult socialization is needed is the occupational role; an adult must learn what others will demand of him in his role and what he will come to demand of himself.
>
> *Kramer, 1974, pp. 137–138*

Anyone entering a new and complex role experiences a process of role development before being able to function with maximum effectiveness. This chapter will focus on the developmental process experienced by clinical nurse specialists (CNSs). Both novice CNSs and those who are experienced but in a new position go through a process of role development, although the experienced CNS's path varies from that of the neophyte CNS. Understanding this process is important for educators to adequately prepare nurses for their expanded role and for both CNSs and administrators to set realistic performance expectations. Role development is a fluid, dynamic process; understanding this can be of immense comfort to CNSs experiencing the daily turbulence of most "real world" practice settings.

## REVIEW OF THE LITERATURE

The concept that role development occurs in sequential phases has been examined within nursing as well as in other professional groups. In a study of scientists, engineers, accountants, and professors, a grouping categorized as "knowledge workers," Dalton, Thompson, and Price (1977) observed four career stages: apprentice, colleague, mentor, and sponsor. Within nursing, CNS role development as a process of skill acquisition and changing the focus of practice has been the approach of P. Baker (1987) and Holt (1987). Baker noted changes in her practice focus as she gained experience in the CNS role. Based on this experience, Baker developed model activities clustered according to the number of years in the role, with the first two years focusing on establishing role identity through direct care functions. Years three and four of CNS practice were directed to change agent activities, and years five and six focused upon the consultant subrole.

Holt proposed developmental stages that could serve as guidelines for evolving expertise. She noted that individual differences in the CNS and the uniqueness of each setting affect developmental patterns. However, she proposed that the focus of the CNS's role evolves in seven sequential phases: (1) increasing confidence through individual direct patient care, (2) direct care and/or planning for groups of patients, (3) working with staff to change the nursing care of specialty patients, (4) conducting and sharing small clinical research projects, (5) planning for patient care delivery changes based on research and experience, (6) enlarging influence to a higher level of the health care system, and (7) integrating all role components with increasing confidence.

Dreyfus and Dreyfus (1980) presented a model of skill acquisition which delineated predictable phases in such diverse groups as pilots and chess players. Applying the model to the clinical skill development of registered nurses, Benner (1984) described Dreyfus' five levels of proficiency: novice, advanced beginner, competent, proficient, and expert. While Benner's work did not focus specifically on the CNS, one could anticipate that the process of clinical knowledge acquisition is the same for this group of nurses as for the general population. According to Benner, the expert practitioner is one who no longer needs to rely on analytic principles (rules, guidelines, maxims) to transform an understanding of the situation into appropriate action. Expert performance is fluid, flexible, and highly proficient. The expert nurse utilizes analytic problem-solving methods only when faced with a new situation or when the initial grasp of the problem proves to be incorrect. In a subsequent study, Benner and Tanner (1987) found that experts used intuitive judgment to quickly assess and intervene in patient situations.

Another approach to understanding role development has focused on the experience of the new CNS and the feelings engendered, as competence and confidence in practice are developed. On the basis of interviews with four clinical specialists, V. Baker (1979) identified four phases of role development: orientation, frustration, implementation, and reassessment. As previously noted by Hamric (1983), these bear an interesting resemblance to Kramer's (1974) phases of reality shock: honeymoon, shock, recovery, and resolution. In addition, Oda (1977) described three phases of specialized role development which parallel three of Baker's stages: role identification, role transition, and role confirmation (Table 3–1).

It is the authors' view that CNS role development is a complex and emotional process. The CNS is a nontraditional nurse with expanded boundaries. The role does not fit the usual conceptions of staff nurse, head nurse, or supervisor, and as a consequence, the CNS does not "belong" in the same way that staff nurses belong to a nursing unit. Many nurses, administrators, and physicians continue to misunderstand the CNS role and may view the specialist with suspicion or hostility. Furthermore, the nature of the role itself and the complex and rapidly changing health care environment dictate continuous change in CNS role enactment. Consequently, role development is an ongoing and challenging process for CNSs.

Despite considerable discussion and speculation, little systematic investigation of this phenomenon has occurred. Instead, most writing is anecdotal in nature (P. Baker, 1987; Holt, 1984; Kwong, Manning,

**TABLE 3–1.  Descriptions of Role Development**

| V. BAKER | M. KRAMER | D. ODA | CHARACTERISTICS |
|---|---|---|---|
| Orientation | Honeymoon | Role Identification | New CNS, enthusiastic, optimistic, anxious; eager to prove self, make change; clarifying role to self and setting. |
| Frustration | Shock | — | Depression and frustration in the face of overwhelming problems, slow change, and resistance; conflict between school-bred and work-world values. Feelings of inadequacy in role. |
| Implementation | Recovery | Role Transition | Rethinking and clarifying role to self and setting; modifying activities in response to feedback; specific projects with tangible results; returning perspective; sense of humor. |
| Reassessment | Resolution | Role Confirmation | Acceptance and reinforcement of role definition; renewed enthusiasm and optimism; risk-taking; further role refinement. |

Data compiled from Baker, V.: Retrospective explorations in role development. *In* Padilla, G.V. (ed): The Clinical Nurse Specialist and Improvement of Nursing Practice. Wakefield, MA, Nursing Resources, 1979; from Kramer, M.: Reality Shock: Why Nurses Leave Nursing. St. Louis, C. V. Mosby, 1974; and from Oda, D.: Specialized role development: A three-phase process. Nurs Outlook *25*:374–377, 1977.

and Koetters, 1982), or based on very small or unknown sample sizes (V. Baker, 1979; Oda, 1977; Ayers, 1979). Furthermore, most discussion of role development is limited to novice CNSs. It is imperative, therefore, to collect data as a foundation for an empirically based formulation of CNS role development, while considering the broad range of CNS experience. The purposes of the study described in this chapter were to describe the role development of CNSs, to compare experienced and inexperienced CNSs in regard to their role development, and to identify barriers and facilitators to successful role development.

## METHODOLOGY

### Procedure

Names of practicing CNSs and five organized CNS groups were identified from the professional network of the authors. Potential participants were invited to complete a questionnaire at their convenience and return it by mail. Informed consent was assumed by questionnaire return. In several situations, organized CNS groups were requested to copy the questionnaire and distribute it further to their own professional networks. No instructions were given about returning undistributed questionnaires; therefore, it is not possible to ascertain the precise number of questionnaires actually distributed. One hundred and seven (107) responses were received. Seven were not usable, resulting in a study sample of 100 currently practicing full-time CNSs.

### Instruments

The entire 16-page questionnaire was developed by the authors specifically for the purposes of the current study. Instruments were created to measure each of the conceptual areas: clinical practice characteristics, job satisfaction, the process of CNS role development, barriers and facilitators of role development, and challenges of the CNS role. A general demographic data section was also included in the questionnaire. A review of literature in each of the major conceptual areas assisted with item construction and provided the basis for face validity. During the instrument development phase, the entire questionnaire was critiqued by a nurse researcher colleague and pilot-tested with 15 practicing CNSs for format and clarity. These CNSs critiqued the instruments representing the major conceptual areas in the study in order to establish content validity.

First, the Clinical Practice Inventory obtained information on the characteristics of the CNS's current practice setting as well as other selected information such as practice history, career orientation, and self-assessment of clinical expertise.

The Advanced Practice Job Satisfaction Survey listed 23 specific factors that could be considered sources of both satisfaction and dissatisfaction for nurses in advanced practice. Respondents were asked to review the list, first rating the extent to which each factor contributed to job satisfaction and then the extent it contributed to dissatisfaction.

The Role Development Process Assessment was based on conceptual themes from V. Baker's four developmental phases for CNSs with less than three years of experience. First, a brief summary of each of Baker's phases was presented, followed by the question: "To what extent did you experience this phase?" Responses were on a five-point scale from "not at all" to "a great deal." Then, participants were asked: "If you did experience this phase, why do you think you did? If you did not experience this phase, why do you think you did not?" Respondents were asked to indicate when the phase began and ended, calculating from their first month of employment.

The second part of this section was directed toward CNSs with more than three years of experience in their present positions. These CNSs were asked: "How would you describe your current phase of role development?" To encourage the participants to write their thoughts and feelings in detail, each question was followed by approximately one half page of blank space. CNSs who have had more than one position were asked whether they experienced role development differently in each position.

The Barrier/Facilitator Assessment consisted of two open-ended questions with large blank spaces provided for subject responses. The questions were: "Considering all your CNS positions, what **single** factor do you consider to be the most helpful/greatest barrier or obstacle in your role development?"

Finally, the Challenge Assessment was directed toward experienced CNSs. It consisted of one open-ended question: "How do you remain challenged in your CNS role?" A large blank area was provided for subjects to write in their responses.

## Sample

While responses were received from widely separated geographic locations, 83 per cent of the respondents live in Virginia, Illinois, California, and Canada. Ninety-eight per cent of the survey respondents were white females, varying in age from 29 to 63 years. The majority were employed in large teaching hospitals. Table 3–2 outlines the

**TABLE 3–2.   Demographics of Respondents**

| Total Number of Respondents | Number/Percent |
| --- | --- |
| 0–3 total years as a CNS | 42 |
| 3–16 total years as a CNS | 58 |
| Total | 100 |

### RESPONDENTS BY YEARS IN CURRENT POSITION

| | |
| --- | --- |
| 0–0.9 years | 19 |
| 1–1.9 years | 24 |
| 2–2.9 years | 13 |
| 3–3.9 years | 10 |
| 4–4.9 years | 9 |
| 5–5.9 years | 8 |
| 6–9.9 years | 10 |
| Over 10 years | 7 |

### RESPONDENTS BY TOTAL YEARS AS A CNS
(all positions)

| | |
| --- | --- |
| 0–0.9 years | 16 |
| 1–1.9 years | 18 |
| 2–2.9 years | 8 |
| 3–3.9 years | 8 |
| 4–4.9 years | 9 |
| 5–5.9 years | 10 |
| 6–9.9 years | 18 |
| Over 10 years | 13 |

### RESPONDENTS BY GEOGRAPHIC AREA

| | |
| --- | --- |
| Northeast | 12 |
| Southeast | 19 |
| Southwest | 1 |
| South | 4 |
| Midwest | 27 |
| West | 18 |
| Northwest | 0 |
| Canada | 19 |

### RESPONDENTS BY SEX

| | |
| --- | --- |
| Female respondents | 98 |
| Male respondents | 2 |

### RESPONDENTS BY AGE

| | |
| --- | --- |
| Under 25 | 0 |
| 25–35 | 55 |
| 36–45 | 30 |
| 46–55 | 11 |
| Over 56 | 3 |
| No Response | 1 |

### RESPONDENTS BY ETHNIC ORIGIN

| | |
| --- | --- |
| Caucasian | 99 |
| Other | 1 |

### CERTIFICATION STATUS OF RESPONDENTS*

| | |
| --- | --- |
| Certified | 40 |
| Noncertified | 60 |

*Figures may be skewed because Canada does not use United States certifying examinations.

demographic characteristics of respondents including years of experience. The participants reported a mean of 4.53 years of total CNS experience and a mean of 3.43 years in their current positions. The respondents generally appeared to be both hard working and committed to their careers. Most reported working more than 40 hours a week, varying from 40 to 72 and averaging between 45 and 50 hours per week. Overall, the CNSs were more satisfied than dissatisfied and considered their careers very to extremely important. Forty per cent were certified by either the ANA or a specialty organization. (It is important to note that Canadian CNSs do not use the United States certification process, although some of them reported being certified. However, the majority of Canadians were not, which increased the number of uncertified respondents.)

Participants reported that their time was distributed among five role components in descending order of frequency: patient care and consultation; education; administrative activities such as committee work; research; and professional development activities including publications, organizational activities, and self-learning. Preliminary data analysis did not identify marked differences between experienced and inexperienced CNSs related to the distribution of time spent in each of the components. These findings appear to be consistent with those of another study (ANA Clinical Nurse Specialists: Distribution and Utilization, 1986).

## RESULTS

Survey data indicate that the experience of role development is a highly variable and complex phenomenon. Seven definable phases were identified from the descriptions of both novice and experienced CNSs (Table 3–3). However, there was no one sequence—rather, respondents moved from phase to phase in a highly fluid, individual fashion. Some CNSs in positions for less than three years noted being simultaneously in different phases with different nursing units. Four of these subjects experienced an overlapping of the first four phases, with one CNS noting, "Surprisingly, perhaps, there are elements of all phases still present to varying extents." Only one respondent did not experience any distinct phases.

The majority of respondents did describe their experiences in terms of phases. Baker's first three phases were experienced by almost all the CNSs who had been in their positions for three years or less, although there were differences in the intensity of experience (Table 3–4). Significant variation in the length of the phases was reported, as

**TABLE 3–3.   Phases of Role Development**

| PHASE | CHARACTERISTICS | DEVELOPMENTAL TASKS |
|---|---|---|
| Orientation | Enthusiasm, optimism, eager to prove self to setting<br>Anxious about ability to meet self- and institutional expectations<br>Expects to make change | Learn formal and informal organizations<br>Learn key players; begin establishing relationships and power base<br>Explore expectations to see if compatible with own<br>Identify and clarify role to self and others |
| Frustration | Discouragement and questioning due to unrealistic expectations (either self- or employer); difficult and slow-paced change; resistance encountered<br>Feelings of inadequacy in response to the overwhelming problems encountered, pressure to prove worth | Develop more realistic expectations<br>Work on time management and setting priorities<br>Develop short-term goals or projects to get tangible results/feedback<br>Develop support system within and/or outside work setting |
| Implementation | Returning optimism and enthusiasm as positive feedback received and expectations realigned<br>Organization and reorganization of role tasks, modified in response to feedback<br>Implementing and balancing new subroles<br>Regaining sense of perspective<br>*May* focus on specific project(s) | Enhance visibility and power base within informal and formal organizations; build coalitions and networks<br>Identify tangible accomplishments<br>Complete transition to advanced practice level, if necessary<br>Continue to reassess and refocus direction |
| Integration | Self-confident and assured in role<br>Rated self at advanced level of practice<br>Activities reflect wide recognition, influence in area of specialty<br>Continuously feels challenged; takes on new projects; expands practice<br>Either moderately or very satisfied with present position<br>Congruence between personal and organizational goals and expectations | Continued role evolution and skill development to strengthen subroles and competencies (see Ch. 1)<br>Share expertise and experience with others through publications, research, professional activities<br>Maintain flexible approach<br>Be alert for signs of complacency or boredom |
| Frozen | Self-confident, assured in role<br>Rated self at intermediate or advanced practice level<br>Experiencing anger/frustration reflecting experience<br>Conflict between self goals and those of organization/supervisor<br>Report sense of being unable to move forward due to forces outside of self | Obtain feedback from supervisor and peers<br>Re-evaluate self goals in relation to CNS role and organization<br>Objective assessment of organization: is there potential for compatibility?<br>Attempt to redesign or renegotiate the role<br>If unsuccessful consider change in position/career direction |
| Reorganization | Reported earlier experiences that represent integration<br>Organization experiencing major changes<br>Pressure to change role in ways that are incongruent with own concept of CNS role and/or self goals | Open discussion with change agents<br>Attempt compromise to preserve integrity of role and still meet needs of organization<br>If unsuccessful, change position/title or negotiate job change |
| Complacent | Experiences self in role as settled and comfortable<br>Variable job satisfaction<br>Questionable impact on organization | Need to re-energize<br>Reconfigure role to allow growth by identifying new need of client population or institution |

**TABLE 3–4.  Role Development Phases**

| | | "TO WHAT EXTENT DID YOU EXPERIENCE THIS PHASE?" | | | | | | |
|---|---|---|---|---|---|---|---|---|
| PHASE | Not Yet | Not at All 1 | 2 | Moderate Amount 3 | 4 | A Great Deal 5 | Range of Month Began | Range of Duration (months) |
| *First Position CNS (N=42)* | | | | | | | | |
| Orientation (N=42) | — | — | 5% | 36% | 16% | 43% | 1st–2nd | 2–10 |
| Frustration (N=41) | 1 | 5% | 12% | 34% | 15% | 34% | 1st–16th | 1–18 |
| Implementation (N=32) | 11 | — | 16% | 28% | 31% | 25% | 1st–24th | 1–12 |
| *Second Position CNS (N=12)* | | | | | | | | |
| Orientation (N=12) | — | 8% | 25% | 17% | 17% | 33% | 1st–3rd | 1–8 |
| Frustration (N=12) | — | 17% | 32% | 17% | 17% | 17% | 1st–12th | 2–7 |
| Implementation (N=11) | 1 | 18% | — | 55% | 18% | 9% | 2nd–15th | 1–22 |

49

well as in the ordering of phases. The first three phases generally occurred in order, but were not necessarily discrete—38 per cent of first position CNSs and 50 per cent of second position CNSs reported overlap between phases, noting that they experienced some elements of the next phase before moving into it completely.

Responses to the question of why the phase was or was not experienced were coded into the following categories derived from the data: situational characteristics (such as factors within the institution, type of patient, presence of administrative or peer support), role characteristics (comments relating directly to the CNS role itself), and personal characteristics (comments based on the individual CNS's personality or affective reactions to a given phase).

Those respondents who had been in their current positions for more than three years were given an open-ended question about their present developmental phase. First the data were examined for degree of congruence with Baker's four phases. It was apparent that some of the more experienced CNSs were reporting their developmental phases in different terms than the neophyte CNSs. Content analysis was used to create coding categories. Seven phases of role development emerged. Three of these were analogous to Baker's categories (see Table 3–3).

For each phase of role development, the authors identified a list of characteristics to describe the phase more specifically. A series of "developmental tasks," i.e., the goals that must be achieved if the next phase is to be reached (see Table 3–3), were derived by the authors, based partially on the comments of respondents and on the strategies they reported as helpful in moving on to the next phase. From this perspective, CNSs may not progress from one phase to the next without sustained and directed effort.

Because of the distinctive differences between novice and experienced CNS role development, the following discussion will address each group separately.

## Initial Role Development: The CNS in First Position

### *Orientation Phase*

The orientation phase is a natural developmental step in learning a new role. It began immediately and was experienced by all respondents in positions for less than three years (Table 3–4). As with each phase, the duration was highly variable among respondents, lasting from 2 to 10 months, with a mean duration of 4.6 months. Orientation is characterized by enthusiasm and optimism. The new CNS expects to make changes that would benefit the organization, but lacks an established network or the acceptance necessary to make change happen and may feel some anxiety about the ability to meet personal and institutional expectations. Typical descriptions of this phase included, "I was eager to put knowledge and skills gained in master's preparation into practice"; "I was enthusiastic about making an impact on nursing care"; "I was new to the position, new to the hospital, and the first CNS the hospital had ever employed. I was very excited about the possibilities and challenges and wanted to make a positive impression."

Situational characteristics, specifically the newness of the institution and city, were most commonly cited as reasons for experiencing an orientation phase. Almost half of the CNSs in their first position reported that the CNS role was new to their institutions. Characteristics related to the CNS role were also mentioned as reasons for this phase: "I was filled with positive expectations for what I felt was an almost perfect job." The opportunities and scope of the CNS role are both exciting and overwhelming. Regarding personal characteristics, some CNSs commented on feeling insecure about their skills or inadequate in the face of potential difficulties, while others were eager to begin working after being in school.

Factors that appear to diminish the strength of this phase include familiarity with the setting and staff or previous experience in positions with some of the same characteristics as the CNS position. In these situations, expectations were more realistic, resulting in a decreased feeling of orientation.

The developmental tasks of the orientation phase include: learning about the formal and informal organization and the influential individuals in the organization, establishing relationships, and building a power base. The CNS must explore the expectations of key leaders to ascertain compatibility with self-expectations. The CNS must identify and clarify the role to self and others, especially if the role is newly created. And importantly, CNSs in an orientation phase must begin to internalize their own worth in the role.

Inhibitors to moving quickly and successfully through the orientation phase include the lack of previous role models in the setting, lack of guidance or clear expectations from administration, and changes in the reporting relationship for the CNS during the orientation experience.

### Frustration Phase

As can be seen in Table 3–4, 95 per cent (40 out of 41) of first position respondents with less than three years experience went through the frustration phase; 83 per cent of experienced CNSs also experienced this phase when beginning a new job. The sense of frustration began immediately for some CNSs, and as late as the 16th month of employment for others. For most respondents, it followed orientation, although one CNS commented that she "falls in and out [of this phase] periodically." Again, duration was highly variable, from 1 to 18 months in length. The frustration phase is a powerful and disconcerting experience, characterized by feelings of discouragement and inadequacy as the CNS's initial assessment reveals unrealistic personal or organizational expectations, overwhelming problems, and the realization that making change is more difficult and slower than originally expected (one CNS remarked on the "glacial speed" with which change occurs). The CNS can be discouraged by resistance encountered and may feel inadequate in the face of pressure to prove worth in the role. The questioning of one's expertise and ability is one of the most difficult components of this phase.

Situational characteristics contributed most often to a sense of frustration. These included lack of clear role definition in the institution, confusion and conflict between self- and hospital expectations, staff resistance to new ideas, lack of administrative support and feedback, and lack of sufficient CNS resources to meet demand, with resulting time pressures. "As I became more familiar with the work setting I began to see all the areas that needed work—while this is challenging, it also became overwhelming at times. Certain areas were full of resistance." CNSs commented on the lack of administrative support or even understanding of the potential uses of the role. Role characteristics, especially role ambiguity, were also noted. Personal factors listed include impatience, insecurity, feelings of inadequacy due to either the inexperience or the competence of nursing staff, or "ridiculous self-expectations." One CNS seems to have all three characteristics (situational, role, and personal) in her response: "I used the words 'inadequate and overwhelmed' frequently to describe myself to friends. Had been an expert ICU staff nurse . . . then felt I was an expert at nothing. Although I covered the surgical areas, I was not a *specialist* in any of these areas . . . . Compared to my peers (who were experienced) I really felt substandard. I cried a lot, too! I believe it [the frustration phase] lasts much longer than reported [18 months for this CNS] and is a very powerful stage." In contrast, two respondents believed the frustration phase was normal and natural, with one commenting, "It's part of living and working in a challenging job."

It is important to emphasize that this phase is not inherent in the experience of CNS role development. The seven CNSs who did not experience frustration or who experienced it only mildly seemed to have positive situational characteristics as a major determinant. A supportive environment, receptive staff, strong role models, and a clear project focus helped to diminish or eliminate this stage. In two respondents, there was a strong match of expectations between the individual and the institution. One of these CNSs noted "great relief by [the health care] team at having someone coordinate and problem-solve [for] this patient population." The flexibility and stimulating nature of the role were also mentioned.

How does one cope with the difficult feelings engendered during the frustration phase and emerge successfully through this period? Patience and persistence were noted frequently, one respondent stating, "I can't change this system; too big for an individual to change—have to be patient." Some CNSs were helped by the realization that this phase would pass with time and that the implementation phase was worth waiting for. Another important coping strategy was to participate in activities to increase self-esteem, such as talking with colleagues, writing an article, or speaking at a conference away from the institution. Other individuals concentrated on areas in which they could make tangible progress or focused on a specific project in order to see results from their work and increase their positive feelings. Others decreased their expectations, developed allies within the setting, or found someone knowledgeable about the role (CNS peer, administrator, faculty member, CNS at another institution) with whom they could talk. One mentioned having an "escape hatch," a personal way to relieve stress.

The developmental tasks of this phase follow from these strategies for coping. They include developing more realistic expectations, setting priorities and managing time more productively, developing satisfactory working relationships with significant others in the setting, learning to make the system work for one's own goals, and building some positive sense of self as *specialist*. A crucial task is to develop a support system, especially if the CNS does not already have one. While peers are clearly helpful in supporting the frustrated CNS, other persons both within and outside the work environment can also provide support for the CNS. The CNS needs to develop a perspective based on the realities of the setting and to begin working toward short-term goals or projects that can provide immediate gratification, while waiting for results on more complex issues.

### Implementation Phase

The increased stress of the frustration phase can be a motivating force in moving the CNS into the implementation phase. This phase was commonly experienced, beginning immediately for one CNS and as late as two years for another. Again, duration was highly variable, from 1 to 12 months in length (one experienced CNS in her second position said this phase lasted for 22 months). Implementation is affectively characterized by returning optimism and feelings of self-worth as one begins experiencing comfort with the role. There may be a sense of hope and accomplishment gained from having "made it" through the frustration phase. Characteristically, the CNS is more capable of objectively assessing the situation and modifying approaches in response to feedback, resulting in some reorganization of role tasks. New role components are added in practice; the four subroles are implemented with more balance and fewer incidences of feeling over-whelmed. There may be a focus on short-term projects that can yield tangible results, but this was not experienced by all respondents. More universal was the clarification of role definition and priorities, which took into account a more realistic perspective. One CNS characterized this phase as one of "reassessing direction; [I am] more proactive . . . than reactive . . . . Feeling secure enough in the environment that I can take risks in development."

There were numerous situational characteristics identified as re-sponsible for the experience of this phase. The most frequent was positive feedback and support from colleagues, supervisors, staff, phy-sicians, and patients and families. Other factors that increased confi-dence were learning the resources and politics of the system, receiving referrals from nurses and physicians, and stabilizing relationships so that they require less energy. Personal characteristics of self-confidence in skills, determination to focus, and acceptance of the slowness of system change were identified. Role characteristics mentioned included clarification of role definition and structuring and prioritizing time more effectively. While some CNSs experienced this phase immediately, the mean beginning point for this phase was 8.8 months after employ-ment (Table 3–4).

Developmental tasks for this phase include the need to continue to reassess direction and focus activities, reorganize and modify ap-proaches, identify tangible accomplishments, incorporate subrole com-ponents, and balance them without feeling overwhelmed. In this phase, CNSs learn how to make the system work for their own goals and build coalitions and networks to facilitate change and solidify their power base. An important task of this phase is to assess one's level of clinical expertise and complete the transition to the level of advanced practi-tioner if not already there.

The issue of practice level deserves further attention. One of the survey questions asked: "How would you assess your current clinical skills for the CNS role?" Four levels of practice were listed: novice, beginner, intermediate, and advanced. No definitions were given for these various levels, so that respondents offered a personal assessment of their level of practice, using criteria unknown to the investigators. The results showed a marked difference in assessed level of practice by total years as a CNS (Table 3–5). Seventeen per cent of the CNSs with less than three years of experience rated themselves as novices, while another 19 per cent rated themselves at the beginner level, and only 26 per cent at the advanced level. Some CNSs with as much as five years of experience in the role did not rate themselves as being at an advanced clinical skill level. Perhaps respondents interpreted the question as referring to skills in all the CNS subroles rather than specific clinical skills. Further study would be necessary to determine the extent to which this kind of self-assessment may approximate Benner's levels of clinical expertise. These results, however, are disturbing. Advanced clinical skills need to be a top priority for the new CNS, in order to progress to the integrated phase.

REASSESSMENT? Analysis of data from the current study did not support reassessment as a distinct phase. For many CNSs, the implementation and reassessment phases as defined by V. Baker were difficult to distinguish. The term "reassessment" is misleading, because reassessing one's performance is a characteristic of the implementation phase. In addition, the major feature of risk-taking that Baker attributed to this phase occurs in all phases. Consequently, some respondents classified themselves in reassessment after a very short time in the role. Baker's work was based on interviews with four CNSs who had been in the role 12 to 18 months. It is questionable whether her subjects had reached the integration phase, although it appears that they were experiencing some elements of it. Using the defining characteristics, most respondents in this study who categorized themselves in reassessment were actually in implementation.

**TABLE 3–5.  Stated Levels of Practice by Total Years as CNS**

| Years as CNS | Novice # | % | Beginner # | % | Intermediate # | % | Advanced # | % | Total # | % |
|---|---|---|---|---|---|---|---|---|---|---|
| 0–0.9 | 6 | 37.5 | 6 | 37.5 | 1 | 6.0 | 3 | 19.0 | 16 | 100 |
| 1–1.9 | 1 | 6.0 | 2 | 11.0 | 11 | 61.0 | 4 | 22.0 | 18 | 100 |
| 2–2.9 | — | — | — | — | 4 | 50.0 | 4 | 50.0 | 8 | 100 |
| 3–3.9 | — | — | — | — | 7 | 87.5 | 1 | 12.5 | 8 | 100 |
| 4–4.9 | — | — | — | — | 5 | 55.5 | 4 | 44.5 | 9 | 100 |
| 5–5.9 | — | — | — | — | 3 | 30.0 | 7 | 70.0 | 10 | 100 |
| 6–9.9 | — | — | — | — | 2 | 11.0 | 16 | 89.0 | 18 | 100 |
| Over 10 | — | — | — | — | — | — | 13 | 100.0 | 13 | 100 |
| Total | 7 | 7.0 | 8 | 8.0 | 33 | 33.0 | 52 | 52.0 | 100 | 100 |

## The Experienced CNS

As was previously noted, CNSs with more than three years of experience used descriptors that fell outside of Baker's phases. Based on the survey findings, four additional phases of role development were identified. These will be described and discussed, with special attention given to their application for CNSs who have been in the role for more than three years.

### *Integration Phase*

Integration is characterized by self-confidence and assurance in the role, high job satisfaction, an advanced level of practice, and signs of recognition and respect for expertise within and outside the work setting. While productivity could not be specifically assessed in a questionnaire, it can be hypothesized that the integration phase is the most productive. Applying the defining characteristics of this phase to respondents with less than three years of experience revealed that four of them appeared to be in this phase; however, most respondents did not reach the integration phase until after three years in the CNS role (Tables 3–6 and 3–7).

In this phase, the role has "come together," with struggles and conflicts characteristic of earlier phases largely resolved. Among the respondents, the percentages of CNSs who met the criteria for the integrated phase varied from 10 per cent for those with less than five years experience in the role to 50 per cent of those with more than six years total experience in the role. When comparing length of time as a CNS versus length of time in present position (Tables 3–6 and 3–7), it can be seen that the experienced CNS can achieve the integrated phase in a shorter period of time than her novice colleague. In fact, evidence in respondent comments indicates that a change in position actually facilitates the developmental progression in some instances. As one CNS stated, "When I started my first job I was really not an expert . . . . By the second job I could really move in at the expert level."

Integrated CNSs described a high level of satisfaction with themselves, their institutions, and their accomplishments. Typical comments include: "[I feel] experienced, valued and supported . . . have a track record and no longer have to prove myself . . . able to focus more quickly on problem areas . . . almost always use theory in current activities." A CNS with 15 years' experience wrote: ". . . the role is well established . . . seen as 'ideal' by other CNSs . . . . Role components understood by nurses, physicians and other health care professionals . . . . Administration allows freedom and flexibility . . . knowledge base

TABLE 3–6. Developmental Phase by Total Years as a CNS

| | Total Years as aCNS (all positions) | | | | | | | | | | | | | | | | | |
| | 0–0.9 | | 1–1.9 | | 2–2.9 | | 3–3.9 | | 4–4.9 | | 5–5.9 | | 6–9.9 | | Over 10 | | Total | |
| | # | % | # | % | # | % | # | % | # | % | # | % | # | % | # | % | # | % |
|---|---|---|---|---|---|---|---|---|---|---|---|---|---|---|---|---|---|---|
| Orientation | 2 | 12.5 | — | — | — | — | — | — | — | — | — | — | — | — | — | — | 2 | 2 |
| Frustration | 8 | 50.0 | — | — | 1 | 12.5 | 2 | 25.5 | 1 | 11.0 | — | — | — | — | — | — | 12 | 12 |
| Implementation | 6 | 37.5 | 16 | 89.0 | 3 | 37.5 | 4 | 50.0 | 6 | 67.0 | 5 | 50.0 | 1 | 5.5 | — | — | 41 | 41 |
| Integration | — | — | 2 | 11.0 | 2 | 25.0 | — | — | 1 | 11.0 | 1 | 10.0 | 8 | 44.5 | 8 | 61.5 | 22 | 22 |
| Complacent | — | — | — | — | — | — | — | — | — | — | — | — | 2 | 11.0 | 1 | 7.5 | 3 | 3 |
| Frozen | — | — | — | — | 1 | 12.0 | — | — | 1 | 11.0 | 2 | 20.0 | 3 | 17.0 | 2 | 15.5 | 9 | 9 |
| Reorganization | — | — | — | — | — | — | — | — | — | — | 1 | 10.0 | 2 | 11.0 | — | — | 3 | 3 |
| No Response | — | — | — | — | 1 | 12.5 | 2 | 25.0 | — | — | 1 | 10.0 | 2 | 11.0 | 2 | 15.5 | 8 | 8 |
| Totals | 16 | 100.0 | 18 | 100.0 | 8 | 100.0 | 8 | 100.0 | 9 | 100.0 | 10 | 100.0 | 18 | 100.0 | 13 | 100.0 | 100 | 100 |

**TABLE 3–7. Developmental Phase by Years in Current Position**

| | YEARS IN CURRENT POSITION | | | | | | | | | | | | | | | |
|---|---|---|---|---|---|---|---|---|---|---|---|---|---|---|---|---|
| | 0–0.9 | | 1–1.9 | | 2–2.9 | | 3–4.9 | | 5–5.9 | | 6–9.9 | | 10–16 | | Total | |
| PHASE | # | % | # | % | # | % | # | % | # | % | # | % | # | % | # | % |
| Orientation | 2 | 11 | — | — | — | — | — | — | — | — | — | — | — | — | 2 | 2 |
| Frustration | 8 | 42 | 1 | 4 | 1 | 8 | 2 | 11 | — | — | — | — | — | — | 12 | 12 |
| Implementation | 6 | 31 | 20 | 84 | 5 | 38 | 8 | 42 | 2 | 25 | — | — | — | — | 41 | 41 |
| Integration | 3 | 16 | 2 | 8 | 4 | 30 | 2 | 11 | 2 | 25 | 5 | 50 | 4 | 57 | 22 | 22 |
| Complacent | — | — | — | — | 1 | 8 | — | — | 1 | 13 | 1 | 10 | — | — | 3 | 3 |
| Frozen | — | — | 1 | 4 | 1 | 8 | 2 | 11 | 2 | 25 | 1 | 10 | 2 | 29 | 9 | 9 |
| Reorganization | — | — | — | — | — | — | 1 | 4 | 1 | 12 | 1 | 10 | — | — | 3 | 3 |
| No Response | — | — | — | — | 1 | 8 | 4 | 21 | — | — | 2 | 20 | 1 | 14 | 8 | 8 |
| Total | 19 | 100 | 24 | 100 | 13 | 100 | 19 | 100 | 8 | 100 | 10 | 100 | 7 | 100 | 100 | 100 |

has earned respect and recognition . . . have been in the institution long enough to know all the 'ins and outs.'"

Characteristics that define this phase include recognition and validation of the CNS's advanced knowledge, as evidenced by being regularly consulted by nursing administration, physicians, staff, and peers, as well as by outside organizations, and giving workshops and conferences outside and within the work setting. Those CNSs categorized as being integrated consistently reported continued challenge in the role and in their current position. Many indicated that they were challenged by the clinical problems confronted, by changes in technology, and by new projects within the institution. Many also reported being challenged by greater involvement in professional activities, by expanding the research component of the role, by publishing, or by other outside activities. This is consistent with Holt's (1987) premise that the focus of development of the experienced CNS is to improve the care of all patients within the specialty by enlarging the sphere of influence beyond the bounds of the immediate workplace. Holt's hypothesis that the CNS achieves this phase after seven years in the role is not supported by this survey. CNSs are able to achieve this phase more quickly, some after only one year in the role (see Table 3–6).

From the foregoing discussion, it becomes evident that for those CNSs who achieve and fulfill the integration phase, the CNS role provides a satisfying and rewarding career. Furthermore, the employing agency derives maximum benefit from the implementation of the CNS role. This positive state of affairs is most likely to result when the philosophy and goals of the CNS are compatible with those of the employing agency.

For the experienced CNS, continued growth in the role seems to be facilitated by certain setting characteristics: the availability of continuous feedback to validate role performance, freedom to develop the role without unnecessary restrictions or impediments, encouragement and support for broadening the sphere of influence, and recognition of the contributions the CNS makes to patients and the institution. The multifaceted nature of the role itself and the challenges of practice also seem to account for this phase for some CNSs.

### Frozen Phase

Some experienced CNSs used terms such as "stuck," "stifled," or "frozen" to describe one phase of development. Although they expressed feelings of anger and frustration, these responses seem to reflect a realistic appraisal of themselves and their institutions. Typical of this group is the comment from one CNS who has been in her current position for 10 years: "I feel stuck trying to meet the organizational needs . . . have been unable to pursue research interests, program development . . . lack of clear goals . . . ." A 15-year veteran stated, "Administration is not supportive of my interest in doing research in a particular area . . . . I am frustrated and need to move on to a position where the objectives of the institution would match mine . . . . I am at the peak of my career and see myself not able to accomplish my professional goals."

The most striking difference between integrated and frozen CNSs appears to be the inability of the frozen group to achieve satisfaction within the role and/or the position in which they found themselves. Like the integrated CNSs, those who are in the frozen phase have been in their present positions for several years, reporting feelings of confidence and self-assurance, and most have achieved the advanced level of practice. These nurses indicate that work is moderately to extremely important to them; they report activities that would indicate some recognition within their own institutions. However, these CNSs report major conflict between their own goals and the organization's goals or constraints. Most indicated a poor relationship with their supervisor or general lack of administrative support for the programs or goals valued by the CNS. These CNSs sensed that they were not achieving their maximum potential and tended to attribute their frozen state to factors outside of themselves and external to the CNS role.

The developmental tasks of this phase center around reassessment and renegotiation of both the role and position within the organization. While the respondents attributed their dissatisfaction and lack of growth to factors outside of themselves, it is essential that the reassessment include an objective self-evaluation. Philosophy and personal goals may be incongruent with the stated purposes or philosophy of the organization. A clash of personal styles may account for conflicts with a supervisor or others within the organization. When such self characteristics are seen to be the barriers to continued role development, the CNS may need to seek feedback and counseling from trusted peers, a supervisor, and other colleagues within or outside of the organization to determine how to resolve the problems.

An equally objective assessment of situational characteristics should be undertaken. Questions that may need to be asked include:

1. Is there administrative support for the CNS role? (Does the nursing department value nursing practice? Do other CNSs also feel frozen? Are CNSs regularly appointed to appropriate committees and consulted in matters affecting them or influencing practice?)

2. Is the CNS job description and position within the organization

congruent with the title as described in the literature and practiced within the community?

3. Is placement within the organization conducive to full implementation of the role?

4. Is the scope of the job and the workload realistic in terms of time and energy expended? Or is the CNS spread so thin that there is little visible accomplishment or sense of satisfaction?

When the reassessment of self and organization has been completed, the CNS may want to initiate a full and frank discussion with the supervisor, or perhaps with other administrative staff, in an effort to resolve conflicts or redesign the job to enhance job satisfaction and further role development. If such discussions are unproductive, and no resolution appears to be possible, the CNS must consider whether to remain in the organization, move to a different setting, or choose a new career direction.

No data are available to indicate the fate of these frozen individuals; it is intriguing to speculate that they may be analogous to the "lateral arabesquers" Kramer described (Hamric, 1983). If they stay in their CNS positions, one wonders whether they will remain frustrated or slide into a permanently complacent group of specialists. In either case, it would appear that both the institution and the CNS will be the losers if progression to the desired phase of integration does not occur.

### Reorganization Phase

The reorganization phase is typically experienced by CNSs who are in organizations that are undergoing major changes in nursing or hospital administration or in funding for the institution. These changes often necessitate a reorganization in the CNS's practice, which can create conflict for the CNS. Individuals affected by such change reported earlier experiences in the same work setting which seemed to represent the phase of integration, but they now report that changing expectations in their setting conflict with personal goals. Typical of this group was one who said, "I believe that as the first clinical specialist in this institution I have significantly influenced patient care and the level of nursing practice . . . we now have many more CNSs . . . [but] now as a direct result of budget cuts the CNSs have had to assume new responsibilities not in keeping with the CNS role. I'm not happy with the way I see the role changing . . . more administrative responsibilities . . . filling in as staff." Another CNS with eight years of experience said, "Due to demands of the hospital financial situation, I have had to move from a strictly CNS position to one of Staff-Developer-Coordinator . . . . The former Director supported the CNS role . . . now the financial situation dictates the role." These CNSs seem to be expressing a sense of personal hurt and loss, as past successes and accomplishments are no longer recognized, and continued success in the organization appears to depend upon conforming to organizational requirements incongruent with previously valued performance.

The dilemma of the CNS facing major role reorganization is particularly difficult. Organizations and their needs do change, especially in these turbulent financial times. When changes occur there is often a realignment and refocusing of both traditional and nontraditional jobs. The CNS may be particularly vulnerable to internal disruptions because the role is relatively unstructured and because the skills developed in CNS subroles are readily applicable to many nonclinical functions. Furthermore, the long tenure of the CNS in the institution and the carefully nurtured power base the CNS has achieved may be viewed by the organization's leaders as an impediment to the fulfillment of new organizational goals.

An important developmental task for the CNS caught in unwelcome organizational change is to engage in open dialogue with the effecting change agent(s) in an effort to find a nonacrimonious resolution. The CNS needs to establish whether the projected changes are temporary owing to immediate financial or other constraints or are permanent reflections of a changed philosophy or organizational direction. If the change is temporary, it may be possible for the CNS and administrator to reach a satisfactory compromise, in which the CNS assumes additional duties or responsibilities with the expectation that the preferred role activities can be resumed at some time in the foreseeable future.

If the role change is expected to be permanent, the CNS must decide whether or not the new role is acceptable or whether it can be renegotiated to incorporate elements that preserve the integrity of the CNS role, allow for job satisfaction, and meet the new needs of the organization. If no compromise can be found, a career move for the CNS may be indicated.

### Complacent Phase

A small number of CNSs seemed to be in a category they described as being "settled into a comfortable position," or "plugging along." These respondents were either somewhat satisfied or very satisfied with their positions. They characterized themselves as stable in the role based on their experience. One remarked, "I've done it all—the challenge is gone—looking for something to make it exciting again." One was returning to school for a Ph.D. It is possible that this survey sample had few complacent CNSs because these would be less motivated to participate. While complacency is not necessarily negative (in fact, it may be a very helpful temporary phase for high-energy CNSs who need to "recharge their batteries"), some question exists about the extent to which the complacent CNS influences the institution. In the authors' experience, CNSs who remain in the complacent phase for long periods are not seen as change agents but rather have constructed their practices to meet selected, narrowly focused needs. This steady-state phase, while helpful to the CNS in some ways, may be deleterious to both the CNS and the institution if continued over time.

Developmental tasks of this phase focus on the need to re-energize. The CNS may need to change some aspect of practice, or focus on a new unmet need of the client population or institution. Returning to school may also help re-energize the CNS. In some way, the CNS must alter role enactment to allow for growth.

## Role Development of the Experienced CNS in a Second Position

Twenty-nine respondents had been in more than one CNS position; two had had three CNS positions. Seventy-nine per cent of these subjects experienced role development differently in each position. Fifty per cent of this group experienced overlap between phases, compared with 38 per cent of novice CNSs. As with inexperienced specialists, the onset and length of each phase was highly variable. However, the first three phases were generally shorter for experienced CNSs than for novices (Figures 3–1 and 3–2). Importantly, the frustration phase was clearly shorter for CNSs in second positions. In addition, in most cases experienced CNSs achieved the integrated phase more rapidly than inexperienced specialists.

One-third of the sample (32 per cent) only stated that the experience was different because of different colleagues, expectations, and focus. It was not possible to assess from these respondents' descriptors whether their role development was more or less difficult.

For over one-third of the experienced group (36 per cent), role development was smoother the second time around. For these CNSs, their self-confidence, knowledge of the role, and independence made movement through the phases faster and more fluid (i.e., there was more overlap between phases). Some specialists had left a troublesome first position, so that the second position seemed wonderful by comparison. As one CNS commented, "In my first position, I got stuck in frustration. Looking back, I could see that the role was not workable at that time."

The process of role development was not necessarily easier, how-

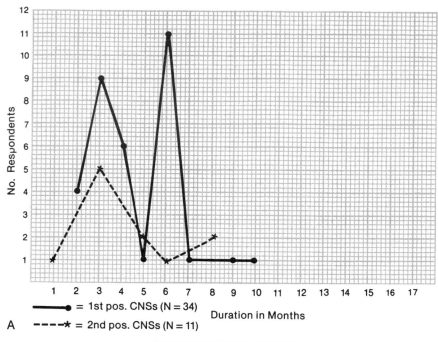

A

**ORIENTATION PHASE**

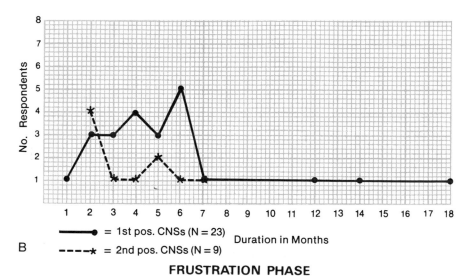

B

**FRUSTRATION PHASE**

**Figure 3–1.** Duration of phases—orientation (A), frustration (B), and implementation (C).

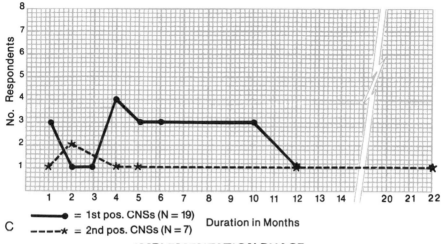

Figure 3–1 *Continued*

ever. For less than one-quarter of the sample (23 per cent), the experience was more negative. These respondents noted lack of peer support in the new setting, more time demands, and less clarity from their administrators regarding expectations. One respondent noted that she had had four bosses in five years, requiring continuous renegotiation and shifts in focus.

What can one conclude about role development for the experienced CNS? While the CNS's own sense of confidence and role clarity does appear to assist the process, it is clear that variables in the setting, especially peer and administrative support, are key factors influencing role development for both novice and experienced CNSs. Many administrators are more interested in hiring experienced CNSs, presumably because they believe these specialists will be more productive more rapidly. These data show that administrators need to be equally concerned about factors in the environment which support advanced practice and about their own support for the role. Experience alone will not guarantee a smooth transition, as evidenced in the following discussion.

## Facilitators and Barriers to Role Development

### Facilitators

Respondents were asked to identify those factors most helpful to their role development as well as those considered to act as barriers.

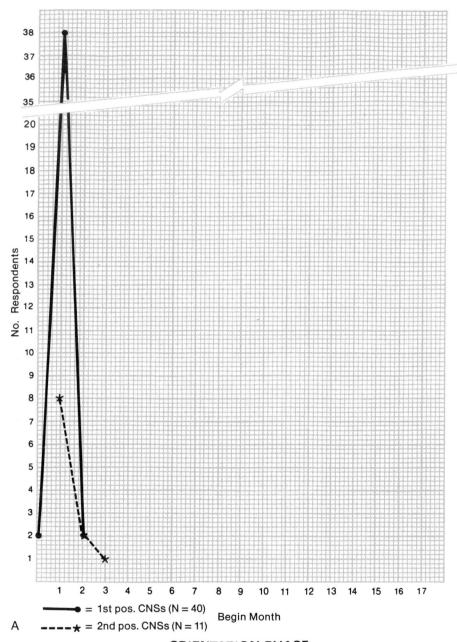

**ORIENTATION PHASE**

**Figure 3–2.** Month phases begin—orientation (A), frustration (B), and implementation (C).

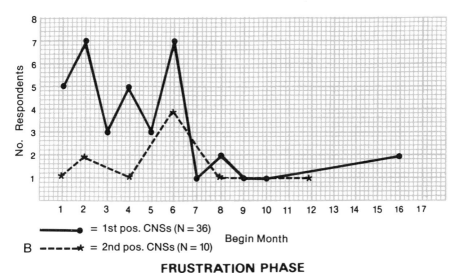

B ————• = 1st pos. CNSs (N = 36)
  — — —✳ = 2nd pos. CNSs (N = 10)

Begin Month

**FRUSTRATION PHASE**

**Figure 3–2** *Continued*

*Illustration continued on following page*

There were no identifiable differences in responses between novice and experienced CNSs. Among both groups, peer support from other CNSs and administrative support for the role were considered most helpful (Table 3–8). More specifically, peer support included the presence of other CNS colleagues in the institution, contact with graduate faculty and/or former classmate peers, structured discussions about the role with other CNSs, and general support from others in a regional CNS interest group. One CNS noted, "Most helpful is having peers—they are the best sounding boards; supportive; we gain from each others' experience and risk taking. We collaborate on projects. Those who have had more experience in the role really can help the novice." The concept of CNS peer support is discussed at length in Chapter 14.

The person supervising the CNS is clearly a key individual in facilitating the developmental process. Administrative support takes many forms: having a nursing administration willing to share knowledge of the system, identify key leaders, and describe future plans; seeking the input of the CNS in administrative decision-making; recognizing the CNS's accomplishments; providing guidance; allowing freedom and flexibility to develop the role; and giving the CNS authority in the practice setting. These findings are consistent with nursing literature relating to the importance of administrative support for the CNS role (see Chapter 13).

The high value placed by CNSs on the availability of peers and

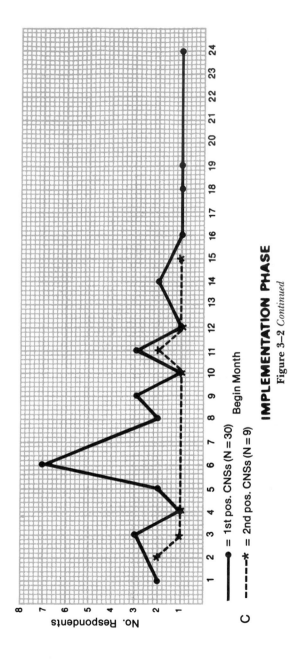

**IMPLEMENTATION PHASE**

Figure 3–2 *Continued*

**TABLE 3–8.   Factors Most Helpful in Role Development***

| FACTOR | PERCENT LISTED |
|---|---|
| Peer support | 28 |
| Administrative support | 25 |
| Self characteristics | 18 |
| Role characteristics | 9 |
| Mentor | 7 |
| Experience | 4 |
| Colleagues from other disciplines | 3 |
| Other | 6 |

*N = 114 responses.

role models noted in this study has not been previously documented. It is interesting to note that nearly all of the respondents indicated that they belonged to a peer group, either in the work setting or in the community, and that the peer group met regularly. While the network sampling strategy may have increased the prominence of this theme, even CNSs who were the only ones in their setting or city also actively sought peer support and feedback.

Other factors facilitating the CNS's role development were categorized as self characteristics and included the specialist's own clinical competence, self-confidence, sense of humor, "a stubborn streak that would not allow failure," motivation, flexibility and interpersonal skills. For example, one respondent noted, "Clinical competence is the most important factor in leading to socialization in the role; if competence and commitment to quality are evident, the role naturally develops."

Other facilitators included having a mentor; qualities of the role itself, such as flexibility, independence, and patient contact; experience; the support of colleagues in other disciplines; political awareness; positive feedback; having clear goals within one's specialty; and a "true desire by all disciplines to improve the quality of patient care."

Two themes interwoven with several of the previously discussed categories were flexibility and commitment. Flexibility appeared in administrative, self, and role characteristics as facilitating role development. Commitment to quality care and a sense that commitment was shared by nurse and physician colleagues, administrators, and other team members was also a strong facilitator of the process.

### Barriers

As might be expected, many of the obstacles to role development are the opposite of the facilitators (Table 3–9). One set of obstacles, however, represented one-third of the negative responses. This major category related to administrative problems. Lack of administrative support and guidance from the specialist's supervisor was frequently

**TABLE 3–9.   Greatest Barrier To Role Development***

| FACTOR | PERCENT LISTED |
|---|---|
| Administrative problems | 32 |
| Lack of other's understanding the role | 14 |
| Intraprofessional problems | 13 |
| Time pressures | 12 |
| Self characteristics | 7 |
| Lack of peer support | 5 |
| Interprofessional problems | 4 |
| Role characteristics | 3 |
| Other | 9 |

*N = 92 responses.

mentioned, with one respondent noting, "verbal support does not always translate into behavioral support." There were other problems, however, including administrative limitation and misuse of the role, lack of recognition of the CNS, poor leadership, and administrators not believing in the worth of the role.

The negative effects of this lack of administrative support and the positive effects of a strong coalition between administration and specialists are illustrated by this comment: "My department of nursing has been through a great deal of stress over the past few years. There was no support for the CNS role and I entered the phase of frustration very quickly and stayed there. Now, with new nursing administration there is much stronger support for the role and soon our numbers will increase. I feel I'm starting over again, but actually am refocusing my direction and being allowed to have input into appropriate administrative processes—am no longer seen as superfluous by administration. With administrative support, I am able to focus on the things I have assessed as being important and needy of my intervention."

Lack of understanding of the CNS role was the second most frequent barrier. When nursing staff do not understand the role, they tend to limit the CNS to certain activities or see the role as a physician substitute. Physicians may also misunderstand the role and may have the same reactions noted in staff nurses.

CNSs also identified intraprofessional conflicts, specifically staff resistance to change, apathy, and nurses unaccustomed to consulting other nurses as experts. One CNS stated that her greatest barrier was that experienced staff considered themselves specialists and felt threatened by her.

The magnitude of job expectations, multiplicity of demands placed on the CNS, and general time pressures were obstacles noted in 12 per cent of the responses. A number of CNSs with less than three years experience indicated that personal characteristics of impatience, insecurity, and perfectionism act as barriers.

Lack of role models and peer support were mentioned less frequently than expected, given the importance of this factor in facilitating role development. Conflicts with physicians and other team members, unclear role definition, and other factors such as politics within the institution, size of the hospital, incompatibility with organizational goals, and inability to document cost-effectiveness were also listed.

## Challenges in the Role

The authors were interested in what keeps the CNS challenged and growing. Those respondents who had been in their current positions for more than three years were asked: "How do you remain challenged in your CNS role?" Whether a CNS for three years or sixteen, most respondents reported continual stimulation. Typical of the challenges indicated by specialists with three to five years experience were "always trying to define the needs and meet them . . . relationships with patients and families . . . [my] role as clinical preceptor . . . having something new added each year to the components of the role." Some CNSs with more than five years experience also commented on their relationships with patients and families, the continuing stimulation from peers and colleagues, and the learning of something new every day. Many CNSs were challenged by reaching out professionally into greater involvement in professional organizations, into research or publication. A few were developing private practices as an adjunct to their full-time positions. Some indicated an interest in pursuing a higher degree.

There were no significant differences in the challenges as reported by CNSs within the various developmental phases. Even those categorized as frozen or complacent apparently found an interest either within or outside of the primary work setting which proved professionally challenging. Correlated with this finding is the fact that 91 per cent of all respondents reported that their careers were very or extremely important to them. Thus, a picture emerges of a group of highly involved professionals who seek and find challenging activities, even when the primary work setting is frustrating or disappointing.

Since there are no comparable data relating to other nursing professionals, no conclusions can be drawn from this study about what keeps CNSs from moving into positions that might provide greater opportunities for upward mobility. It is acknowledged, of course, that some CNSs do change career direction. Are these the individuals who viewed themselves as frozen in the CNS role? Are they the ones who became complacent? Do some of those who find themselves facing unwelcome role reorganization accept or seek nonclinical positions? Some CNSs change jobs or directions for reasons unrelated to satisfaction with the particular position. Like other nurses, they may return to school, relocate, or assume new personal or family responsibilities. Further study is needed to determine whether there are differences between those who remain in CNS positions throughout their careers and those who at some time move into other fields.

It is also important to note here that the respondents' high degree of involvement in their roles may reflect the attrition bias common in all professions: those who fail to find continued challenge in the profession may drop out and find employment in other positions. Despite this, however, there was a striking theme of the inherent challenge available in the CNS role. In some ways this is not surprising, given the changing nature of the health care environment and advanced nursing practice.

## LIMITATIONS

An obvious limitation of this study is the self-selection method used to identify respondents and the lack of information about nonrespondents. Because of the method of distribution, most of the respondents were from large urban teaching hospitals with established CNS groups. Their experiences may not reflect the experiences of those who work in smaller community hospitals or in nonhospital settings.

A further limitation is that the findings are based only on experiences as reported by the CNS, with no corroborating information from other sources. Thus, the subjects' inherently subjective perceptions of their phase of development, level of practice, or other factors were the sole source of data. The authors designed a section to validate V. Baker's phases of role development. It could be argued that this approach may have biased the respondents toward these particular phases.

Despite these limitations and others inherent in exploratory, descriptive research, a fascinating, complex, and richly varied picture of CNS role development emerges from the data. The authors are deeply indebted to the CNSs who gave generously of their time and thoughts to aid in understanding this important phenomenon.

## DISCUSSION

### Strategies for Enhancing Positive Role Development

Based on this description of role development phases, facilitators, and barriers, how can one strengthen positive role enactment and specifically encourage progression into the integration phase? The following discussion of strategies to enhance role development will begin with the graduate student experience.

### Role Socialization in the Graduate Program

Role development begins in graduate school. "The clinical nurse specialist program is seen as a process of socialization in which the student as nurse is helped to modify current perceptions and enactment of the nurse role to one that has ben defined by the faculty as the role of the clinical nurse specialist" (Cason & Beck, 1982, p. 26). Intending to assess role change in students, these authors examined the role expectations of entering and exiting students as compared with expectations of CNSs, faculty, and administrators. Although the sample size was small and the data involved only one institution, the findings are noteworthy. Changes did occur in the students' priorities, with exiting students' profiles most closely resembling those of practicing CNSs and least resembling those of faculty. "The findings of this study suggest that students chose as role models those persons overtly exemplifying the role, i.e., those actually practicing the clinical nurse specialist role" (Cason & Beck, 1982, p. 38). Two serendipitous findings from this study included "the degree of agreement regarding relative importance of these [CNS] behaviors is greater between practicing clinical nurse specialists and nursing service administrators than it is between clinical nurse specialists and faculty. Graduate faculty and nursing service administrators differed significantly in their ranking of clinical nurse specialist role behaviors" (p. 38). The role conflicts created by such disagreement are noted by the authors as potential contributors to the "reality shock" experienced by the graduate.

Preparing graduate students for the realities of the CNS role, or "anticipatory socialization" to use Kramer's terminology, is an important initial step in enhancing positive role enactment. There are many components of this process. It is important to prepare students to be expert clinicians, as well as help them remain mindful of the limits of their knowledge base. However, clinical expertise is not sufficient. Graduate students must also be exposed to theoretical and practical aspects of the CNS role. They need to challenge assumptions and develop realistic expectations of CNS practice. Analyzing existing CNS job descriptions and developing interview questions and strategies for beginning one's work as a new CNS should be expected elements of the curriculum. Students need to be prepared for the possible slowness of movement through developmental phases, especially in the first year.

CNS students need to experience the subroles directly, rather than simply observe a preceptor demonstrate them. Watching and analyzing a skilled specialist in practice can give students valuable insight into role enactment. However, students must then practice the role behaviors to be adequately prepared for assuming a CNS position upon graduation. This "role immersion" can be monitored by faculty, with anticipatory guidance and assistance offered in applying relevant theory to situations and analyzing difficult encounters to help the student "process" the experience.

In a summary of recommendations for directions in oncology nursing, a group of oncology nursing leaders noted that clinical immersion experiences were needed in graduate curricula to prepare oncology CNSs (OCNSs). They further stated that these experiences should clearly include development of expertise in direct care, discussions of OCNS role development, and practice with other OCNS role functions, not just observation. They recommended that "the clinical immersion occur over time with the opportunity to reflect on this experience with an expert coach" (Donoghue & Spross, 1985, p. 71).

Requiring students to develop a record of their clinical experiences with the CNS role (a clinical log) for faculty review can serve many purposes. Initial experiences with advanced practice can be reflected upon and analyzed with faculty guidance. The strong emotional reactions to advanced practice, with its related ethical and interprofessional issues, can be chronicled and processed with the help of faculty expertise. Clinical logs also help the student to identify actual or potential activities for the CNS interacting with patients and staff. Logs can help students anticipate variables to assess when seeking a position after graduation. The record can continue to be a source of information and self-support after graduation.

Follow-up discussions of the experiences recorded in the clinical logs should occur as part of the CNS practicum course. Most students encounter many of the issues identified in individual logs. Faculty can use the log data as examples for class discussion, can suggest related readings to increase students' knowledge regarding issues, and can discuss strategies for dealing with problems encountered.

An important aspect of graduate role preparation involves learning to exist creatively within the system. Theoretical material can be very helpful in preparing students to analyze problem situations that they will encounter in practice. Specifically, readings on leadership, problem-solving, motivation, power, learning theory, change, organizations, stress and burnout, and conflict resolution can all be useful when applied to specific problem situations. Faculty need to model the application of theory to troublesome practice situations initially, as students may need help seeing the relevance of theory to specific practice problems.

It is important that the process and factors impeding CNS role development are discussed in graduate programs. Students need to understand the inevitability of encountering staff, physician, and administrative resistance and to learn some strategies to use in overcoming it. Exercises such as formulating and prioritizing short- and long-term goals for a certain position as well as developing evaluation criteria for these goals can be helpful. A clinical/change project in which the student plans, implements, and evaluates the project is a helpful activity. Such exercises enhance the student's own clarity regarding the role. In addition, realistic objectives for a position can be an important aid in the job interview.

Clinical competence, including relevant technical skill, is essential for anyone using the CNS title. To enter a CNS position with less knowledge or skill than that of the staff nurses working within the specialty is courting failure. Consequently, students should have sufficient positive clinical experience to have mastered staff nursing in their specialty before entering a graduate program. Graduate education can then focus on deepening clinical knowledge, practicing various CNS roles, and increasing use of independent judgment and autonomy. Students who have not mastered staff nursing should have extensive work experience related to the specialty they wish to pursue prior to beginning graduate school. In addition, these individuals should look for graduate programs that emphasize clinical practice experiences. It is possible for such graduates to negotiate positions that will allow development of this mastery and exercise of leadership ability as well. Such positions must be carefully negotiated and expectations clarified so that the neophyte CNS has the time to strengthen clinical skill.

### Orientation Phase Strategies

CNSs at every level indicated that a major facilitator of role development was strong administrative support, and the major deterrent was the lack of such support. Padilla and Padilla (1979) discussed the need for CNSs, as change agents, to firmly establish their legitimate and expert influence over those who will participate in the desired change. Thus, their authority base and leadership position must be clearly visible and known to the staff with whom they work. Since CNSs in staff positions lack the direct authority to implement change, they are highly dependent on "borrowed" authority to achieve agreed-upon goals. The supervisor, who has formal authority, must make it clear that the CNS is authorized to fulfill the assigned functions. Administrative support both for the CNS role and for the activities and programs of a particular CNS needs to be clearly articulated, not only to the CNS but to others who are affected by the role. Further discussion of administrative support can be found in Chapter 13.

Table 3–10 offers a list of important questions for administrators who contemplate hiring a CNS. If the answers to these questions are affirmative, an institution is ready to provide the administrative support so crucial to successful CNS practice.

Whether beginning or experienced, the newly employed CNS needs a structured orientation plan. The CNS needs the time and opportunity to become acquainted with the organizational structure, philosophy, goals, policies, and procedures of the institution. Administrators should identify key individuals for the CNS to meet, should share departmental objectives, and should help the CNS identify skill deficits that need attention. Organizational visibility, the establishment of a power base, and role tasks during the orientation phase depend to a large extent upon the opportunities the CNS has to be present when decisions are being made that will affect either the CNS role or the specialty area.

The CNS and the supervisor also need to spend time exploring and agreeing on role expectations. Some priority setting to achieve a realistic performance level may be necessary. The initial focus should be on immediate objectives and short-term goals. Measurable changes in staff behavior or outcomes of new patient care programs rarely occur within the first year. Thus, evaluation of performance should emphasize structure and process achievements (see Chapter 4). The supervisor should see progress toward the advanced level of practice as demonstrated by successful interventions with individual patients. Beginning CNSs need consensual validation and feedback frequently during the

**TABLE 3–10.    Questions to Ask in Preparation for Hiring a CNS**

Has the institution thoughtfully identified where it is in its development and what a CNS is needed for to contribute to that development?

Are the expectations realistic and achievable by one individual?

Do structural and system factors allow for success, or do certain changes need to occur before the specialist will be able to be effective?

Can administration clarify the CNS's position within the organization?

Do the skills and personal goals of the individual specialist being hired match/ complement the institution's needs?

Has the CNS been given sufficient authority and control of practice to match the responsibility for changing practice?

Is there a system for evaluating performance and productivity in terms of agreed-upon, clear criteria that are valued by the institution?

first year, preferably a minimum of every three months. Specifically, they need help with setting limits, with understanding how to cope with problem situations, and with maintaining a sense of perspective. Anticipating and preparing for the frustration phase may modify its course and duration.

Supports both outside and within the work setting helped the CNSs in this study to cope with frustrations and problems. If there are other more experienced CNSs in the setting, it might be helpful to assign a preceptor, particularly to the neophyte CNS, to act as a role model and to be available for objective analysis of problems. If there are no other CNSs or if all of the CNSs are neophytes, they may be encouraged to meet with their counterparts in neighboring institutions or to join a CNS support group in the community.

As stated earlier, the experienced CNS beginning a new job experiences the same phases of development as the neophyte, except that the phases are likely to be shorter. Thus, regular feedback and opportunities for validation are critical to any CNS in a new position.

### Frustration Phase Strategies

Both the CNS and the supervisor need to remain alert for signs of frustration. As noted in the survey, the phase may come and go, overlapping with other phases as the CNS discovers the flaws in the institution and experiences resistance to programs and activities. Neophyte CNSs, particularly, may have a tendency to blame either themselves or the institution.

The CNS supervisor and the peer group can be extremely helpful in dealing with the painful affective responses experienced during the frustration phase. Comparing notes with others who have had similar experiences and having a confidant help relieve tension. Identifying someone to interpret the institution's history can give insight into the intractability of certain problems. Administrators who ensure that the CNS is apprised of what is being done about known problems can make a partner rather than an adversary of the frustrated CNS. The first author has worked with new CNSs through monthly role development sessions. Having the opportunity to share frustrations with a group of peers and an administrator who has institutional perspective is one strategy for helping novices to anticipate and move through this phase.

A number of techniques or actions were identified by survey respondents as helpful in facilitating movement from frustration to implementation. These are listed in Table 3–11. It was interesting to note that these actions were usually initiated by the CNS, rather than by someone else in the setting.

**TABLE 3–11.    Strategies for Reaching the Implementation Phase**

Initiate conflict resolution and role clarification discussions with individuals with whom the CNS is experiencing role conflict.

Set limits on performance expectations.

Increase visibility within the institution via educational programs and speaking, consultation, research activity and publication.

Modify approaches and try new ones.

Take time to assess where one is in development and what has been accomplished, and deliberately plan the next steps.

Develop good relationships with peers and colleagues.

Look for and begin to see the results of patient care interventions in complicated cases.

The new CNS also needs help in dealing with feelings of inadequacy. One subject reflected, "It is helpful to remind neophyte CNSs that 'change' occurs very slowly in the 'real world.' Also, it is very easy to become frustrated by comparing yourself to experienced CNSs. Beginning CNSs feel that they must offer 'five new programs per week.' Initially, the important thing is to establish credibility and comfort within the role."

Time management is also a problem for many neophyte CNSs. If this is the first position in which the individual was expected to be self-directed, set priorities, and use time effectively without direct supervision, there may be a sense that time is flying and little is being accomplished. Or the CNS may feel that the effort to accomplish everything that needs doing becomes overwhelming. These CNSs will need help in reassessing priorities and setting realistic expectations. It is often helpful for the CNS to focus on one or two short-term projects that can be successfully completed. The resultant positive feedback can help the CNS feel good about self and job again.

As during the phase of orientation, evaluation of the CNS may need to focus on process and accomplishment of short-term goals, since tangible results may not yet be apparent.

### Implementation Phase Strategies

In this phase the CNS moves from the intermediate to the advanced practice level if not already there. This is demonstrable by increased recognition and acceptance by staff, other CNSs, physicians, and those in other disciplines, and by increased patient referrals. Nursing and hospital administration recognize the CNS, for example, through appropriate committee appointments or teaching assignments. Individuals and groups within and outside the setting seek consultation.

In this phase, the CNS subroles are incorporated into practice with greater confidence and less stress. However, there is danger that the old sense of frustration may recur as time and energy fail to keep up with increased demands. Again the CNS and the CNS's supervisor need to be alert for the signs of impending burnout. There may be a need to reassess the demands being made on the CNS and jointly determine which are most important in terms of organizational needs and CNS role development. It may again be helpful to focus on one or several short-term projects or goals.

Positive signs of practice expertise should be evaluated during this phase. There should be evidence that staff and patients are benefitting from the CNS's involvement. Small studies may be undertaken, both to provide research experience and to validate CNS effectiveness. Feedback from those with whom the CNS works most closely may be a part of the evaluation, to provide information about areas of strength and weakness.

### Integration Phase Strategies

It appears that positive resolution of the earlier developmental phases is essential if integration is to take place. Survey data suggest that the integrated CNS most significantly maximizes the role's potential. Therefore, efforts to retain promising individuals in such positions appear to be worthwhile and cost-effective.

CNSs as a group view themselves as autonomous, highly motivated, self-directed professionals who, as experts in their fields, are entitled to considerable latitude in defining goals and objectives to guide their activities. When the supervisor's or organization's imperatives are seen as restrictive or incompatible with the CNS's personal goals, role development may become frozen, halting further growth. At every phase of role development, there may be resistance from staff, head nurses, or members of other disciplines. Conflicting or competing demands are made for the CNS's time and attention. When such circumstances arise, even the most experienced and integrated CNS needs visible administrative support and advice, as well as objective, constructive counsel from a trusted mentor.

Thus, the integrated CNS expects and needs a great deal of freedom and independence but also needs a safe sounding board, feedback, constructive criticism, and advice. The integrated CNS needs to continue learning and to cultivate increased expertise in practice as well as in the various subroles. The CNS should seek (and the supervisor should promote) appointment to key committees, and the CNS should expand the role in a planned way over time. Encouragement and, if possible, organizational support (such as clerical assistance and time away from clinical duties) for research, writing, and other outside professional activities foster the CNS's professional growth. CNSs in this phase are ideal preceptors for graduate students.

Conceptually, the CNS role was devised to provide expert practitioners a means to advance professionally without moving out of the practice role. In theory, the CNS should have the same opportunities for advancement within nursing practice as are available to teachers and administrators. In practical terms, this has not been the case, as the CNS generally enters the position at the top of an institution's clinical ladder. One challenge to administrators and CNSs is to develop a promotional system in the spirit of the clinical ladder which offers the ongoing stimulation experienced CNSs need to maintain growth.

There are other ways to reward the successful CNS with tenure in the organization. Salary, of course, is the most tangible reward and should keep pace with the salaries of administrative and teaching staff of comparable education and experience within the institution. Other benefits and privileges should also be equal to those of individuals in nonclinical positions. To a large extent, the value an institution places on excellence in practice will be measured by the organizational position of the CNS relative to those in other positions.

### Frozen and Reorganization Phase Strategies

For CNSs in the frozen and reorganization phases, supportive and nonjudgmental counseling from an objective outsider may be helpful in resolving the role conflict. The issues that need to be resolved include an appraisal of whether or not the goals of the CNS are realistic given the exigencies of the situation. The CNS who feels overwhelmed by the immediate needs of the organization may need assistance in formulating strategies to convince administration of the merit of the CNSs priorities. For example, putting a desired program or plan in writing with an emphasis on how the program may help to resolve organizational problems or fit in with organizational goals may provide an opportunity for active renegotiation of the CNS role. Similarly, a desire to do research may not be appropriate at a time when the organization is in the midst of crisis or is undergoing rapid change. The CNS may then need to decide if the research goal can be postponed temporarily, and discuss with administration the likelihood of there being a future time when the goal might be realizable.

While the CNS may recognize the frozen state, there may be times when the CNS's supervisor or others in the setting first become aware of the CNS's frustration and lack of progress. As part of the ongoing dialogue between the CNS and the supervisor, discussion of plans, goals, and future directions of the CNS within the organizational framework should be helpful in preventing the "freezing" or in redirecting the CNS's activities so that role development can continue. Supervisors need to be open to renegotiating role expectations to allow for this growth.

When such situations develop, both the CNS and the administrator can play a part in finding a satisfactory resolution. Those individuals responsible for promulgating changes should discuss the proposed changes with the CNS as early in the change process as possible. If the necessary realignment of role responsibilities is to be temporary, a definite plan for resumption of the former role may be incorporated into the discussions. If the change necessitates ongoing role change, together the CNS and supervisor must carefully consider whether the new responsibilities are consistent with the CNS role definition. If not, the CNS will need to consider whether the new role (which should carry a different title) is acceptable and plan accordingly.

If no compromise between the organization's needs and the goals of the CNS can be found, the administration and CNS might find it mutually beneficial for the CNS to make a career move. The contributions the CNS has made to the organization should be fully appreciated and the leave taking eased, both for the CNS and for those within the organization who will be affected by the CNS's departure. Allowing time for the CNS to find another position, demonstrating appreciation for contributions made to the organization, providing appropriate references, and maintaining open communication throughout the process can make the transition as painless as possible. In seeking a new position, the CNS should carefully assess career goals and job expectations to be certain that the new position will offer an opportunity for job satisfaction.

## SUMMARY

The evolution of the CNS role is characterized by continued defining, refining, and refocusing. Because the role is designed to meet changing needs of patients and institutions, role expression must also change. It is clear that role development must be an ongoing, dynamic process for the CNS to be effective. CNS role development can be characterized into phases and developmental tasks. The findings reported in this chapter can help CNSs, administrators, and educators to assess, analyze, and facilitate role enactment. Each individual CNS's experience is dependent upon many personal, setting, and role variables. These differences make role development a rich and diverse process for the advanced nursing specialist.

## Acknowledgment

The authors wish to thank Dr. Marie Annette Brown at the University of Washington, Seattle, for her excellent assistance in developing the questionnaire used in this survey.

## References

American Nurses Association. Clinical Nurse Specialists: Distribution and Utilization. Kansas City, ANA, 1986.

Ayers, R.: Effects and role development of the clinical nurse specialist. *In* Padilla, G.V., (ed): The Clinical Nurse Specialist and Improvement of Nursing Practice. Wakefield, MA, Nursing Resources, 1979, pp. 14–21.

Baker, P.: Model activities for clinical nurse specialist role development. Clinical Nurse Specialist *1*(3):119–123, 1987.

Baker, V.: Retrospective explorations in role development. *In* Padilla, G.V. (ed): The Clinical Nurse Specialist and Improvement of Nursing Practice. Wakefield, MA, Nursing Resources, 1979, pp. 56–63.

Benner, P.: From Novice to Expert. Reading, MA, Addison-Wesley, 1984.

Benner, P., & Tanner, C.: Clinical judgment: How expert nurses use intuition. Am J Nurs *87*(1):23–31, 1987.

Cason, C.L., & Beck, C.M.: Clinical nurse specialist role development. Nurs Health Care *13*(1):25–38, 1982.

Cooper, D.: A refined expert: The clinical nurse specialist after five years. Momentum *1*:1–2, 1983.

Dalton, G.W., Thompson, P.H., and Price, R.L.: The four stages of professional careers—a new look at performance by professionals. Organizational Dynamics *6*(1):19–42, 1977.

Donoghue, M., & Spross, J.A.: A report from the first national invitational conference: The oncology clinical nurse specialist role analysis and future projections. Oncol Nurs Forum *12*(2):35–73, 1985.

Dreyfus, S.E., & Dreyfus, H.L.: A five-stage model of the mental activities involved in directed skill acquisition. Unpublished report supported by the Air Force Office of Scientific Research (AFSC), USAF (Contract F49620-79-C-0063), University of California at Berkeley, February, 1980.

Hamric, A.B.: Role development and functions. *In* Hamric, A.B., and Spross, J. (eds): The Clinical Nurse Specialist in Theory and Practice. New York, Grune & Stratton, 1983, pp. 39–56.

Holt, F.M.: A theoretical model for clinical specialist practice. Nurs Health Care *5*(8):445–449, 1984.

Holt, F.M.: Executive practice role editorial. Clinical Nurse Specialist *1*(3):116–118, 1987.

Kramer, M.: Reality Shock: Why Nurses Leave Nursing. St. Louis, C.V. Mosby, 1974.

Kwong, M., Manning, M.P., and Koetters, T.L.: The role of the oncology clinical nurse specialist: Three personal views. Cancer Nurs *5*(6):427–434, 1982.

Oda, D.: Specialized role development: A three-phase process. Nurs Outlook *25*:374–377, 1977.

Padilla, G.V., & Padilla, G.J.: Nursing roles to improve patient care. Nurs Dig *6*(4):1–13, 1979.

Yasko, J.M.: Variables which predict burnout experienced by oncology clinical nurse specialists. Cancer Nurs *6*:109–116, 1983.

Yasko, J.M.: A survey of oncology clinical nursing specialists. Oncol Nurs Forum *10*:25–30, 1986.

# A Model for CNS Evaluation

*Ann B. Hamric*

## INTRODUCTION

Evaluating the effectiveness of the CNS role continues to be problematic. Although the literature is replete with pleas for more thorough evaluation of the CNS, and cost containment pressures and limited nursing budgets continue to threaten the number of CNSs and their influence (Hamric, 1983; Harrell & McCullough, 1986), there have been few attempts to evaluate either the effectiveness of the CNS role or the practice of an individual CNS. There are a number of reasons why CNS evaluation is difficult.

First, the CNS is a self-directed practitioner whose practice is constantly changing to meet the diverse needs of patients, nurses, and institutions. These independent characteristics have resulted in a lack of consensus regarding performance criteria. In the absence of consensus, CNSs and their administrators may not feel competent to specify measurable standards for the CNS. Performance objectives developed for a particular focus of practice may be obsolete by the time they are annually reviewed owing to changes in the work setting which may dictate changes in the CNS's activities. In most action-oriented clinical environments, structured time to develop evaluation methodologies is not available or sanctioned. As Abramson noted, "Evaluation and service frequently make competing demands, and the requirements for a well-substantiated evaluation of effectiveness may be difficult to meet in 'the turbulent setting of the action program'" (1979, p. 215). It is difficult to structure time for evaluation either before or after an activity. Many CNSs become immersed in the next patient problem or project before the results of their previous interventions can be evaluated. When difficulties become apparent, it is tempting to move to a different intervention or to abandon the project without undertaking a systematic

**83**

assessment of what went wrong. Even if such assessment is performed, the CNS is unlikely to take time to document the results, and valuable evaluation data are lost.

Compounding these problems is the tendency of many CNSs and administrators to move too quickly to outcome evaluation. Evaluation of outcomes is the most difficult type of evaluation and requires many organizational supports and resources. If time is not taken to build these supports, the outcome data may be flawed. For example, a CNS who developed a teaching program for diabetic patients was interested in evaluating the impact of the program on patients. She was continually frustrated in her evaluation attempts because of structural problems with the program: patients were not brought on time to the sessions, some patients were missed, there were problems with speakers from other disciplines. Structural evaluation was much more helpful at this stage of the project than outcome evaluation.

The issue of who should evaluate the CNS has been a stumbling block. Most institutions have a system of performance appraisal, sanctioning the administrator to whom the CNS reports with evaluating the CNS. However, some CNSs prefer self-evaluation or peer review because they believe that only other CNSs understand the role enough to evaluate it. Peer review systems have been slow to develop (see Chapter 14). Evaluation by nursing staff, physicians, or patients may seem threatening to CNSs. Discussions of who is qualified to evaluate the CNS have in some instances obscured the central issue of identifying relevant criteria of effectiveness.

Finally, role ambiguity continues to be a factor complicating evaluation. Role descriptions are broad and CNS practice is diverse. While individual institutions may have achieved role clarity, there continues to be divergence in the literature regarding CNS practice.

If the CNS role is to survive and thrive, sound documentation of the effect of this practitioner on nursing practice and patient care must replace individual conviction that the role is viable. The need for sound evaluation has been noted previously (Hamric, 1983). This chapter will discuss a model for evaluating the CNS, with strategies for developing an evaluation plan. The focus will be on evaluating the individual CNS and on reviewing reported CNS evaluation studies. Issues in researching the impact of the CNS role are essentially the same as reported earlier (Hamric, 1983; Hamric, 1985).

Any evaluation system for the CNS must meet certain criteria. First, evaluation must spring from practice to be meaningful. That is, whatever method is developed must be filtered through the CNSs' understanding of their practice (Hamric, 1985). Second, because of the varied role components and changing nature of CNS practice, it is doubtful that there will ever be one global instrument to evaluate the CNS. Some generic job descriptions have been developed (Chambers, et al., 1987; Colerick, Mason, and Proulx, 1980), but they have limited usefulness as evaluation tools. One advantage of Donabedian's model (discussed below) is the three levels from which to approach evaluation. This gives flexibility as well as a means to organize and critique the variety of evaluative modes available to CNSs (Hamric, 1985).

# DONABEDIAN'S MODEL FOR PATIENT CARE EVALUATION

Donabedian (1966) identified three areas of patient care which can be used as foci for evaluation: structure, process, and outcome. Bloch (1975) discussed these same categories in relation to nursing care, and both models have been related to the CNS by Hamric (1983) (see Table 4–1).

The first of Donabedian's categories, structural evaluation, focuses on the setting or system in which health care occurs and on the attributes of care providers in the system. For the CNS, factors such as numbers, qualifications, and utilization of caregivers (e.g., nurse-patient ratios; numbers of RNs, LPNs, and aides on staff), and presence of support services (e.g., physical therapy) are structural variables. Interest in

**TABLE 4–1. Donabedian's Model for Patient Care Evaluation as Applied to Nursing by Bloch, and to the CNS by Hamric**

| Donabedian and Bloch | | |
|---|---|---|
| *Structure* | *Process* | *Outcome* |
| Care Providers | Care | Care Recipient |
| Characteristics of:<br>  setting<br>  system<br>  care providers | Appropriateness and<br>  completeness of care<br>  delivery<br>For nursing, the quality of<br>  nursing process | End result of care in<br>  terms of change in<br>  patient's:<br>  • physical health state<br>  • cognitive state<br>  • psychosocial state<br>  • behavioral state |
| **Hamric** | | |
| *Structure* | *Process* | *Outcome* |
| CNS effect on selected<br>  institutional practices (ex.,<br>  RN turnover) | CNS ability to perform in<br>  subroles:<br>  • direct practice<br>  • educator<br>  • consultant<br>  • researcher | CNS impact on patient<br>  outcome:<br>  • health state<br>  • cognitive<br>  • psychosocial<br>  • behavioral |
| CNS level of professional<br>  activity | CNS impact on nursing staff<br>  performance | |
| CNS time documentation | | |
| Characteristics of system in<br>  which CNS practices | CNS self-evaluation of<br>  professional growth | |

structural variables is based on the assumption that proper settings and supports will result in quality health care (Donabedian, 1966, p. 170). The second facet of evaluation, process evaluation, focuses on the care provided. It examines the processes of care delivery, such as technical competence and quality of the nursing process employed by the CNS. The final facet, outcome evaluation, focuses on the care recipient—the patient. In most studies of medical care, outcome has been measured in terms of patient recovery, restoration of function, and survival (Donabedian, 1966, p. 167). Bloch referred to these parameters as measuring the patient's "health state" and identified others that could be used to measure outcomes. These additional parameters are cognitive outcome (the patient's knowledge of the disease and treatment); psychosocial outcome (the patient's attitudes toward care, motivation, family participation in treatment); and behavioral outcome (the patient's compliance with recommended health practices and other observable health-related behaviors). Bloch argued that there was no question that these variables are valid outcome variables, even though they have an "admittedly tenuous relationship to health state" (Bloch, 1975, p. 258).

Numerous strategies have been developed to evaluate the CNS. Many combine elements, especially structure and process variables. One must look at the content of the questions in a given instrument to know whether the instrument is focused on structure, process, or outcome.

## Structural Evaluation

Structural evaluation is an important place to start when designing a CNS evaluation plan. As noted, this facet of evaluation examines administrative factors within the institution and characteristics of caregivers. Examples of structural variables relative to the institution would include numbers of registered nurses (RNs) and other staff members; patient-nurse ratios on unit(s) where the CNS practices; number of committees to which a CNS belongs; the CNS job description and position within the organization; and presence of adequate services to support nursing practice. Structural variables related to characteristics of the caregiver would include such items as qualifications of the CNS, the CNS's attendance at continuing education programs, and the CNS's use of time and leadership style. Structural evaluation gives information about the environment in which the CNS practices and the CNS's level of professional activity. See Table 4–2 for examples of structural evaluation strategies.

It is important to start with structural evaluation because "a sound structure undergirds the CNS role within an institution; it is the sine qua non of CNS effectiveness. Examining structural variables such as

**TABLE 4–2.   Structural Evaluation Strategies**

- Time documentation of CNS activities (Robichaud & Hamric; Nevidjon & Warren; Crigler, et al.)
- Evaluate aspects of system which support (or do not support) CNS activities (e.g., presence of secretarial support, position in organization)
- Evaluate whether appropriate activities occurred to meet goals identified (Malone)
- Structural performance standards (Colerick, Mason, and Proulx; Chambers, et al.)

organizational placement, presence of administrative support, RN:patient ratio and RN mix can assist administrators and CNSs to determine whether conditions exist that allow CNSs to practice effectively" (Hamric, 1985, p. 63). Structural variables allow one to assess the climate within which the CNS practices.

The advantage of this form of evaluation is that data are concrete and relatively easy to obtain. One of the best examples of useful structural data is a time record of a CNS's activities (Robichaud & Hamric, 1986; Crigler, et al., 1984; Nevidjon & Warren, 1984). The CNS records time spent in subroles as well as in administrative activities and time away from the institution. Percentage of time spent with role components, quantitative use of services (numbers of patients seen and consultations), distribution of time by geographic area, and time necessary to achieve specific goals and objectives are examples of structural information that can be obtained from time documentation (Robichaud & Hamric, 1986). One needs to see whether appropriate activity occurs in sufficient quantity to allow for desirable outcomes. Time documentation is a useful first step in evaluating CNS performance, especially when a CNS is beginning a new role. "The objective data provided through time documentation can assist the CNS's administrator in guiding both the time management and the continuing role development of a CNS" (Robichaud & Hamric, 1986, p. 35).

Structural variables may point out the constraints on CNS practice (such as excessive requirements for administrative duties) and may identify factors that facilitate or hamper CNS effectiveness. For example, presence of administrative support has been shown to be a critical factor contributing to CNS job satisfaction and presumably to performance (see Chapters 3 and 13). Staff nurse satisfaction and turnover are two other structural variables that may relate to CNS effectiveness, depending upon CNS placement and objectives. Finally, structural components such as number and type of caregivers on the CNS's unit(s) and accessibility of other health team members have a bearing on the milieu in which a CNS functions and thus may influence that CNS's impact.

Chambers and her colleagues developed structural standards of performance to use in evaluating the CNS (Chambers, et al., 1987).

Examples of these structural statements include: "meets quarterly with nurse manager(s) regarding standards of care for specific client population; conducts at least one major yearly workshop or course; responds to requests for consultation from staff regarding patient care; maintains a system for recording consultations" (p. 127). These performance standards are structural because they assess whether activity occurs at a determined frequency. They do not assess either how well the activity was performed (process) or the result of the activity (process or outcome depending upon whether the result was nurse- or patient-directed). Although helpful in determining whether appropriate CNS activities have occurred, these performance standards do not directly measure effectiveness.

While structural variables may yield helpful data, the assumption underlying structural evaluation, i.e., that provision of a proper setting will result in high-quality care, is particularly tenuous when examining an environment as complex as the one in which most CNSs practice. For example, one can determine the amount of time a group of CNSs spend in direct practice, consultation, and education. One cannot tell from these data, however, whether they are functioning effectively in these subroles. Although structural evaluation should be an integral part of an individual CNS's annual evaluation, it cannot stand alone as an evaluation method.

## Process Evaluation

Process evaluation, or the study of what the caregiver does, yields data regarding the CNS's ability to perform in each subrole. Most studies examining individual CNS effectiveness have concentrated on process variables. Examples of strategies for making process evaluations include staff or head nurse evaluation, in which members of a nursing staff and/or head nurses who observe CNSs evaluate their performances, using behavioral criteria (Hamric, Gresham, and Eccard, 1978; Girouard & Spross, 1983). Evaluation by the staff is predominantly a process strategy, as it focuses on how well the CNS implements the role. Process standards include statements such as "She performs patient activities with a high degree of clinical competence" and "She provides effective health teaching to select patients." Structural standards such as "She regularly schedules in-service programs and is responsive to our ideas for topics" are also contained in these instruments.

Administrative review is a widely used process strategy. In this design, the CNS and supervisor establish mutual goals and objectives and evaluate them together at regular intervals. Administrative review can also use the CNS's job description as an evaluative guideline.

A third type of process evaluation is that undertaken by other health care professionals or consumers. In this instance, individuals are questioned regarding processes of care as a means of evaluating the effectiveness of the caregiver. Physicians, other health care professionals such as social workers or physical therapists with whom the CNS works, and patients and their families can be asked to evaluate the CNS's delivery of health care.

A fourth type of process evaluation focuses on improvements in various components of nursing process. Most formal research on the effectiveness of the CNS role has utilized this method. Examples in the literature include the work of Georgopoulos and Jackson (1970) and Georgopoulos and Sana (1971), who examined nursing Kardex behavior and content of intershift report, respectively, as measures of the quality of nursing process. Ayers (1971) studied the "clinical insight" of nursing staff on units with CNSs. Little and Carnevali (1967) looked at nurse behaviors of CNSs as compared with behaviors of staff nurses. Girouard (1978) studied the preoperative teaching and documentation activities of nurses on two units, one of which had a CNS. Each of these studies showed positive correlation between the introduction of the CNS role and the improvement of the nursing staff's ability to perform some aspect of nursing, according to the measures studied. Although dated, these studies are methodologically sound and have yielded the most positive findings.

A more recent study also found significant improvements in nursing staff processes after introduction of a CNS in a state psychiatric hospital (McBride, et al., 1987). The CNS worked with nursing staff to encourage greater care in nursing documentation, particularly assessment. After only six months, the investigators found statistically significant differences in both the quality and quantity of nurses' notes. "The staff became more likely to document both the patient's behavior and physical appearance, to note discharge planning with the liaison, and to make summary statements. These findings become especially important if one considers that the nursing staff had no idea about how the nursing notes were being analyzed" (p. 59). This project, undertaken with numerous practical constraints, could serve as a model for other CNSs and researchers. Taken as a group, these process studies constitute the strongest support of the impact of the CNS role in improving nursing practice.

A fifth type of process evaluation is that of peer review. This strategy is explored in Chapter 14. Self-evaluation, according to stated goals and objectives or job description, is also a useful process strategy. Certainly, self-evaluation is an important component of any individual CNS performance appraisal. Depending upon the goals established, it may be more or less important than other strategies. In practice, however, it is difficult for CNSs immersed in a role to objectively evaluate their own activities. Because of this inherent subjectivity, self-evaluation should be coupled with other methods to achieve a balanced evaluation.

There are numerous advantages to process evaluation. Although it is an indirect measure of the CNS's impact on quality of care, process evaluation directly examines the activities of the caregiver, which may be especially relevant to the question of whether proper practice has occurred (Donabedian, 1966, p. 169). For the individual CNS attempting to implement a broad, unstructured role, process evaluation can give needed validation of the scope, appropriateness, and effectiveness of CNS practice. Presently, the process method is the most practical means of CNS evaluation. A number of instruments are available (Table 4–3). Use of written records, direct observation, and questionnaires are relatively straightforward data collection methods. In addition, most nurse administrators and CNSs are familiar with evaluation according to objectives and goals.

The major disadvantage of process evaluation is that it is not a direct measure of the quality of care rendered. For example, simply influencing a staff's perception of quality nursing care (a classic process measure) does not automatically raise the level of care which that staff provides. There is insufficient research correlating patient care processes with outcomes to permit one to conclude that positive changes in nursing process result in positive patient outcomes. These drawbacks point to the fact that an accurate, comprehensive evaluation of the CNS role requires the use of all three of Donabedian's evaluation categories. In spite of these problems, however, process evaluation alone can yield relevant data concerning CNS effectiveness, especially in the indirect functions of consultation and education.

## Outcome Evaluation

Outcome evaluation examines the results of care in terms of changes in the recipient of the care; for the CNS, outcome evaluation

**TABLE 4–3.   Process Evaluation Strategies**

- Peer review (Malone; Chapter 14)
- Staff and/or head nurse evaluation of CNS activities (Hamric, Gresham, and Eccard; Girouard & Spross)
- Performance review of goals and objectives; job description (Davis, et al.; Malone)
- Consumer or other health care professional evaluation of CNS expertise
- Audit of improvements in nursing process
- CNS self-evaluation of goals and objectives; job description

measures CNS impact on patient care outcomes. (The reader should note that CNS activities such as consultant can lead to positive changes in knowledge, attitudes, and behavior of staff nurses which could technically be considered outcomes for the CNS whose objective was to change staff practices. Because such changes are measured by process strategies, and because Donabedian's model deals only with *patient* outcomes, the author has chosen to consider the CNS effect on nursing staff as part of process evaluation, rather than outcome evaluation.)

The most obvious example of an outcome evaluation is one that measures changes in the patient's health status. In this type of evaluation, physical parameters such as presence or progression of disability or alleviation of symptoms are measured. Length of stay and number of hospital readmissions have been used as outcome measures, with a reduction in both indicating improvements in the patient's health status. As previously noted, Bloch (1975) identified additional categories of cognitive, psychosocial, and behavioral outcome. An example of evaluation according to cognitive objectives would be measuring the increase in patient knowledge after institution of a teaching program. Psychosocial variables such as improved social interaction or family understanding and participation in a patient's treatment may also be the focus of an outcome evaluation. In behavioral evaluation, items such as patient adherence to a therapeutic regimen or health-related behaviors such as quitting smoking are examined.

Classically, outcome evaluation represents the most important measure of the quality of nursing care. When an individual CNS works intensively with one client group, it should be possible to use outcome measures to document impact. Indeed, for CNSs contemplating independent practice or fee-for-service consultation to patients, this type of evaluation is especially important (Hamric, 1985).

If the CNS's institution has a strong quality assurance program that evaluates patient outcome criteria, outcome evaluation may be practical. Correlating such outcome data with concurrent process information would be ideal. If no such program exists, it may be unrealistic to attempt a large-scale outcome evaluation, regardless of its advantages. It may still be possible to obtain statistics from the business office, such as patient length of stay prior to the beginning of a CNS project and after completion. Such information could be correlated with other data to yield information related to the CNS's effect on patient outcomes.

While outcome criteria for a variety of patient problems have been developed, measurement of these criteria has proven to be difficult. There are other barriers to implementing an outcome evaluation specifically for the CNS. In the tertiary health care setting where most CNSs practice, many variables other than the quality of nursing care influence the patient's health state. It is difficult to identify outcome criteria solely attributable to nursing care, much less to one CNS's intervention. Cognitive, behavioral, and psychosocial variables can be more difficult to measure than health state but may often be the realm in which nursing makes its unique contribution to patient welfare. Reliable outcome criteria in the complex patient with chronic disease and multisystem involvement are the most difficult to develop, yet this is the client population with which most CNSs deal. Given these difficulties, outcome evaluation may need to be undertaken selectively, after structure and process criteria are in place. Combining process and limited outcome measures is certainly feasible, however, and is preferable to evaluation by process measures alone.

One further problem deserves mention. It is difficult for a health care provider to conduct an outcome study. Specifically, the CNS working with a patient group may experience conflicts between the clinician role and the researcher role. Experimenter bias may also be difficult to overcome. CNSs change interventions to meet changing patient conditions, which could compromise the integrity of the research. It may be advisable to have someone removed from actual patient care conduct formal research on outcomes for an individual CNS.

In a review and critique of nurse practitioner (NP) evaluation studies, Prescott and Driscoll (1980) identified similar problems with the use of outcome variables. They noted that patient satisfaction was the most frequently used outcome variable in the 26 studies they reviewed. Other measures included patients' knowledge about their plan of care, patient complaints, tendency of patients to seek care, patients' adherence to diet and correct compliance with medication regimen, and health state variables such as blood pressure, blood sugar, and labor and delivery complications. They recommended that short-term outcomes associated with specific illnesses or conditions offered the most potential sensitivity to provider processes. CNSs might well be able to use similar measures in evaluating their practices.

In the current competitive health care climate, patient satisfaction with services is a potent variable. Hospitals are vying with each other for insured patients, with product lines oriented toward consumer comfort and accessibility. CNSs may wish to use patient satisfaction with health care services as a measure of effectiveness, and this may be positively viewed by administration. Caution must be exercised when using patient satisfaction as an indicator of nursing care quality, however. Eriksen (1987) found a predominantly inverse relationship between quality of nursing care and patient satisfaction, specifically in the areas of physical care and teaching patients to deal with their illness (two clear practice domains for the CNS). She noted, "The findings of this research would suggest that professional nursing values and administrative concerns are at times in opposition to those of the patient" (p. 34). Eriksen concluded that "data regarding patient satisfaction with nursing care should not be used as the sole evaluation mechanism regarding quality of nursing care" (p. 35).

One study examined specific patient perceptions in addition to general satisfaction and found significant differences between patients cared for by a CNS compared with those being followed by a physician. Bartucci (1985) found that patients' perceptions of adequacy of time spent with them, display of concern toward them as individuals, and accessibility of the primary care provider between visits were significantly higher for post-renal transplant patients being followed in a clinic setting by a CNS. The investigator also asked a general patient satisfaction question; the results were not significantly different between groups. CNSs interested in patient perceptions of care should work to identify discrete issues important to patients rather than query patients about overall satisfaction with care. It is likely that more discriminating measures would yield more positive findings.

Although it is clearly recognized that improved patient outcomes should be an important result of CNS practice, measuring this relationship has proven to be technically difficult. Two older studies found positive relationships between CNS interventions and patient outcomes. Pozen, et al. (1977) found a significantly increased return-to-work rate, a decline in smoking, and increased knowledge in a randomized trial of patients with acute myocardial infarction. They attributed these findings to the CNS's teaching and individual counseling interventions. Linde and Janz (1979) studied the effect of a comprehensive patient teaching program on knowledge and compliance of 48 patients undergoing valve replacement and coronary bypass surgeries. Half of the patients (25) were taught by CNSs and half (23) by nurses with less than master's preparation. Patients were tested for knowledge and compliance preoperatively, at discharge, and during the first two postoperative visits. Of patients taught by the CNSs, the investigators found significantly higher test scores at discharge. One difference in these studies as compared with others that found no difference in patient outcome related to CNS intervention (Little & Carnevali, 1967; Murphy, 1971) is the careful selection of nurse-dependent outcome measures. Specifically, these authors used behavioral and cognitive objectives rather than health state, which was used in the studies that found no difference attributable to CNS intervention.

Recent research is even more encouraging. One of the strongest demonstrations of the impact of CNS practice on patient outcomes was reported in 1986. Brooten, et al. studied the effects of early hospital discharge on low birthweight infants whose families received CNS support. Infants were randomly assigned either to a control group (discharged according to routine nursery criteria) or to an early-discharge group (discharged before they met the weight required for the control group). The early-discharge group received instruction, counseling, home visits, and daily on-call availability from a perinatal CNS. Infants in the early-discharge group did as well in numerous outcome measures as the control group infants, while costing the institution 27 per cent less in mean hospital charges. The investigators concluded that "early discharge of very-low-birthweight infants, with follow-up care in the home by a nurse specialist, is safe and cost-effective" (Brooten, et al., 1986, p. 934). The authors clearly indicated that specific CNS processes were major determinants of infant outcome. "The continued home monitoring of the infant's physical status, the parents' ability to cope, their compliance with specialized medical procedures, and their use of any equipment required for high-risk infants discharged early mean that home follow-up care must be provided by nurses who have specialized in high-risk neonatal care" (Brooten, et al., 1986, p. 937). The interdisciplinary group that conducted this research is also noteworthy. Such collaborative efforts between CNSs, nurse researchers, physicians, and hospital administrators can result in methodologically strong evaluation research such as was achieved by Brooten and her colleagues.

## PROCESS RELATED TO OUTCOME EVALUATION

The most thorough evaluation correlates process to outcome by examining relationships between caregiver practice and patient outcome. In process-outcome evaluation, outcomes should be explicit, measurable, and based on clearly desirable, predetermined goals. These requirements have proven to be difficult for CNSs to meet. Benner's important work on clinical expertise reveals some of the reason for this difficulty. As clinical experts, CNSs perceive clinical situations intuitively and holistically. The meanings of a particular patient situation are based on a deep background understanding and contextual cues present in the particular circumstance. Benner noted that while the use of formal models to teach new knowledge has been valuable, "formal models never capture the complexity of the real situation" (Benner, 1985, p. 41). Most attempts to develop quantitative outcome criteria in nursing have been, of necessity, more formal and context-free than actual practice. CNSs as clinical experts may legitimately believe that such measures cannot adequately reflect the impact of their practice on patients' lived experiences.

While there are numerous examples of process-outcome studies in different clinical specialties, they do not specifically address CNS processes. One such general study relating process to outcome is especially noteworthy. Knaus, Draper, Wagner, and Zimmerman (1986) studied treatment and outcome in 5,030 patients in intensive care units at 13 tertiary care hospitals. They found that the processes of interaction and coordination of care between physicians and nurses were significantly related to patient mortality rates. One hospital did significantly better than the other 12 in actual versus expected mortality rates. In reporting the characteristics of this institution, the investigators noted, "This hospital also had the most comprehensive nursing educational support system. Clinical specialists with master's degrees and extensive experience in intensive care units had as their primary responsibility the orientation and development of the nursing staff . . . . Excellent communication between physicians and nursing staff was ongoing to ensure that all patient care needs were met" (Knaus, et al., 1986, p. 415). They concluded, "Our results support the belief that involvement and interaction of critical care personnel can directly influence outcome from intensive care" (p. 416). While not specifically focusing on CNS processes, this study lends powerful support to the impact of collaborative practice on patient survival.

One recent account of a demonstration project attempted to determine the effect of a CNS on home health nurses' processes of care as well as on patient outcomes (Oleske, Otte, and Heinze, 1987). Home health agencies were randomized into one of three study groups: those receiving CNS consultant services and continuing education on cancer, those receiving just continuing education, and those who were only observed. All three groups showed improvement in nurses' assessment and patient management skills. Nutritional assessment skills significantly improved in the group of nurses receiving the CNS's services, but this was the only significant difference among groups. Patient outcomes were not significantly different, even though an effort was made to select patient outcomes that related to nursing judgment and were believed to be largely achievable with appropriate nursing intervention. The authors questioned whether the CNS's services may have been spread too thin (she covered three to four agencies) to have had a noticeable effect.

Another process-outcome study examined the relationship between a comprehensive discharge planning protocol implemented by a gerontological CNS (GCNS) and hospital costs and revenue. Using a double blind experimental design, Neidlinger, Scroggins, and Kennedy (1987) demonstrated a significant decrease in hospital costs and an increase in hospital revenues in patients receiving the GCNS's discharge planning intervention as compared with those noted for a control group of similar patients. Hospital costs for the experimental group averaged $60 less per patient day than those for the control group. The researchers commented, "The net savings of $34,707 amounted to more than the salary costs for the GCNS for that entire year" (p. 229). They speculated that if the GCNS continued to see the same number of patients monthly as she did during the study period, the potential annual savings to be realized by the hospital would approximate $0.5 million. This study is noteworthy for the attempt to relate a common process strategy, that of discharge planning, to outcomes related to hospital costs.

The methodology involved in conducting process-outcome studies is complex and problematic. Prescott and Driscoll (1980) offered four suggestions for strengthening this type of evaluation: using process variables that have a known relationship to the desired outcome; using numerous structure, process, and outcome variables that will reflect the full range of role activities; using outcome variables that have enough sensitivity to detect differences among providers; and comparing practice against explicit criteria and standards rather than against another provider (Prescott & Driscoll, 1980, p. 32). Although referring to NP evaluation, these recommendations are useful for CNSs as well.

Benner's recommendation of clinical ethnography as a research strategy for understanding the illness experience is a helpful vehicle for individual CNSs who wish to describe and evaluate their practice. Taking time to record paradigm cases and describe nursing interventions and patient responses can aid nursing's understanding of how CNS processes affect patient outcomes. "Clinical ethnography is an ideal research strategy for providing knowledge for the expert coach because it focuses on the content and context of the illness experience as well as the disease processes" (Benner, 1985, p. 41). Such narrative documentation can be strong support for the impact of advanced practice on patient care.

Since the advent of DRGs, hospitals gather volumes of patient-specific data that could be useful for CNSs. For example, relating the process of discharge planning to patient length of stay is a possible strategy, since hospitals keep length of stay data recorded by DRG. There has been some research in this area (Marchette & Holloman, 1986), and many CNSs have discharge planning as an important responsibility. Identifying strategies such as this one with clear institutional cost implications is a good approach for CNSs embroiled in cost-effectiveness debates.

Process-outcome evaluation is not for the novice CNS. Indeed, it should be undertaken only by experienced specialists who have developed structural and process evaluation modes for their practices. For these individuals, however, examining outcome criteria and relating them to CNS processes may offer a means to strengthen evaluation as well as expand nursing's knowledge base.

## USE OF THE MODEL IN EVALUATING CNS PRACTICE

Evaluation must spring from practice. Any evaluation strategy should be based on role components that the CNS has emphasized in practice. A newly hired CNS endeavoring to establish clinical credibility in a hospital unfamiliar with CNSs will need quite a different evaluation plan from an established CNS working to strengthen discharge planning on a given unit. The flexibility and multifaceted role of the CNS mean that there is no one right way to evaluate this nurse. Use of Donabedian's categories allows one to select from a variety of strategies to tailor an evaluation plan to an individual CNS.

When CNSs are acting as consultants or teachers, their effect on patients is mediated through other nurses or other health care professionals; consequently, they may be too far removed to measure selected patient outcome. In these situations, one would be more interested in examining changes in nursing behavior, knowledge, or attitude attributable to CNS intervention. As mentioned previously, one would use process strategies to evaluate these subroles.

Process methods require direct observation of the CNS's practice. If a CNS is not observed enough for the evaluator to get some sense of the CNS's skills and priorities, the evaluation cannot be completed fairly.

It is critical that CNSs and administrators do the preplanning necessary to support evaluation. They should take the time to deliberately design evaluation methods before beginning a new project or practice emphasis. "Preplanning by setting goals and determining appropriate methods, measures, evaluators and time intervals for measurement can provide tangible documentation that enables the CNS to analyze failures critically as well as take credit for successes" (Hamric, 1985, p. 65).

There are a number of methods one can use in implementing this evaluation model. One is the "goal-action-evaluation format" described by Malone. "The goals were stated as proposed outcomes; actions included specific steps or programs for reaching the targets; and the evaluation section provided mutually agreed upon indicators for measuring outcome achievement" (Malone, 1986, p. 1375). This format was used in preparing a bimonthly report of progress toward each identified goal.

Evaluating successful achievement of a particular goal may involve structure, process, and outcome measures. For example, a CNS was asked to work with the staff of a surgical unit to implement primary nursing. Both the unit's head nurse and the CNS believed that primary nursing would affect such patient factors as incidences of wound infection and length of stay (Table 4–4). In this example, the measures followed from the goal. One must be careful that evaluation criteria match goals and that goals are measured by other than strictly structural criteria.

Malone noted the importance of documentation: "Like others, CNSs often have difficulty consistently documenting their practice. Some document compulsively. Those who leave no tracks for analysis of their work, however, endanger the CNS role. With no trail for evaluation, accountability is impossible, and no budgetary defense exists for maintaining well-paid clinical experts . . ." (Malone, 1986, p. 1377).

**TABLE 4–4.   Use of Donabedian's Model in Evaluating CNS Goal**

Goal:  To facilitate discharge planning and continuity of care through implementing primary nursing on a surgical unit.

**Structure**

(Focus: Did the intervention occur? In this case, did primary nursing get implemented?)

*Objectives:*
1. Educational sessions on primary nursing are held.
2. Guidelines are developed for primary nurses and associate nurses.
3. The unit employs sufficient numbers of RN staff to implement primary nursing.
4. Patients are able to identify their primary nurse.
5. The primary nurse is identified on the patient's chart and an assessment is made of each patient within 24 hours of admission.

**Process**

(Focus: What is the quality of the primary nursing model? How well is primary nursing being practiced?

*Objectives:*
1. Staff satisfaction improves after introduction of primary nursing.
2. Quality of staff's use of nursing process improves after model is implemented.
3. Staff evaluations of educational sessions are positive.
4. Staff turnover and absenteeism both decrease after introduction of primary nursing.
(See Kent and Larson [1983] for additional structural and process measures.)

**Outcome**

(Focus: What difference did the model make for patients?)

*Objectives:*
1. Patients on the primary unit have a decreased length of stay compared with similar patients (controlling for such variables as acuity and age) on the unit before primary nursing was implemented.
2. Patient satisfaction with nursing care increases compared with satisfaction before implementation.
3. Patients demonstrate more knowledge about their home care requirements than did similar patients on the unit before primary nursing was implemented.
4. The number of postoperative complications experienced by patients decreases after the introduction of primary nursing.

Table 4–5 suggests a procedure for developing a method for evaluating individual CNSs. The first step is to identify the focus (or foci) of the CNS's practice. This focus can easily change over time; therefore, an evaluation procedure utilized in the first year of one's practice might not be appropriate by the third year. On the basis of these practice emphases, one can then define the desired goals or end products, as well as the measurable objectives for each goal. These objectives will determine whether structure, process, outcome, or a combination of these categories should be employed in making the evaluation and what measures or standards would be appropriate. Finally, it needs to be determined who should conduct the evaluations and at what intervals.

Use of such a procedure can enable one to consider the following points. First, what is the focus of the evaluation? It is as unrealistic to expect that any one evaluation measure can encompass all aspects of the CNS role as it is to expect that one CNS can simultaneously practice all aspects. In individual performance appraisal, it is more reasonable to select a few components that a given CNS has emphasized and evaluate them thoroughly. Different measures and different evaluators may be indicated depending upon one's goals. It is important to carefully match measures to objectives. It is similarly important that the evaluator have the relevant information needed to conduct a meaningful evaluation. An administrator who does not observe the CNS other than in individual meetings cannot conduct an objective performance appraisal without gathering data from those with whom the CNS interacts in the clinical setting. Strategies discussed here should be employed to gather data related to specific objectives from a variety of sources to ensure a balanced evaluation.

The second point to consider is the time required to implement an evaluation method. It is important to determine which data related to an individual's performance are easily accessible. Outcome evaluation is generally a slower method because of the time elapsed before patient outcomes manifest themselves. If a program for CNS performance appraisal must be quickly implemented, structural or process strategies may be more feasible in the short run. Other practical constraints, such as expense or numbers of people involved in evaluation, may dictate the method chosen by the individual CNS. For example, a non–unit-based CNS interested in staff evaluation must elicit the cooperation of a group of staff nurses and spend adequate time with them for the method to yield reliable data (Hamric, Gresham, and Eccard, 1978). It may be more realistic for this CNS to evaluate the effectiveness of interventions according to outcome criteria for a select client group.

The CNS should have significant input in determining both the method and the content of any performance appraisal. Constructing

**TABLE 4–5.   Guidelines for Developing an Evaluation Strategy
for Individual CNSs**

| Steps in Process | Example #1<br>(One Major Focus) | Example #2<br>(One of a Number of Foci) |
|---|---|---|
| 1. Select focus (or foci) of practice | 1. CNS to develop teaching program for spinal cord–injured patients | 1. CNS to identify educational needs of surgical nurses and provide appropriate in-service education for all shifts |
| 2. Set goals, desired end results | 2. CNS sets two goals:<br>a. Nursing staff will accept and implement program (nursing staff outcome)<br>b. Patients will have increased knowledge and increased ability to perform self-care (patient outcome) | 2. 80% of all staff will participate in in-service programs at least once a month |
| 3. Determine whether structure, process or outcome evaluation is indicated | 3. a. Structure<br>b. Process<br>c. Outcome—cognitive and behavioral objectives | 3. a. Structure<br>b. Process |
| 4. Determine appropriate method and measure(s) | 4. a. Record of numbers of staff available for program<br>–Administrative support— materials, time, etc.<br>–Audit reward system of unit— positive reinforcement for staff implementation<br>b. Questionnaire to staff—to determine attitude(s) about program<br>–Evaluate nursing records (process audit)—to determine number of staff implementing and number of documented teaching sessions<br>c. Questionnaire to patients—test knowledge<br>–Test self-care abilities and compare with patients before the program was implemented | 4. a. Time schedule— adequate staffing to allow attendance<br>–Administrative support—materials, setting<br>b. Audit nursing records—program topics, attendance; questionnaire to staff—to evaluate topics appropriate for their educational needs |
| 5. Determine appropriate evaluator(s) | 5. CNS to collect audit data, business office data; survey nursing staff; and test patients | 5. CNS to collect audit data, survey nursing staff |
| 6. Determine appropriate intervals for measurement | 6. One year after program implementation | 6. Six-month intervals |

an evaluation tool is a valuable exercise in self-analyzing role performance. It also allows for modification as one matures and priorities change within the position, thus preserving flexibility to meet the needs of one's client population. A thorough self-evaluation should be part of the CNS's performance appraisal.

Given the current state of the art, an annual evaluation consisting of a number of methods at various levels of the model is probably the most valid means of evaluation for the individual CNS. Performance appraisals should occur at least once a year to document performance for the individual's record and the institution and to provide directions for professional growth.

## GETTING STARTED IN CNS EVALUATION

One cannot jump immediately into process-outcome evaluation. Indeed, the evaluation research reported in this chapter is too complex to be feasible for the individual CNS seeking to strengthen performance evaluation. For these individuals the question becomes: how does one begin to evaluate the role?

Initially, the CNS and administrator should discuss what each needs from an annual evaluation. Supervisors may be content with a structural record of time in various subroles; they may wish to have goals and objectives (which may be process and/or outcome oriented) as well. If a major program is being developed, the CNS and supervisor may wish to identify outcome criteria to measure the program's success and devote some planning time to designing a thorough evaluation. If both are novices at CNS evaluation, it is wise to start with structural parameters. It is also advisable to focus process and outcome measures on individual CNS subroles or on specific patient characteristics likely to be affected by CNS intervention. Ensuing chapters give specific strategies for evaluating each CNS subrole. It is important that, whatever evaluation plan is developed, there is consensus that the evaluation is appropriate and useful. The data gathered should give both the CNS and administrator meaningful feedback about the individual's performance. Too many administrators are content with a cursory annual performance evaluation, which will not give a CNS the meaningful feedback needed for growth in the role.

Evaluation has been described as a continuum moving from chance, sporadic performance feedback, through periodic evaluations progressively incorporating structure, process, and outcome objectives, to process-outcome evaluation research (Hamric, 1985). If a CNS is currently at the less structured end of the continuum, it is wise to start small and build upon one's own work.

Collaborating with others can be a useful means of strengthening evaluation. Working with a physician colleague to identify patient outcomes indicative of successful intervention is one possibility. Non-unit-based CNSs may wish to do time-limited contracting with nursing staff of a particular unit to identify specific interventions the staff need and then gather data regarding effectiveness (Hamric, Gresham, and Eccard, 1978). Collaborating with a nurse researcher to evaluate the role more systematically is another possibility. Several of the studies reported were the result of such collaboration.

Begin the year by preplanning for evaluation. Take time to think through each goal in relation to structure, process, and outcome objectives (see Table 4–4). How can these objectives be measured? What data need to be collected during the year to allow for a meaningful evaluation? There are no simple answers to these questions; the answers must be discovered for each individual CNS. But deliberately designing the evaluation component at the beginning of the year can have real benefits in terms of valid data at the end of the year.

Another strategy for getting started in evaluation is for CNSs with similar interests to join together to examine a particular problem. By pooling resources and sharing the tasks, more sophisticated evaluation may be possible than would be achieved by individual effort. Novice CNSs would do well to team with CNSs more experienced in evaluation.

CNSs who are feeling pressure to justify advanced practice in their settings would be well advised to design projects and activities addressing areas of greatest concern within their institutions. Improved discharge planning, decreasing procedural costs, reducing the number of outlier patients in a particular DRG category, and generating revenue are examples of some possible CNS projects (Hamric, 1985). An editorial by a nursing administrator demonstrated the strong advocacy of CNSs who are influencing the practice environment. "In virtually every survey of nurses, the professional practice climate is identified as one of the key attractions in selecting a place to work. Managers alone cannot develop that climate. Clinical experts are essential in creating the excitement in the practice environment that attracts and retains nurses" (Fralic, 1988, p. 6). Fralic noted successful new program implementation, more effective recruitment and retention, efficient staff training, and developing the nursing staff's reputation for excellence with physicians, patients, and families as important CNS processes. She stated of the CNS positions in her institution, "Are these all cost-effective and financially justified positions? Absolutely" (Fralic, 1988, p. 6). All of these areas have potential for individual CNSs seeking to demonstrate the worth of advanced practice in terms valued by the institution.

## SUMMARY

An article describing an informal interview of CNSs regarding evaluation highlights a point of concern: "Approximately 80 percent of the nurses I interviewed either had no job description or had a job description but had never been evaluated. Their mission to produce results was not articulated in a form which was measurable or would hold the CNS accountable. Evaluations tended to be diffuse and subjective" (Morath, 1988, p. 72). Even though this reported interview was conducted in 1982, concern remains that many CNSs are in a similar situation today. A variety of strategies have been presented which can be used by individual CNSs to strengthen their annual performance appraisal, which in turn should strengthen the CNS role within the institution.

In the current health care climate, demonstrating positive changes in patients and nursing behaviors attributable to CNS intervention is not only desirable, it is a necessity for survival of this advanced practice role. Thorough evaluation of CNS effectiveness cannot be demonstrated by structural parameters alone. If CNSs are to demonstrate the worth of the role, evaluation must move beyond structure to incorporate process and outcome measures as well. Recent studies documenting CNS impact on patients and nurses have been encouraging. Individual CNSs can use Donabedian's framework to design evaluations that demonstrate their effectiveness in improving patient outcomes as well as nursing staff behaviors.

### References

Abramson, J.H.: The four basic types of evaluation: Clinical reviews, clinical trials, program reviews and program trials. Public Health Rep 94:210–215, 1979.
Ayers, R.: Effects and development of the role of the clinical nurse specialist. In Ayers, R. (ed): The Clinical Nurse Specialist: An Experiment in Role Effectiveness and Role Development. Duarte, CA, City of Hope National Medical Center, 1971.
Bartucci, M.R.: A comparative study of outpatient care as perceived by renal transplant recipients. ANNA J 12(2):119–124, 1985.
Benner, P., & Wrubel, J.: Clinical knowledge development: The value of perceptual awareness. Nurs Educ 7:11–17, 1982.
Benner, P.: The oncology clinical nurse specialist: An expert coach. Oncol Nurs Forum 12(2):40–44, 1985.
Bloch, D.: Evaluation of nursing care in terms of process and outcome: Issues in research and quality assurance. Nurs Res 24:256–263, 1975.
Brooten, D., Kumar, S., Brown, L.P., et al.: A randomized clinical trial of early hospital discharge and home follow-up of very-low-birth-weight infants. N Engl J Med 315:934–939, 1986.
Chambers, J.K., Dangel, R.B., Germon, K., et al.: Clinical nurse specialist collaboration: Development of a generic job description and standards of performance. Clin Nurs Spec 1(3):124–127, 1987.
Colerick, E.J., Mason, P.B., and Proulx, J.R.: Evaluation of the clinical nurse specialist role: Development and implementation of a dual purpose framework. Nurs Leadership 3(3):26–34, 1980.
Crigler, L., Hurt, L., Burge, S., et al.: Quantifying the clinical nurse specialist role: A pilot study. VA Nurs 52(3):37–42, 1984.

Davis, D.S., Greig, A.E., Burkholder, J., and Keating, T.: Evaluating advance practice nurses. Nurs Management 15(3):44–47, 1984.

Donabedian, A.: Evaluating the quality of medical care. Milbank Mem Fund O 44:166–206, 1966.

Eriksen, L.R.: Patient satisfaction: An indicator of nursing care quality? Nurs Management 18(7):31–35, 1987.

Fralic, M.F.: Nursing's precious resource: The clinical nurse specialist. J Nurs Admin 18(2):5–6, 1988.

Georgopoulos, B.S., & Jackson, M.: Nursing kardex behavior in an experimental study of patient units with and without clinical nurse specialists. Nurs Res 19:196–218, 1970.

Georgopoulos, B.S., & Sana, M.: Clinical nursing specialization and intershift report behavior. Am J Nurs 71:538–545, 1971.

Girouard, S.: The role of the clinical specialist as change agent: An experiment in preoperative teaching. Int J Nurs Stud 15:57–65, 1978.

Girouard, S., & Spross, J.: Evaluation of the CNS: Using an evaluation tool. In Hamric, A.B., and Spross, J. (eds): The Clinical Nurse Specialist in Theory and Practice. New York, Grune and Stratton, 1983, pp. 207–218.

Hamric, A.B., Gresham, M.L., and Eccard, M.: Staff evaluation of clinical leaders. J Nurs Admin 8(1):18–26, 1978.

Hamric, A.B.: A model for developing evaluation strategies. In Hamric, A.B., and Spross, J. (eds): The Clinical Nurse Specialist in Theory and Practice. New York, Grune and Stratton, 1983, pp. 187–206.

Hamric, A.B.: Clinical nurse specialist role evaluation. Oncol Nurs Forum 12(2):62–66, 1985.

Harrell, J.S., & McCullough, S.D.: The role of the clinical nurse specialist: Problems and solutions. J Nurs Admin 16(10):44–48, 1986.

Kent, L.A., & Larson, E.: Evaluating the effectiveness of primary nursing practice. J Nurs Admin 13(1):34–41, 1983.

Knaus, W.A., Draper, E.A., Wagner, D.P., and Zimmerman, J.E.: An evaluation of outcome from intensive care in major medical centers. Ann Intern Med 104:410–418, 1986.

Linde, B.J., & Janz, N.M.: Effect of a teaching program on knowledge and compliance of cardiac patients. Nurs Res 28(5):282–286, 1979.

Little, D.E., & Carnevali, D.: Nursing specialist effect on tuberculosis. Nurs Res 16:321–326, 1967.

Malone, B.L.: Evaluation of the clinical nurse specialist. Am J Nurs 86:1375–1377, 1986.

Marchette, L., & Holloman, F.: Length of stay: Significant variables. J Nurs Admin 16(3):12–19, 1986.

McBride, A.B., Austin, J.K., Chesnut, E.E., et al.: Evaluation of the impact of the clinical nurse specialist in a state psychiatric hospital. Arch Psych Nurs 1(1):55–61, 1987.

Morath, J.M.: The clinical nurse specialist: Evaluation issues. Nurs Management 19(3):72–80, 1988.

Murphy, J.F.: If P (additional nursing care): then Q (quality of patient welfare)? WICHE Commun Nurs Res 4:1–12, 1971.

Neidlinger, S.H., Scroggins, K., and Kennedy, L.M.: Cost evaluation of discharge planning for hospitalized elderly. Nurs Econ 5(5):225–230, 1987.

Nevidjon, B., & Warren, B.: Documenting the activities of the oncology clinical nurse specialist. Oncol Nurs Forum 11(3):54–55, 1984.

Oleske, D.M., Otte, D.M., and Heinze, S.: Development and evaluation of a system for monitoring the quality of oncology nursing care in the home setting. Cancer Nurs 10(4):190–198, 1987.

Pozen, M.W., Stechmiller, J.A., Harris, W., et al.: A nurse rehabilitator's impact on patients with myocardial infarction. Med Care 15(10):830–837, 1977.

Prescott, P.A., & Driscoll, L.: Evaluating nurse practitioner performance. Nurs Prac 5(4):29–32, 1980.

Robichaud, A.M., & Hamric, A.B.: Time documentation of clinical nurse specialist activities. J Nurs Admin 16(1):31–36, 1986.

# PART II

# SUBROLES AND COMPETENCIES OF THE CNS

# Clinical Practice and Direct Patient Care

Theresa L. Koetters

## INTRODUCTION

### Putting Direct Care into Perspective

Although the Clinical Nurse Specialist (CNS) role has existed for about two decades and has been implemented in a variety of ways in many settings, the function of expert practitioner remains a crucial subrole. The belief that expert practice and a focus on patient care are the first and foremost responsibilities of CNSs was described as early as 1966 (Reiter, 1966; Johnson, 1967). Despite many changes in health care and in the nursing profession, this belief continues to be espoused by nursing leaders (Baird, 1985, Tarsitano et al., 1986) and the American Nurses' Association (ANA, 1980; 1986). In the *Social Policy Statement* issued in 1980, the ANA emphasized clinical expertise in the role and described one characteristic function of the CNS as "direct care of selected patients or clients in any setting, including private practice." In addition, the 1986 ANA document, *The Role of the Clinical Nurse Specialist,* stated that, "The CNS takes a comprehensive approach to nursing practice, demonstrating the ability to foresee and discuss care options and potential short-range and long-range consequences of that care. . . . The CNS assesses . . . diagnoses . . . plans . . . intervenes . . . and evaluates. . . ."

Historically, the role was established to improve the quality of patient care and nursing practice, regardless of specialty (Georgopoulous & Christman, 1970; Little, 1967). Hawken noted that as patients' needs "in hospitals and homes become more complex and as the care patients receive increases in sophistication, the education and knowledge of the person they turn to for help and information also needs to be specialized and timely" (1987, ix). Issues of changing demographics, increasing technology, and shifting financial responsibility for health care all reflect the complicated environment within which CNSs are challenged to practice and contribute to the present and future justification of the direct care subrole.

## Definition of Clinical Practice

The direct care subrole of the CNS often consists of two components. One is direct care that is regularly and systematically provided. Such direct care may focus on a specific clinical problem. An example of this is a neuroscience CNS who evaluates all head injury patients in order to identify and treat specific behavioral sequelae resulting from head injury. In another situation, an oncology CNS might negotiate to maintain a caseload of three outpatients for whom the CNS provides nursing care including assessment, symptom management, education, and chemotherapy administration.

The second aspect of direct care is episodic and is provided to meet a specific need or solve a particular problem. For both types of direct care the range of activities are numerous, as reflected in Table 5–1. The difference is the regularity with which the direct care is performed. The direct care component of CNS practice should include regular and systematic care. The nature of the practice setting will dictate the extent of episodic direct care. For example, a unit-based CNS will probably provide more episodic care than an institution-based CNS; and the care provided by the CNS in private practice is unlikely to have an episodic component. The amount of time spent in the clinical area, regardless of the types of activities, will also vary. Practicing CNSs have stated that anywhere from 25 to 50 per cent of a work week should be devoted to direct care/clinical practice (Craft & Pfiederer, 1982; Welch-McCaffrey, 1986).

Indirect care activities focus on the caregiver or the care processes.

**TABLE 5–1.   Range of Direct Care Activities of the CNS**

Primary nurse for small group of patients
Associate nurse for small group of patients
Providing total patient care during a shift
Providing care to one or two complex patients for part of a shift
Doing complex discharge planning
Administering treatments and/or medications on a team once or twice a month
Providing patient education—individual or group
Facilitating a patient and family support group
Developing a care plan for a complex or unusual patient
Developing a care plan for a specific clinical problem
Crisis intervention

Such activities have been identified by Hamric and Fenton (1983; 1985) among others. Indirect care activities of the practitioner subrole are listed in Table 5–2.

# CHARACTERISTICS OF DIRECT CARE

It is a challenge to describe the characteristics of care rendered by specialists. One needs to visualize the most expert of nurses and how that nurse practices, then list traits, qualities, or properties that describe the nurse's care. The care is expert and thoroughly skilled; it is delivered and performed confidently and in a timely manner. Other nurses will describe the CNS's care as excellent; they may be able to appreciate the expert role modeling. Upon closer examination, the CNS is actualizing the nursing process in an expert way (Benner, 1985; Fenton, 1985). Another nurse can easily identify when the CNS is assessing, interviewing, questioning, and observing. The depth and breadth of information that the CNS is able to obtain exemplifies the wealth of the CNS's own knowledge and skills.

Problem identification or nursing diagnosis is usually done swiftly. Compared with a staff nurse, the CNS will probably identify more potential problems by virtue of experience with and specialized knowledge of a particular population of patients. The CNS will consistently be aware of prevention of complications regardless of the disease process or diagnostic entity. In the past, preventive measures were taken to increase and improve patient well-being and physical health. Today, CNSs are also asked to be cognizant of length of stay (LOS) and how they can help to shorten it (Eisenberg, 1987).

Nursing interventions are performed easily by the CNS, whether it is bedside care, administering a particular therapy, providing emotional support, or facilitating patient teaching. CNSs actively learn new and innovative therapies to be incorporated into nursing practice. What should become fairly obvious is how well the CNS can also function as a competent, if not expert, staff nurse. A very important message is

**TABLE 5–2.   Range of Indirect Care Activities of the CNS**

Facilitating a staff support group
Collaborating with a staff nurse to develop a patient care plan
Participating in clinical rounds (e.g., discharge planning, medical, interdisciplinary)
Developing standards, standard care plans, protocols, patient education materials
"Breaking the rules" and "Massaging the system" (Fenton, 1985)
Participating in quality assurance activities
Recommending/initiating referrals to other health care providers
Participating in interdisciplinary/interdepartmental clinical activities

delivered to staff, administration, and physicians when they see the CNS delivering direct care: that the CNS is a nurse first, with expertise in a particular specialty, as well as a consultant, an educator, or a researcher.

Sometimes there is an attitude of fearlessness about the CNS in patient care situations, as if nothing is beyond the CNS's knowledge and skill. In reality, one of the CNS's greatest assets may be the acknowledgment of what the CNS really does not know. By asking for feedback from the staff, the CNS can serve as an example for continuing to strive for personal excellence and quality patient care by seeking new knowledge and learning new skills.

## RATIONALE FOR DIRECT CARE SUBROLE

The reasons for a CNS to provide direct or indirect care to patients or families are numerous and varied. The positive aspects or advantages will be emphasized in this discussion, which will address the CNS, the staff, the patient, the nursing organization, and the nursing profession. Felder (1983) identified many reasons for performing direct care. These are summarized in Table 5–3.

Although Felder enumerated reasons for the CNS to perform direct care functions, the author believes these need further discussion, given changes in health care since Felder's original work. Updating one's knowledge of equipment, devices, new procedures, and new medications is a good reason for the CNS to stay involved with direct care and to maintain and improve already attained knowledge and skills. For example, it may be easy to read a report on a new vascular access device, but until the CNS starts a line or draws blood from that device, it will be harder to talk about it to patients, suggest it to physicians, or teach procedures that its use involves to other nurses.

Another reason for the CNS to stay involved in direct care is to contribute to writing standards of care and to identify opportunities for research utilization and research generation. Having been exposed to the research process during graduate education, the CNS can employ

**TABLE 5–3.  Reasons for Practicing Direct Care**

| | |
|---|---|
| "Learn the routines," orientation | Gain acceptance |
| Demonstrate clinical competence | Enhance CNS's visibility and accessibility |
| Function as a role model | Assert autonomous nursing role |
| Assess constraints under which staff work | Experience reality |

(Adapted from Felder, L.: Direct patient care and independent practice. *In* Hamric, A. B., and Spross, J. (eds): The Clinical Nurse Specialist in Theory and Practice. New York, Grune and Stratton, 1983.)

critical thinking in evaluating patient care and systems problems. Keeping an idea list of questions or concerns from the clinical area will provide possible research projects or topics for publication.

The increasing acuity of hospitalized patients is common knowledge. Health care providers have written about the phenomenon of being discharged "sicker and quicker." It can be a very good and humbling experience for the CNS to be in the midst of admissions, discharges, and helping with a family of a patient who just experienced a cardiac arrest. The behaviors exhibited by the CNS under as much stress as the staff can defuse potentially explosive situations and can be very supportive. This experience also helps the CNS examine ways to help staff prevent or cope with complex situations. One CNS tried to help staff ease an overwhelming workload by suggesting a plan to change bed linens daily only for those patients who were bedbound, incontinent, or had other problems in which *not* changing the linen daily was a threat to health.

Other reasons for providing direct care can be identified. Direct care may be essential to an individual's sense of job satisfaction. CNSs experiencing considerable organizational stress report that their clinical activities enable them to endure periods of organizational stress and strain. Many CNSs choose the CNS role because it allows them to maintain patient contact while exercising leadership skills. In the past, clinicians who wished to advance could only do so by taking management positions that distanced them from patient care.

In addition, there are practical reasons for maintaining a clinical practice. ANA certification in certain specialties requires a specified number of hours per week in direct care to be eligible for or to renew certification. The nature of a specialty (e.g., critical care, oncology) may be such that many skills require periodic use to maintain competency ("if you don't use it, you lose it"). Skill maintenance through regular direct care activities is particularly important when CNSs are responsible for competency-based assessments of other care providers.

While the coaching functions of the CNS generally benefit the patient, the concepts may also apply to indirect patient care activities because the focus of role modeling expert clinical practice and skills is the nursing staff. Benner outlined the main tasks of a coach in clinical practice: "to interpret the unfamiliar diagnostic and treatment demands; to coach the client through alienated stances; to identify changing relevance; and to ensure that cure is enhanced by care" (1985, p. 43). By virtue of their clinical expertise and in-depth knowledge of a particular clinical population, CNSs can extend themselves to patients as expert coaches while role modeling for the staff at the same time.

Benner did not address the coaching of staff as a CNS function, but the same processes one uses to coach patients apply to coaching staff. When CNSs work beside staff, they can interpret diagnostic and treatment demands that will enhance patient care. They can coach the nurse through "alienated stances" or crises by talking the nurse through a delicate procedure or practicing a conversation with a difficult physician. When a nurse identifies a dropping hematocrit, CNSs can assist in putting that lab value into a context that is relevant to the patient's changing clinical picture. And finally, CNSs can "ensure that cure is enhanced by care" through role modeling "caring behaviors" (Larson, 1986) and giving immediate positive feedback for good care. CNSs can also make concrete suggestions to the staff regarding courtesy, answering call lights, pain management techniques, or whatever is appropriate given the clinical situation.

Staff may tend to take a lot of their own knowledge and skills for granted. Many times staff make significant clinical observations worthy of further exploration or documentation. They may need the encouragement and/or validation that what they know and do is important! By not taking their own knowledge and skills for granted, CNSs do not allow an environment of complacency and stagnation to exist. By carefully examining and reviewing care delivered by the staff, strengths can be acknowledged and weaknesses or learning needs identified. This method of learning and refining skills is known in the mental health disciplines as clinical supervision (Critchley, 1985; Platt-Koch, 1986). Perhaps more of the nursing profession and certainly patients could benefit from nurses learning from mistakes and celebrating successes.

Fenton indicated that another major reason for the CNS to be involved in direct care is to achieve the competency of "building and maintaining a therapeutic team in order to provide optimum therapy" (1985, p. 32). She found that "providing emotional support for the nursing staff, especially in specific challenging situations, was one of the CNS's daily activities" (p. 33). Specific challenging situations could include very emotional situations or ethical dilemmas faced by staff; for example, multiple deaths of very young patients on an oncology unit, repeated cardiac arrests in a viable middle-aged businessman with young children, or disagreeing with the medical plan of care for a mentally incompetent patient and feeling helpless and powerless about serving as the patient's advocate. Whether the CNS identifies what it is like for the staff to try and meet standards of care or assesses obstacles to meeting those standards, the CNS is often in a good position to assume "the role of trying to decrease the stress load of the nursing staff" (p. 33).

When the CNS provides direct care and is "exhibiting behaviors which exemplify progressive and skillful clinical practice" (Calkin, 1984, p. 25), the staff realize that the CNS's goals and those of the staff are more similar than different. By working together over an extended period of time, the staff will begin to improve their skills of assessment and problem identification, intervention, and evaluation and will begin to emulate the care of the CNS.

The CNS may also be able to effect a more positive outcome when the staff identify a patient or family as "difficult." Through tactful, sensitive, and attentive interviewing the CNS may discover the source of the difficult behavior, e.g., the patient's room may be on the "wrong" side of the hospital, the patient's symptoms may be the same as a relative's who died recently, or the patient's diagnosis may symbolize a life of dependency or pain. Whether called in to do crisis intervention or scheduling time with the patient or family for some counseling, the CNS may be able to bring about behavioral or communication changes. For example, one intervention may be teaching the difference between acute and chronic pain for a cancer patient who has just been told that his disease has metastasized to his bones. He has been on the call light all night asking for his pain medication, and the family is irate because he is still uncomfortable. This patient and family become the priority for the CNS while the staff still have to pass medications, answer lights, supervise other staff, and change dressings. What the CNS achieves will benefit the patient, family, staff, and nursing unit.

While the aforementioned reasons for CNS direct care have been primarily focused on patient care and nursing practice, there are a number of benefits the institution's nursing department and ultimately the nursing profession derive from it. First, while the CNS is actualizing the nursing process, there will be interactions with a variety of disciplines. The CNS can identify actual and potential problems early and in a timely manner; as a result of the CNS's interventions, there may be prevention of medical complications, initiation of early discharge planning, or identification of the potential for malnourishment. Such CNS activities require communication with physicians, social workers, and dietitians. This process of collaboration enables the CNS to establish a nursing identity (and, indirectly, nursing autonomy) for these other providers. These interactions benefit the department of nursing and the nursing profession.

Another perspective on the early identification of problem patients or situations relates to the CNS's ability to identify "outliers" in the current DRG system. The CNS can ask questions and plan solutions for patients requiring repeated admissions and for new clinical situations that contribute to increasing the acuity of patients, therefore increasing staffing needs. Tracking problem patients or situations, analyzing incident reports, and monitoring a new treatment or procedure are activities that the CNS could perform while providing direct care. Any one of these activities could further assist the CNS in identifying and developing a new clinical program that could then be marketed by the institution.

CNSs are also in an important position to influence consumers. Although nurses traditionally view patients as consumers of their services, the CNS tends to also view families, visitors, and the community surrounding the hospital as consumers. For example, the CNS may teach daughters of a newly diagnosed breast cancer patient about breast self examination. CNSs can make a good impression on other consumers by interacting with them. Hospital administrators and public relations departments would be wise to view their CNSs as marketing consultants and public relations spokespersons.

Overall, the CNS strives to be accessible and timely in meeting the needs of patients, families, and nursing staff. By spending the critical time in the clinical area, the CNSs' direct care activities contribute to a successful future within the institution.

## DISADVANTAGES AND OBSTACLES TO DIRECT CARE SUBROLE

Felder outlined a number of situations that may be problematic: feelings of resentment and territoriality on the part of staff nurses and other health care providers, time pressures, lack of support, cost to the institution, and narrowing the effects of the CNS's role modeling to one unit or to one nurse (1983). Another problem cited by many authors is role confusion; for example, staff and physicians may be confused when a CNS works a shift in the staff nurse role instead of in the regular CNS role. Administrators and CNSs should negotiate expectations regarding clinical time in order to decrease confusion about the role among staff, physicians, other administrators, other CNSs, and anyone else who may interact with the CNS and question how productivity is being measured.

One author denied that CNSs should have a direct practice role if broad system changes are desired (Everson, 1981). Administrators have questioned the cost-effectiveness of the CNS providing direct care. The challenge for CNSs is to effect system changes in a cost-effective manner through their clinical practice while documenting cost savings or revenue generation for the institution. Some scenarios that concretely address the cost issue include the CNS who teaches nurses through role modeling how averting skin breakdown and decubitus ulcers will prevent outliers from losing money for the hospital; the CNS who assesses wound healing and makes appropriate recommendations regarding products or nutrition can decrease LOS and increase revenue for patients for whom the hospital receives a set amount of payment; the CNS who makes recommendations to modify practice while conserving time and supplies, knowing that certain procedures affect quality of care and patient outcomes; and the CNS who assists with or is actually responsible for patient and family teaching that will enhance a timely discharge can, again, save the hospital money or even make money on patients who are discharged "early" (Mazique, 1987).

Disadvantages have seemed to diminish in recent years as the numbers of CNSs have increased and as the acuity and complexity of different patient populations have increased (Wells, 1985). Sisson studied staff perceptions regarding functions and effectiveness of the CNS in one institution in which the number of positions increased from 1 in 1974 to 16 in 1982 (1987). The overall findings of her study identified a number of unanticipated benefits: "increased value placed on the role . . . increased physician demand . . . an increase in consultation requests initiated by staff nurses" (p. 17). Brown and Wilson have recommended time management strategies to assist the CNS in decreasing time pressures (1987).

Since Woodrow and Bell described impediments to role modeling by the CNS in 1971, the perception of the CNS role as an "oddity" may be decreasing slightly (Sisson, 1987). The role modeling process, however, still needs "(a) the role model, (b) the situation in which the role model may function and (c) someone who seeks or is expected to emulate the model" (Woodrow & Bell, 1971, p. 25). In this author's experience, what may have occurred in the past 16 years is that CNSs have been allowed to function as role models and that staff nurses are not as threatened by CNSs and are more interested in the role modeling process, because of the increased attention being paid to nursing as a profession.

While lack of authority to reward staff who modeled after CNS behavior was identified as an obstacle by Woodrow and Bell, there are other ways for CNSs, in collaboration with head nurses, to build rewards into the system: initiation of a staff support group, acknowledgement of "staff nurse of the month," purchase of new reference books for the unit, or encouraging staff involvement on nursing department committees.

## FACTORS INFLUENCING THE DIRECT CARE SUBROLE

Whether a CNS is new in the role or experienced, there are a number of critical issues to assess when implementing the direct care subrole. It is helpful for the CNS to know the staff mix, i.e., what proportion of staff are RNs, LPNs and nursing assistants. The educational and experiential background of staff will influence CNSs' approaches and entry into the system. This knowledge may influence how the CNS evaluates patient care, teaches classes, or even introduces the CNS role, especially if this is the first CNS in the institution. For example, if the CNS is being introduced at a staff meeting and all of the attendees are aides and LPNs who have never heard of the CNS role, the direct care and resource person aspects of the role rather than the education and research aspects of the role should be discussed. Conversely, with an all RN staff, the CNS may emphasize the nursing process or offer to facilitate the writing of a unit research study.

The nursing care delivery system practiced on nursing units will influence a CNS's direct care subrole. The CNS may use different strategies to implement a direct care role depending upon what system is in place in the department—primary nursing, team nursing, or total patient care. Again, the CNS's expectations of the RN staff may vary considerably, as will the way in which role modeling is done. Primary nursing units may not be as open to the CNS conducting patient teaching or family counseling, whereas the nurse still doing team leading may be accepting of any suggestions in these areas.

The key factor for the CNS to keep in mind regarding these different systems of practice is to clarify how much power or control the nurses have over patient care and then to contribute appropriately. For example, in primary nursing and total patient care, the nurses' scope of practice would seem larger than in team nursing, so suggestions about patient care may be at a higher level. The model of practice may dictate whether the priority for the CNS's activities is the patient or the nurse. Brainstorming with other CNSs in the institution or with the CNS's supervisor may assist in the identification of new and creative ways to reach the nursing staff.

Another critical issue for the CNS is whether the role is unit-based or population-based. A unit-based position limits the environment and the number of nursing staff with whom to become involved. Theoretically, this should positively influence the implementation of the direct care subrole since there are fewer people with whom to interact. In reality, there may be difficulties. Did the head nurse, nursing staff, and medical staff of this unit want a CNS? Does the acuity and the census on this unit warrant a unit-based CNS?

Advantages of being unit-based include being more visible and accessible, being able to be part of and build a therapeutic team, gaining acceptance by unit staff more quickly, and having a finger on the clinical pulse of the unit. The unit-based CNS can make more complete and systematic observations about variables that influence clinical care of patients. It might also be easier to gather data for CNS evaluation from those who interact with the CNS regularly.

Disadvantages of being unit-based include the risk of being over-used to bail the unit out of tough spots (staffing shortages, chronic high acuity, and the like). There is a risk that patients on other units who need the CNS's services may not get them. Some organizations have overcome this by having the CNS be primarily unit-based but available for consultation to other units.

On the other hand, a population-based CNS may be all over the institution trying to influence patient care and nursing practice. This could seem like an uphill battle. However, this flexibility to travel around the institution frees the CNS from unit politics and spreads the wealth of the CNS's expertise. Another advantage to being population-based is that the CNS can assure that every patient who needs CNS evaluation gets seen by the CNS (if one uses admission data/diagnoses rather than relying solely on consultation). The CNS can develop standards to be used throughout the institution rather than for a particular unit.

Disadvantages of this arrangement may include needing to demonstrate competence to many staff; needing to work through several different subsystems (e.g., a variety of head nurses with a variety of managerial styles); and feeling that one's services are spread too thin. The author does not intend a recommendation for or against unit- or population-based CNSs. Differences in expectations for direct care based on placement should be discussed and negotiated by the CNS and supervisor.

Administrative support of the CNS role is addressed in Chapter 13. Emphasis for support of the direct care subrole will be addressed here. The advantages for the nursing administrator to support the CNS in direct care functions are numerous and include obtaining a more accurate picture of the nursing staff's clinical practice; gaining a clearer sense of the acuity of a certain patient population and identification of reasons for changes in acuity (e.g., a new piece of equipment, procedure, or investigational protocol); identifying earlier quality assurance or risk management issues; identifying new clinical problems/concerns and their causes (e.g., outlier populations, lack of staff skills, and so forth); and ensuring role modeling for professional nursing in the clinical areas.

Administrative support logically extends to identifying organizational and/or departmental resources needed by the CNS to accomplish this clinical function. Some questions that may be useful for the CNS and the nursing administrator to ask are: Does the CNS need a beeper or will the nursing office secretary take accurate messages? Does the CNS want to be interrupted by a beeper when delivering patient care? Will the nursing office secretary or the unit secretary answer overhead pages to leave the CNS uninterrupted? Where is the CNS's office and why? Does the staff know how and where to find the CNS for clinical problems? When the CNS is on a clinical unit, who else needs to know where the CNS is and what the CNS is doing and why? Other CNSs may resent the time a colleague spends in the clinical area if their positions have different expectations associated with them. These issues must be addressed in a timely manner and with administrative support and clarification.

The nature of medical practice can influence CNS practice. In a teaching hospital, for example, the CNS (and nursing staff) often have more expert clinical knowledge about a patient population than the house staff who are responsible for the daily medical care of patients. This can pose practice dilemmas in that the CNS runs the risk of supervising and teaching inexperienced or less experienced house staff about the clinical problems of the specialty population, since senior physicians are not readily available. Such experiences may signal the need for protocols jointly developed by senior physicians and clinical specialists. If CNSs find it necessary and worthwhile to engage in medical teaching on a regular basis, they should negotiate a joint appointment to the medical school or department with an appropriate recompense.

A final factor influencing the direct care subrole is the feelings generated in the CNS when performing direct or indirect patient care. CNSs may perceive that they are viewed as extra pairs of hands and may feel used by the nursing staff for an inappropriate reason. The CNS may be performing management functions and feel misused or abused by the head nurse. The nursing staff may act suspicious of the CNS or ignore the CNS when present on the unit. The CNS may be made to feel like a spy or a threat. These feelings and concerns have been described by new CNSs as well as seasoned colleagues (Kwong, Manning, and Koetters, 1982). The CNS should seek assistance to deal with these feelings and attempt to clarify the CNS role for the institution and the nursing staff. Through ongoing communication and clarification of the purpose of the CNS role within the institution, a previously uncomfortable situation will improve.

## STRATEGIES FOR ESTABLISHING/ IMPLEMENTING DIRECT CARE SUBROLE

There is no one right way to implement the direct care subrole. Strategies will vary from institution to institution. The manner in which the subrole is implemented will depend upon whether the CNS is coming to a position directly from graduate school or is changing settings and is thus more experienced in the role. Orientation and getting established may take less time for the experienced CNS because organizational assessment and communication skills may be more polished.

Both new and experienced CNSs may choose to work side by side with staff to become integrated into a system (Felder, 1983). A CNS may choose to interview the whole staff separately on all three shifts, to obtain their perspectives on what they need clinically and where the CNS may fit in. A mistake easily made by seasoned CNSs is to presume to know what staff need and proceed to intervene with inservices or patient care conferences, then wonder why no one will attend or participate.

It is important to schedule time for direct patient care. The CNS needs to schedule clinical time and not let any other commitment interfere. The CNS should attend report at regular intervals and attend rounds to determine which patients or families have the greatest need or are posing the greatest problem to the staff. Sometimes the CNS may choose to take a patient assignment to experience what the staff are going through at a time when census and/or acuity are high.

Some CNSs have clearly defined areas of involvement: enterostomal therapy, cardiac rehabilitation, or gynecologic oncology. These CNSs may experience less ambiguity regarding their roles but may be more accountable. For the staff's sake, these subspecialized CNSs may choose to see every ostomy patient, every myocardial infarction patient, and every newly diagnosed gynecologic cancer patient.

Another component of scheduling direct care deals with sharing the wealth of the CNS's expertise. Patients do not receive care only on the day shift. Most literature regarding implementing the CNS role does not address working or at least meeting all three shifts. While an institution may not require the CNS to meet the needs of the off-shift staff, a discussion between the CNS and the nursing administrator may provide approval or support of such an activity and a new direction for the CNS. Nurses working evening and night shifts have been heard to say that "everything happens on the day shift!" These staff especially appreciate attention from nursing department resource people. Feedback for the CNS who devotes time to off-shift staff can be tremendous.

When an experienced CNS is working with an experienced staff, the strategies to continue direct care activities may have to become more creative. The CNS may choose to subspecialize and work very closely with patients with certain diagnoses. Even though the staff may function at a very high clinical level, the CNS may discover an assessment skill that needs to be upgraded or a symptom that the staff consistently under or over treat. If CNSs really find themselves in the situation of not being needed on a clinical unit, they may search for an appropriate setting where their clinical expertise can be used to assist patients and families, such as a joint practice with a physician colleague located nearby, a senior center that performs health screenings, or time on a different clinical unit that would benefit from the CNSs' role modeling and problem-solving skills.

One small but important factor should be mentioned here. It seems obvious that in wishing to give a strong message of availability, the CNS should occasionally come to work in a nursing uniform. However, many CNSs wear street clothes and a lab coat, even on direct care days. This "CNS uniform" may give staff a message of unapproachability or unavailability.

## EVALUATION OF THE DIRECT CARE SUBROLE

Comprehensive and consistent evaluation of the CNS's contributions in the areas of patient care and improving nursing practice has been a challenge since the inception of the role. Evaluation of the CNS role in general, and peer review as an example, are addressed in Chapters 4 and 14, respectively. Schilke-Davis emphasized that "evaluation of nurses in advanced clinical roles is an excellent opportunity to review progress, encourage professional growth and increase communication between clinicians and administrators" (1984, p. 47). Other authors have tried to capture the relevance of the direct care subrole by a variety of methods: staff nurse evaluation tools (Hamric, Gresham, and Eccard, 1978); self-evaluation (Colerick, Mason, and Proulx, 1980); time documentation (Robichaud & Hamric, 1986); and unit leader evaluation (Girouard & Spross, 1983). The evaluation tool developed by Hamric, Gresham, and Eccard and adapted by Girouard and Spross probably has the best specific questions relating to patient care and the quality and quantity of that care.

Ideally, feedback could be sought from patients and families that the CNS has cared for or influenced. Interviews upon discharge or patient questionnaires given at discharge or mailed to patients' homes can give both qualitative and quantitative data. Questions from the Girouard and Spross evaluation tool could be modified to be directed toward a patient or family member. If the CNS's institution uses patient satisfaction questionnaires, a question could be added regarding meeting and working with a CNS (Welch-McCaffrey, 1985).

Due to the indirect and intermittent nature of many of the CNS's direct care activities, feedback is usually sought from the staff, head nurses, medical staff, and relevant committees, for example, quality assurance, standards, and nursing research. Specific expectations of each group regarding specific job functions of the CNS should be addressed. Major responsibility statements pertaining to direct care should be derived from the CNS job description and developed into questions for the aforementioned groups. For example, staff might be asked if the CNS provides quality nursing care to a select group of patients. Are these patients the most appropriate for the CNS to be following? If not, which group or diagnosis may be more appropriate? For head nurses, is the CNS available enough to provide the kind of role modeling needed by the staff? Has the CNS contributed to improving nursing practice through direct care activities? For physicians, have the direct care efforts of the CNS affected the care of patients on a particular unit? The goal of seeking and documenting this kind of feedback is to identify whether the CNS is making a difference in the quality of patient care and nursing practice, how much of a difference, and what kinds of CNS activities have the greatest impact. Are the expectations of staff, head nurses, and medical staff being met and, if not, how could they be met? Or, if the expectations are unrealistic or inappropriate, how can they be made more congruent? (Propotnik, 1987). This kind of comprehensive evaluation should be done at least annually and more often if there is any question as to the effectiveness of the CNS or the appropriateness of the position.

The CNS must assume responsibility for documenting patient and family contacts and outcomes. Cards on each patient should be maintained with demographics, history, current problems, CNS interventions, and time spent on the case, including follow-up phone calls to patient's home, home health agency, or physician's office. Outcomes could be described by disposition of patient, achievement of nursing goals, success of patient teaching, or the contributions made to a timely and satisfactory discharge. The CNS must develop tools to measure and document changes in nursing practice; for example, a study to document the difference in time needed to start an IV given different pieces of equipment, what happens to patient expectations of bedside care as the technology in a given unit increases, or the necessity of stripping chest tubes.

All CNSs must assume responsibility for collecting data that will contribute to the justification of CNS positions within the nursing department, other health care agencies, and the profession itself. By negotiating for the time needed to collect some of these important data, the CNS can begin to show numbers of patients seen, decreasing LOS for certain diagnoses, contributions made to smooth discharges, and changes in nursing practice. By protecting CNS positions that are currently funded and proving their worth, there will be an inceasing number of CNS positions to continue to improve patient care and nursing practice and contribute to the growing body of relevant clinical research.

## SUMMARY

The CNS role was established to improve the quality of patient care and nursing practice. The expert practitioner subrole must continue to be the central focus for the role in order to achieve the original purpose. CNSs must be prepared to negotiate, justify, and maintain a strong clinical practice that will include direct and indirect care activities. While "CNSs cannot be all things to all people" (Hamric & Spross, 1983, p. 304), they are in key positions to potentially influence many aspects of the current health care delivery system.

*References*

American Nurses' Association, Congress for Nursing Practice, Nursing—A Social Policy Statement. Kansas City, American Nurses' Association, 1980.
American Nurses' Association, Council of Clinical Nurse Specialists, The Role of the Clinical Nurse Specialist. Kansas City, American Nurses' Association, 1986.
Baird, S.: Administrative support issues and the clinical nurse specialist. Oncol Nurs Forum 12(2):51–54, 1985.
Benner, P.: The oncology nurse specialist an expert coach. Oncol Nurs Forum 12(2):40–44, 1985.
Brown, M. M., & Wilson, C.: Time management and the clinical nurse specialist. Clin Nurs Specialist 1(1):32–38, 1987.
Calkin, J. D.: A model for advanced nursing practice. J Nurs Admin 14(1):24–30, 1984.
Colerick, R. J., Mason, P. B., and Proulx, J. R.: Evaluation of the clinical nurse specialist role: Development and implementation of a dual purpose framework. Nurs Leadership 3:26–34, 1980.
Craft, M. J., & Pfiederer, D.: Practice setting and the successful pediatric clinical specialist. Ped Nurs 8:187–189, 1982.
Critchley, D. L.: Clinical supervision. *In* Critchley, D. L., & Maurin, J. T. (eds): The Clinical Specialist in Psychiatric Mental Health Nursing: Theory, Research, and Practice. New York, John Wiley & Sons, 1985, pp. 495–510.
Eisenberg, P., Spies, M., and Metheny, N. A.: Characteristics of patients who remove their nasal feeding tube. Clin Nurs Specialist 1:94–97, 1987.
Everson, S. A.: Integration of the role of the clinical nurse specialist. J Cont Educ Nurs 12(2):16–19, 1981.
Felder, L.: Direct patient care and independent practice. *In* Hamric, A. B., and Spross, J. (eds): The Clinical Nurse Specialist in Theory and Practice. New York, Grune and Stratton, 1983.
Fenton, M. V.: Identifying competencies of clinical nurse specialists. J Nurs Admin 15(12):31–37, 1985.
Georgopoulous, B., & Christman, L.: The clinical nurse specialist: A role model. Am J Nurs 70(5):1030–1039, 1970.
Girouard, S., & Spross, J.: Evaluation of the CNS: Using an evaluation tool. *In* Hamric,

A. B., and Spross, J. (eds): The Clinical Nurse Specialist in Theory and Practice. New York, Grune and Stratton, 1983.

Hamric, A., Gresham, M. L., and Eccard, M.: Staff evaluation of clinical leaders. J Nurs Admin 8:18–26, 1978.

Hawken, P. L.: Foreword. *In* Menard, S. W. (ed): The Clinical Nurse Specialist Perspectives on Practice. New York, John Wiley & Sons, 1987.

Johnson, D. E., Wilcox, J. A., and Moidel, H. D.: The clinical specialist as a practitioner. Am J Nurs 67:2298–2302, 1967.

Kwong, M., Manning, M. P., and Koetters, T.: The role of the oncology clinical specialist: Three personal views. Cancer Nurs 5(6):427–434, 1982.

Larson, P.: Cancer nurses' perceptions of caring. Cancer Nurs 9(2):86–91, 1986.

Little, D.: The nurse specialist. Am J Nurs 67:552–556, 1967.

Mazique, S.: Personal communication, 1987.

Menard, S. W., & Wabschall, J. M.: Evaluation of the clinical nurse specialist. *In* Menard, S. W. (ed): The Clinical Nurse Specialist Perspectives on Practice. New York, John Wiley & Sons, 1987.

Paulen, A.: Practice issues for the oncology clinical nurse specialist. Oncol Nurs Forum 2:37–39, 1985.

Platt-Koch, L. M.: Clinical supervision for psychiatric nurses. J Psychosocial Nurs 26(1):7–15, 1986.

Propotnik, T.: Personal communication, 1987.

Reiter, F.: The nurse-clinician. Am J Nurs 66:274–280, 1966.

Robichaud, A. M., & Hamric, A. B.: Time documentation of clinical nurse specialists' activities. J Nurs Admin 16(1):31–36, 1986.

Sisson, R.: Co-worker's perceptions of the clinical nurse specialist role. Clinical Nurse Specialist 1(1):13–17, 1987.

Schilke-Davis, D., Greig, A. E., Burkholder, J., and Keating, T.: Evaluating advance practice nurses. Nurs Management 15(3):44–47, 1984.

Spross, J., & Hamric, A. B.: A model for future clinical specialist practice. *In* Hamric, A., and Spross, J. (eds): The Clinical Nurse Specialist in Theory and Practice. New York, Grune and Stratton, 1983.

Tarsitano, B. J., Brophy, E. B., and Snyder, D. J.: A demystification of the clinical nurse specialist role: Perceptions of clinical nurse specialists and nurse administrators. J Nurs Educ 25(1):4–9, 1986.

Welch-McCaffrey, D.: CNS evaluation methods. A presentation for Collaboration for Clinical Excellence in a Cost-Conscious Environment. San Francisco, UCSF CNS Conference, 1985.

Welch-McCaffrey, D.: Role performance issues for oncology clinical nurse specialists. Cancer Nurs 9(6):287–294, 1986.

Wells, D. L.: Gerontological nurse specialists: Tomorrow's leaders today. J Gerontol Nurs 11(5):36–40, 1985.

Woodrow, M., & Bell, J. A.: Clinical specialization: Conflict between reality and theory. J Nurs Admin 6:23–28, 1971.

# The CNS as Consultant

*Anne-Marie Barron*

## INTRODUCTION

Consultation is an important aspect of the clinical nurse specialist (CNS) role. Tarsitano, Brophy, and Snyder (1986) studied perceptions of nurse administrators and clinical nurse specialists regarding components of the CNS role. Both groups perceived being a consultant to the nursing staff as the most valued function of the role. Fenton (1985) studied areas of competencies demonstrated by CNSs. She added "the consulting role" as a new area of skilled performance demonstrated by CNSs to the seven areas of skilled performance outlined by Benner (1984). O'Connor and Malone (1983) discussed the consultation model for the CNS staff at the University of Cincinnati. They described the organizational emphasis on the consultative role as opening new opportunities for financial support, measurement of results, and accountability. In the current economic climate, these findings are particularly meaningful.

CNSs in psychiatric liaison positions have had considerable experience with consultation. Consultation-liaison nursing (liaison nursing, for short) is described in the literature (Hitchens, 1973; Lipowski, 1974, 1981, 1983; Robinson, 1974; Nelson & Schilke, 1976; Lehman, 1979; Lewis & Levy, 1982; Barron, 1983; Simmons, 1985). In this chapter, liaison nursing is often the frame of reference for practice. It is hoped that the description of the process and issues related to consultation will be relevant to the consultative component of CNS practices regardless of specialty.

The degree of importance placed on the consultative component of CNS practices depends upon many factors. It is related to the needs of the staff and patients with whom the CNS is working; the expertise of the staff; the philosophy, goals, and priorities of nursing administration; and the goals and priorities that the CNS has established. The emphasis placed on the consultative subrole may fluctuate over time, but nursing consultation will remain an essential and valued activity for most CNSs. This chapter will discuss practical implementation of the consultative role. The author draws from the literature, from her experiences as a psychiatric liaison nurse, and from the experiences of CNS colleagues.*

## DEFINING CONSULTATION

Caplan (1970) defined consultation as a process of communication between professionals which can be systematically taught, applied, and analyzed. While the content of consultation varies widely depending upon the specialized knowledge of the consultant, the process and techniques of consultation are similar regardless of the consultant's specialty area.

Caplan's description of the consultation process is summarized in the following paragraphs. During consultation, communication occurs between the consultant, who is a specialist, and the consultee. The consultee identifies a work-related problem, recognizes that a consultant may have useful, specialized expertise to apply to the problem, and initiates the consultation. Very commonly in nursing and in mental health (which was Caplan's area of specialization), the problems relate to the care and treatment of patients. The consultant may offer education, clarification, diagnostic formulation, and additional problem-solving strategies. The professional responsibility for the patient remains with the consultee. The consultee is free to accept or reject the recommendations of the consultant. The consultant is not administratively responsible for the consultee, and a collaborative relationship rather than a supervisory relationship is maintained. (The unusual situation in which the consultant assumes responsibility for the patient as clinical expert, because care is being seriously compromised, is discussed in detail later in the chapter.)

The dual goals of consultation are to improve the consultee's skill in handling a work-related problem and to enhance the consultee's ability to master future problems of a similar type. The consultant responds to specific, circumscribed issues raised in the consultation and does not seek to remedy other problems of the consultee's practice. The privacy of the consultee is respected in relation to the exploration

*The author wishes to acknowledge her appreciation to three CNS colleagues—Virginia Kilpack, R.N., Ph.D., Judith A. Spross, R.N., M.S., C.S., and Harlene Caroline, R.N., M.S.—for their open reflection and examination of their work as consultants and for their candid, enthusiastic sharing of those experiences as contributions to this chapter.

of personal feelings and problems, which are discussed only to the extent that they are overtly displaced onto, or are interfering with, the consultation situation. While the consultation may have the effect of enhancing the consultee's sense of self-esteem, through the successful mastery of a problem, the focus remains on the current work-related difficulty rather than on the consultee's sense of well-being.

Caplan described four types of consultation. Client-centered case consultation has as its primary goal assisting the consultee to develop an effective plan so that the patient can receive the best care. The consultee seeks the specialized expertise of the consultant for assistance with patients who have particularly difficult or complex problems. In consultee-centered case consultation, improving patient care is also a concern, but the focus is directly on the consultee's problem in handling the current situation, and the goal is to assist the consultee to overcome the deficits. The problem may be related to lack of knowledge, skill, confidence, or professional objectivity. In program-centered administrative consultation, the focus is on planning and administration. Consultee-centered administrative consultation considers the consultee's (or group of consultees') problems or difficulties as they interfere with the objectives of the organization. This chapter will focus on client-centered case consultation.

Lipowski (1983) developed a comprehensive model of psychiatric consultation which incorporates both client- and consultee-centered situations. In this model, consultation encompasses an evaluation of the referred patient, the patient's interaction with staff, and the specific needs of the consultee. The patient's family and social supports are also considered. The consultant carefully discusses the patient with the consultee and clinical team, providing regular follow-up for the duration of the patient's hospitalization. Although the model was developed for psychiatric specialists, it can be useful to any clinical consultant. CNS consultants often engage in this type of comprehensive consultation, considering the needs and interactions of both patient and staff.

## The Process of Consultation

The process of consultation is conceptualized by the author in terms of the nursing process—that is, in terms of the four steps of assessment and diagnosis, planning of care, implementation, and evaluation. This schema relates to the steps of consultation outlined by Caplan: (1) assessment of the consultation problem following the consultation request, (2) the consultation report, (3) implementation of the consultant's recommendations, and (4) follow-up. Conceptualizing and describing the process in terms of a model that is familiar to the nursing staff may make the process more easily communicated and understood.

Most commonly, staff nurses request consultation because they have identified problems with patients or families and would like assistance with them. The consultant and consultee together consider the experiences of the patient and the staff in relation to the problem, thereby often merging the categories of client-centered case consultation and consultee-centered case consultation.

## Assessment

This initial phase of consultation involves clarifying with the consultee the specific nature of the problem and the major variables contributing to it. Questions to be answered initially are: What is the specific problem? Why is it now a problem? What is the patient or family experiencing? How are the consultee and other members of the staff affected by the problem?

Initially, the consultee and consultant together consider the nursing assessment thus far completed and try to come to an understanding of the patient's experience. If, after discussing it, they recognize that their assessment is incomplete, they jointly decide on a plan to complete the assessment. If consultees are not confident of their skills in the area of nursing assessment, the consultant can assess the patient directly. It is often ideal to see the patient together with the consultee; this can offer an opportunity for teaching and role modeling for the consultant and a sense of continuity in nursing care for the patient. However, if the problem seems to represent significant staff-patient conflict, the consultant and consultee may decide that the consultant should see the patient alone so that the patient may talk openly about what the patient perceives to be the problem. In addition, time demands on staff nurse consultees may make a joint interviewing and assessing of the patient impractical.

## Planning the Intervention

Once the consultee and consultant complete the assessment and clearly formulate the problem, they decide on the best approach for planning interventions. At this point, a nursing conference may be organized to increase the staff's understanding of the problem, to provide a forum for collective problem-solving, and to elicit support for the plan from the team.

In general, it is helpful if the consultant avoids prescribing the best approach to consultees but rather assists them in applying the problem-solving process. The consultant may also enhance consultees' understanding of the situation by informally teaching principles of the specialty as they relate to the problem at hand.

In addition to considering the needs of the patient, it is also important to consider the needs of the consultee and staff. Planning for the staff's needs is an essential aspect of the consultation. Ideally, at the end of the planning phase of the consultation, the consultee, other staff members (if involved), and the consultant will have outlined a practical, workable, mutually agreed upon plan with clear objectives and realistic long- and short-term goals; will have specified who is responsible for carrying out the intervention; and will have established a plan for evaluating or modifying the nursing interventions.

## The Intervention

The overall responsibility for carrying out the nursing intervention formulated during consultation remains with the consultee. If the consultant is to be involved directly in the intervention, that responsibility and role should be carefully negotiated and articulated. If, for example, the CNS consultant assumed responsibility for evaluating a given patient's mental status because the staff viewed the situation as particularly complex, the consultant should be clear with the staff about assuming accountability for that assessment. The consultant should document the completed assessment, share this with staff, and help them plan care accordingly. On the other hand, the staff may only need assistance from the consultant with formulating intervention strategies that they would then carry out directly.

## Evaluation and Closure

When the intervention is planned, a method for evaluating its effectiveness should be developed. Outlining in advance specific strategies for measuring whether or not the objectives of care have been attained helps to ensure that these objectives will be realistic. During the planning phase, the consultant and consultee decide what will represent measures of successful intervention. They then set aside a time after the intervention for consideration of those measures. If the objectives of the intervention are not met, the evaluation phase offers the consultant and consultee the opportunity to consider what happened and to modify the intervention plans accordingly.

When the consultation comes to an end, closure of the process should be acknowledged. Such open acknowledgment gives the consultee and consultant the chance to review both the consultation and the relationship that developed during the process. Flynn (1972) eloquently discussed the importance of the relationship between consultant and consultee. Very often consultation occurs because of difficult, complex situations; valued relationships based on trust develop as the consultation process evolves. Recognizing and appreciating that dimension of the consultation process is important. As the consultant and consultee bring the consultation to a close, they may wish to consider possibilities for future consultations.

## DEVELOPING THE ROLE OF CONSULTANT

### Knowledge and Skills Needed

The discussion of knowledge and skills which follows reflects issues and concerns that surfaced within the practices of the author and her colleagues. It is interesting to note that several of these were identified by Fenton as predictors of success for the CNS role (1985).

CNS consultants draw from many theoretical frameworks. While a complete discussion of theoretical considerations relevant to nursing consultation is beyond the scope and purpose of this chapter, knowledge of the following areas is particularly useful: the consultation process, systems theory, communications, change theory, nursing process, problem-solving, conflict resolution, adult learning theory, and group process.

In addition to theoretical understanding, there are cognitive and interpersonal skills important to the development of the CNS consultant role. The following discussion considers some of those skills and qualities.

The CNS consultant must possess high degrees of self-awareness and interpersonal skill. The personal and interpersonal requirements for self-examination within the consultative role are notable. The interpersonal nature of consultative work requires a basic understanding of personal issues and motives and an ability to recognize how one behaves with and is perceived by others. The consultant must also be able to develop positive working relationships and alliances and be able to negotiate the CNS consulting role with nurses and other health care professionals.

Effective time management and the ability to establish priorities are essential. Also the CNS must have the ability to be flexible and tolerate "lack of control." The timing of referrals, the nature of requests, and the needs of staff and patients are variables that, at times, are beyond the consultant's control. There are times when the consultant must move into several situations quickly to assess needs, establish priorities, and plan consultations. Emergency situations may occur which require immediate consultation and re-establishing of priorities (for example, the assessment of a suicidal patient).

Consultants must be able to assess and accept the varying levels of needs and abilities of consultees and plan interventions accordingly and with flexibility. The level of sophistication and clinical expertise of staff can vary widely among different members of an individual unit, or between units, and can greatly influence the quantity and quality of referrals.

Accepting the right of the consultee to act or not act on recommendations is part of the consultation contract. The final decision about implementing consultation recommendations is the consultee's. Except in the unusual situation in which the consultant assumes direct responsibility for the patient as the clinical expert [because to do otherwise would seriously compromise patient care (this issue is discussed in more detail later in the chapter)], the responsibility for care of the patient remains with the consultee. Consideration of factors affecting a decision to disregard the consultant's suggestions becomes part of the overall evaluation of the consultation, but accepting the decision-making power of the consultee is essential.

Fenton identified emotional support of the nursing staff as a primary activity of CNSs. Being able to listen, empathize, and communicate warmth, respect, acceptance, and concern are crucial skills for the consultant. Feelings of anxiety, vulnerability, or inadequacy may precede the consultation request. Among staff, there is a recognition of a problem and a need for help; among patients and families, there are often emotional and/or situational crises to be addressed. If the staff do not feel comfortable with and trust the CNS consultant, they may not request consultation at all. Or, if they do, they may remain detached from or superficial with the consultant. However, if they believe the consultant is genuinely concerned about them and is accepting and nonjudgmental, a deeper examination of the problem with its implications and interventions is possible.

Consultants alone know the scope and limitations of their practices. When consultees make requests, they have no way of knowing the consultant's other commitments and availability. During periods of high demand, the consultant must be able to say no, decline involvement, and refer the consultee elsewhere. There are situations when it is most appropriate for the consultant to decline involvement because the consultee's problem would be more effectively addressed by another professional.

Consulting can be a lonely trade. Consultants often work alone, creating and assuming responsibility for their practices. Day-to-day decisions, priority-setting, problem-solving, and evaluations are accomplished independently. It is essential that consultants establish systems for supervision and support (see Chapters 13 and 14), and it is also essential that they feel comfortable with a significant degree of autonomy.

## Organizational Assessment

Whenever a CNS consultant enters a system, whether as an outside consultant, as a new employee, or as a consultant to a unit in the hospital where the CNS is also practicing, it is important that the variables that actively affect or drive the system be considered. Roy and Martinez (1983) outlined a systems framework for CNSs to use to analyze group behavior (see Figure 2–3). The CNS position in itself is a system operating within larger systems.

Table 6–1 outlines questions stimulated by the Roy and Martinez systems framework, which may be considered by CNS consultants as they view the units to which they are available. Answers to these questions may help the CNS to understand the needs and pressures on those who are expected to seek clinical consultation. And that understanding may help the CNS to develop the consulting role based on an understanding of the unit's strengths, weaknesses, and practical realities.

# IMPLEMENTATION

## Establishing Relationships and Negotiating Roles

Consultation occurs within the context of relationships. The CNS consultant's role interfaces and, at times, overlaps with the roles of other professionals. Establishing positive working relationships, devel-

**TABLE 6–1.  Considering the Unit as a System**

- What does each staff member bring to the unit in terms of experience, motivation, and individual need?
- What are the goals of the group, and how are they accomplished?
- What is the physical set up of the unit, and how adequate are finances, staffing, supplies, and other resources?
- What are the political, economic, and legal realities that influence the unit?
- How does the unit relate to other units and departments within the institution?
- What are the roles, leadership styles, and management philosophies of the nursing leaders on the unit?
- How does group process occur? How does the group communicate, make decisions, manage conflict, develop relationships? Is the group cohesive?
- What has the consultant's experience been with the staff in the past?

oping alliances, and negotiating professional roles so that needs of staff and patients are best served are critical to the implementation of the CNS consulting role.

As CNSs begin to establish the role of consultant, it is important that they meet with key people in the setting to articulate the role and elicit their expectations, goals, and support. In the hospital setting, key people would include the CNS's nursing administrator; physicians within the CNS's specialty area; head nurses, nursing supervisors, and medical directors on units for which the CNS has consultant responsibilities; social workers, other health care providers, and other CNSs. The CNS should meet with staff, defining and describing the role and inviting them to share their expectations and goals for consultation services. Two possible causes of failure of the liaison process are the unrealistic expectations of staff or a distorted view of the purpose of consultation by staff (Lewis & Levy, 1982; Lehmann, 1979). The importance of clearly defining the role to staff and eliciting their expectations cannot be overemphasized.

As the role becomes established, it is important to stay in touch with key people and staff, regularly inviting feedback on their perceptions of the role. This may be done as part of a formal evaluation, and it may also be done less formally in directed discussions. Needs and expectations of consultees change over time. If CNS consultants openly and periodically solicit feedback, they can incorporate current needs and views into their practices, correct distortions and unrealistic expectations, and maintain support for the role. The CNS's role may change in ways that affect the consultative role; such changes should be communicated to consultees.

## The CNS and Administrator Alliance

As with other aspects of the CNS position, it is crucial to be assured of administrative support for one's activities as a consultant (see Chapters 12 and 13). Consultation is an intricate, time- and energy-consuming endeavor. The CNS and nursing administrator must agree that consultation is a valued function for the CNS. One way to assure agreement on goals for CNS practice is for the CNS and administrator to establish goals and priorities for the position. If three-month, six-month, and annual goals are mutually developed, potential areas of conflict can be identified and resolved early in the process, and the CNS can pursue the goals with confidence. If evaluative criteria are developed with the goals, ongoing evaluation can become part of the supervisory and goal-setting process. The nursing administrator's support for consultation can also facilitate the establishment of other important alliances.

## The CNS and Staff Nurse Alliance

The CNS/staff nurse relationship is central to effective CNS consultation. For the new CNS, it is likely that a fair amount of time will be invested in establishing trusting relationships. Anticipating possible negative responses to the consultant role enables the CNS to avoid behaviors that would discourage staff from making referrals. Both CNS behaviors and staff responses that might impair this important alliance are discussed before effective strategies are described.

Initially, it is important that the consultant recognize the potential for being a threat to staff. There are many possible reasons why staff may feel threatened. They may feel intimidated by the educational preparation or the specialty area of the consultant. They may envy the autonomy and independence of the consultant's position. They may feel that the presence of a consultant somehow implies an inadequacy in the performance of their roles. There may be fear that the consultant will take over valued aspects of their work with patients or families. The consultant may be viewed suspiciously as an extension of administration. Somewhat ironically, the consultant can give rise to feelings of anxiety, uncertainty, and inadequacy among staff at precisely the time the consultant is feeling most anxious, uncertain, and self-doubting. It can be very tempting, as a new consultant, to rush in and take over as a "rescuer" in an attempt to prove oneself. Such an approach, however, can validate the fears of the staff that they are somehow inadequate to cope with the situation, and that the consultant will take over their roles with patients and families. It can also serve to foster dependence of staff upon the consultant. Such dependence can feed the ego of the self-doubting new consultant. In the long run, however, the dependency of staff can be counterproductive to the goals of enhancing staff skill and confidence. Direct intervention with selected patients and families is an important part of most CNS consultations. Actively involving the staff in every aspect of the consultation process can both clarify the consultation process and help to avoid dependency of staff upon the CNS.

Perhaps the most important way to minimize threats associated with the role is to allow the staff to get to know the consultant as a human being rather than as an expert. Being visible and available by participating in unit activities such as nursing rounds and reports on patient care, participating in educational conferences, and having lunch or coffee with the staff can be effective ways to facilitate the staff and consultant getting to know one another. The more opportunities that staff and consultant have to get to know each other (both in consultation situations and nonconsultation encounters) the more likely trust and confidence will replace fear and intimidation.

As the CNS is called to consult in a situation, it is important to avoid a "grand entrance." Very often the staff is dealing with simultaneous demands and limited time. By recognizing the constraints influencing staff and arranging with them a mutually convenient, realistic time to discuss a situation, the consultant is communicating respect for staff as well as the collaborative nature of their relationship. For the busy consultant, it can be difficult to take the extra time to recognize and take into account constraints influencing staff. Such an approach, however, is likely to foster and maintain positive relationships and to be met with openness and willingness to work on the consultation problem.

It is also important for the consultant to avoid criticizing staff. There are times when constructive feedback is necessary, but the consultant wants to take care to avoid creating or enhancing feelings of inadequacy or incompetency in the staff. The consultant can openly acknowledge that recognition of the problem indicates an important strength, can underscore the difficult and/or uncommon nature of the problem, and can give credit for the care and problem-solving thus far accomplished. When the consultant recognizes certain behaviors among staff which are adversely affecting the consultation problem, feedback can be offered. Constructive feedback is effective when it focuses on specific, current behavior that can be changed, describes rather than judges behavior, and offers an exploration of alternatives. Feedback offered within the context of a trusting relationship and clearly focused on the behavior rather than on the individual is most helpful.

Determining the needs of staff in relation to the consultation problem, then formulating interventions with them which address their own needs as well as the patient's, are important ways to promote and maintain supportive relationships with staff. Underscoring the importance of Fenton's description of emotional support of the nursing staff as a primary activity of CNSs, one CNS colleague states: "I find out very early on how the staff spells 'S-U-P-P-O-R-T' and then include that as a priority in my interventions." Another colleague stated: "If as the CNS consultant I can support the staff, I believe the staff can then better support the patient." Staff needs can vary widely and may include assisting with difficult patient situations, addressing specific educational needs, offering support groups for the staff, and assisting with more routine nursing care functions. Admittedly, the list of possible needs is incomplete. The process of determining and responding to staff needs can be very useful in developing and maintaining relationships with staff and in actually applying the consultation process.

## The CNS and Physician Alliance

The involvement of CNS consultants in complex care situations mandates that they assertively develop relationships with physicians in their specialty areas as well as with physicians in areas in which they consult. If the highest quality of interdisciplinary care is to be available to patients, CNSs must make their contributions and potential contributions apparent to physician members of the team by actively seeking them out, discussing problems, and sharing their expertise. Strategies for making referrals and requesting consultation between the CNS and physicians should be developed very early in the consultant's practice (see Chapter 16).

## Negotiating Roles With Other Professionals

The ability to negotiate professional roles with other nurse consultants, physicians, and other health care professionals is essential. In the author's experience, initial resistance to the role of liaison nurse was largely the result of "territorial threats."

It is helpful to spend time addressing the purposes and parameters of the consultant's position with professionals whose positions logically interface or overlap with the consultant's. Carefully listening to concerns about the position in terms of the other professionals' positions, while keeping the focus of the CNS consultant's work clearly on the process of assisting the nursing staff in providing nursing care, can also help to clarify role function and prevent ambiguities.

When roles overlap, it is important for there to be open discussion and negotiation between professionals, with an emphasis on mutually deciding how the given responsibilities are to be shared, divided, and assumed. Often, on the surface of a situation, it appears that responsibilities and skills overlap, while more in-depth consideration reveals a complement and synergy of skills between the professionals. For example, a social worker may complete a mental status examination on a patient, while the CNS consultant assists the nursing staff in incorporating the implications of the findings of that examination into the plan of care for the patient. An enterostomal nurse therapist may do the postoperative colostomy care for a patient, while the medical-surgical CNS consultant assists the staff in directing their nursing care toward the physiological and emotional changes in the patient's life which result from the body-altering surgery.

Very often through open negotiation and sharing of responsibilities, collegial, comfortable, and trusting relationships are developed. Once trust and comfort are established, roles and responsibilities can be negotiated based on the actual situation at hand rather than on defense of professional "territory." If, after considerable effort and dialogue, resistance to the CNS consulting role persists, CNSs may want to elicit administrative support to help clarify and problem-solve in relation to the impasse. Having discussed and solicited support for the CNS consulting role with clinical departmental leaders early in the position, the CNS may also have that base of support to draw from if role negotiation becomes problematic.

## Establishing Credibility

An important way to establish credibility as a consultant is to establish effective, mutual relationships with consultees and, within that context, to offer practical, theoretically sound, successful problem-solving strategies and clinical expertise. In some situations, the consultant may wait to be invited into situations in order to demonstrate skills and develop relationships. There are other approaches that CNSs may want to consider, apart from the actual consultation situation, which allow staff to recognize their abilities and get to know them.

Offering timely, practical continuing education programs is a helpful, familiar, nonthreatening way for the CNS to be available to staff. The potential consultant would have a forum from which to be visible, and the staff could appraise the abilities and personality of the CNS from a distance. Some CNSs have found attending change of shift reports or patient care rounds helps them identify potential consultation opportunities. After identifying potential opportunities, the CNS can approach caregivers and offer consultation. Another approach is to work several shifts during which the CNS has a patient assignment similar in workload to that of the staff nurses. Working alongside other nurses, CNSs can demonstrate their competence, get to know and be known by the staff, and gain an understanding of the staff's actual working situation. One colleague found that her offer to work for a staff nurse on a Friday evening shift quickly enhanced her credibility with and acceptance by the staff. The author and other colleagues found that working as staff nurses with patients in particularly difficult or problematic situations gave them initial opportunities to prove their skills as nurses and demonstrate their value as helpful resources.

In the consultation situation, there are strategies that CNSs can employ to create opportunities for enhancing credibility. Lewis and Levy (1982) discussed the importance of initially investing time on units that are most receptive, with the hope of being able to develop a reputation for being helpful. Developing a reputation for being helpful on one unit can serve as an important catalyst to role development and involvement on other units. Prouty called this strategy "creating organizational jealousy" (1983).

One need not have all the answers in order to establish credibility as a consultant. Putting pressure on oneself to have all the answers and then to come across as the all-knowing consultant is counterproductive to promoting consultation and is intimidating to consultees. In fact, consultants are often called into situations for which there are no answers. The goal of consultation may be to assist staff to tolerate a situation in which effective intervention or resolution is not possible (Lewis & Levy, 1982).

In the author's experience and in the experiences of those colleagues interviewed, certain pivotal situations were cited as providing opportunities for CNSs to establish credibility and value as helpful resources. These opportunities seemed to depend in some measure upon luck and good timing as well as the ability of the CNS to identify and create opportunities for establishing credibility. The consultant can be open to such experiences by responding to each request with careful consideration. In retrospect, the consultants did not perceive, at the outset of the consultation, the importance of the situations presented to them. For reasons more complex than initially apparent, ordinary interventions and perspectives of the consultant were perceived as extraordinarily helpful by the staff.

> In the author's practice, such an opportunity presented itself when she was consulted by the Intensive Care Unit (I.C.U.) staff. The staff were caring for a young man who was dying from the toxic effects of an intentional drug overdose. It was a tragic situation. The young man did not present himself for treatment while the effects of the overdose were treatable. When he presented, he was no longer suicidal, but unfortunately, the hepatotoxic effects of the overdose would prove to be lethal several days later. The staff was concerned about psychologically supporting both the patient and the family and requested that the consultant intervene directly. The patient became delirious and then comatose fairly soon after admission to the I.C.U., and the main focus of the consultation became support of the family. Understandably, the family was feeling guilty and stricken with grief. They discussed their feelings with the consultant and with each other and were able to describe some of their own needs in the situation and support one another. They understood the availability of ongoing psychiatric services in their home town and planned to contact their local mental health center. Given the enormous tragedy of the situation, the family actually seemed to be doing as well as could be expected. As the patient's death became imminent, the consultant told the staff that she would extend her availability and come into the hospital during the evening

or night should they feel the family needed additional support. Late in the evening, the staff telephoned the consultant at home stating that the patient was very near to death and that they were concerned about how the family would react at the actual time of his death. The consultant went into the hospital and stayed with the patient and family for several hours. The young man died quietly and peacefully. The family said good-bye to the patient, expressed their appreciation to the staff and the consultant, and left the hospital. The staff expressed much appreciation to the consultant and described her presence late at night, at the time of the patient's death, as being extraordinarily helpful and supportive to them. In the consultant's view, that presence was neither a sophisticated nor an extraordinary intervention, and yet it seemed to represent a turning point in the relationship with the I.C.U. staff. The staff felt supported by that seemingly simple intervention in a meaningful way, which then led to a greater depth in their relationship with the consultant.

Being available to the staff on evenings, weekends, and holidays can be a helpful way to communicate a concern and interest that goes beyond "nine-to-five." The author and the CNSs interviewed found the staff impressed by and receptive to the consultant's availability and the consultant's shared sense of 24-hour responsibility and accountability.

In general, the more visible and available consultants are, the more staff will come to know and utilize them. A cautionary note must be sounded, however, in terms of overextending and managing one's practice. Availability must be balanced with a reasonable workload. In certain situations, there is much to be gained by being extra available, but consultants must use that extra availability judiciously in order to preserve their energy, enthusiasm, and ongoing availability over time. Clearly defining the scope and availability of the consultant's services and establishing a back-up referral system for addressing problems when the consultant is not available are important. Other CNSs, regardless of specialty, can be helpful in terms of applying the problem-solving process to nursing problems. One colleague described a CNS on-call system in which all of the CNSs in the institution shared on-call responsibilities. The staff could always reach a CNS (the specialty area of the CNS would vary) to discuss nursing problems. Physicians within the consultant's specialty can also be helpful resources to staff for assisting with clinical problems and emergencies. Consultants cannot and need not always be available in order be establish and maintain credibility. Identifying other resources can assure staff that problems can be addressed in the consultant's absence.

## Strategies for Promoting Consultation

The first step in promoting consultation involves educating staff about consultative services available to them. The author participated as a speaker in the staff nurse orientation program, explaining the purpose and process of nursing consultation, identifying the CNS consultants available to them, and outlining the procedure of initiating a nursing consultation. She and her CNS colleagues also developed a nursing policy statement regarding consultation. The statement included a definition of nursing consultation and briefly outlined some of the principles and implications inherent in the consultation process. Each nursing unit had a copy of the statement in the Nursing Policy Manual. Other colleagues have developed and distributed brochures that describe the available consultation services and include pictures of the CNS consultants and specific instructions for contacting them.

CNSs may receive requests for consultation in a number of ways. Informally, consultants may simply be approached while on the unit or in the hallway or cafeteria. More formally, they may be contacted through the nursing administration office or hospital paging system. Or, the consultants may have regularly scheduled rounds or predetermined contact times with individual units when they are available to discuss referrals.

## Documenting Consultation

Formal referral forms are used by some consultants. Putting the request in writing encourages consultees to think through and clearly define problems. The forms themselves can be helpful tools for documentation and record-keeping. Forms can ask for concise information such as patient name, date, location, and diagnosis and provide space for the request and consultation report to be recorded. With three-copy forms, the original copy can be included in the patient's record, a copy can be kept for the CNS's records, and the third, if appropriate, could be forwarded to the CNS's nursing administrator. Whether using standardized referral forms or not, CNSs must decide with administrators and consultees how and where documentation of consultations will occur. Documentation in the patient record should be consistent with the institution's policies on nursing documentation. When progress notes are not integrated, the CNS should document on the spcecific form or in the nursing notes. To call the attention of other providers to the consultation report, a brief note in the medical progress notes can be made by the consultant. For the CNS to put the consultation report and follow-up notes in the medical progress notes communicates a social/organizational message to staff that may discourage nursing consultation. Where an integrated progress record is used, this should not be a problem.

## Recognizing the Need to Step Out of the Consultant Role

CNS consultants must be prepared for the unusual situation when they must step out of the role of consultant and, as clinical experts, assume direct responsibility for patients. When the consultant recognizes that patient care is being seriously compromised, and the nursing staff is not able to provide the care necessary in the situation, the consultant must then assume clinical responsibility for the patient (Barron, 1983). Fortunately, in the vast majority of clinical situations, once staff recognize a problem, they are quite willing and able to work with the consultant to remedy it. However, compromised patient care may require that the consultant assume clinical responsibility as the specialist. An example from the author's practice follows.

> A psychiatric liaison nurse was consulted by the nursing staff in the coronary care unit because they were concerned about unusual behavior being displayed by a patient who had had a serious myocardial infarction two days previously. The consultant assessed the patient as delirious. Concerned about the potentially dangerous implications of delirium in this patient, she stepped aside from her consultant role and assumed responsibility for going directly to the patient's intern to stress the importance of evaluating the cause of the delirium. She explained what she was doing, and why, to the staff nurses who had consulted her. The intern minimized the significance of the patient's delirium, stating that he was convinced that the patient's confusion was a psychological consequence of adjusting to the seriousness of his medical situation. Disagreeing with the intern's assessment, the CNS went to the resident and met with the same erroneous conclusion. Explaining that she disagreed with them and that, in fact, she believed that if the cause of the delirium was not evaluated the patient's safety could be compromised, she told them she would discuss the situation with the staff psychiatrist on the psychiatric consultation service and that she would request that he contact the patient's staff physician directly. The CNS initiated a formal psychiatric consultation; the psychiatrist supported the liaison nurse's assessment, and an investigation into the possible cause of delirium ensued. It was determined that the likely cause was the patient's digitalis level, which was found to be higher than the usual therapeutic range. Clearly, a potentially dangerous and correctable condition had been identified.

## Ongoing Development of the Role

With time and positive experience in the role, the consultant ideally has more highly refined knowledge and skills to offer, enjoys the staff's ability to successfully resolve problems for which they once sought consultation, and when consulted, is profoundly stimulated by the sophisticated nature of the request received! Indeed, some nursing consultants find that the number of requests for consultation dwindles over time because staff consultees have utilized the consultant's services so effectively. And many find that over time the nature of requests changes, reflecting higher levels of understanding and development among the consultees. For consultants who "work themselves out of positions," it is important that they recognize the phenomenon that is occurring and identify with consultees new areas to be developed for consultation, such as nursing ethics, nursing research, or other areas of more advanced nursing practice.

Unfortunately, there are influences that frequently interfere with this ideal progression. High turnover among staff, staff shortage, and organizational change are examples of factors that can negatively influence the ongoing development of both consultant and staff practices. Such factors can contribute to a working climate that maintains the status quo (or even fosters regression) among staff members rather than one that supports and stimulates the staff in their growth. In such situations, CNSs must recognize the negative factors, work toward correcting them when possible, and deal with the frustration that can be related to lack of growth or progress.

Workload may change in either direction over time. With wider recognition of skills and knowledge, consultants may find that they are increasingly consulted. Particularly with recognition of clinical expertise, CNS consultants may find that they are consulted more and more frequently to provide direct care to patients and families. Increasing numbers of consultation requests can be reinforcing and flattering to CNSs, but an ever increasing spiral of work can contribute to frustration and burn out. CNSs may find that they must renegotiate their roles or present data to their nursing administrators that more CNS consultant time is necessary in order to realistically meet the demands for their services.

Experienced CNSs must continually monitor their practices making certain that workloads are balanced, that current consultee needs are assessed and addressed, and that they are being stimulated to create exciting and effective practices.

## SUPPORT, REVIEW AND EVALUATION

### Peer Support

CNS consultants often work independently. Peers, defined as other professionals having equivalent academic preparation and engaged in similar work (Lewis & Levy, 1982), can have much to offer in the areas of examining clinical practice, problem-solving, professional development, and support. Simmons (1985) and Lewis and Levy (1982) emphasize the importance for liaison nurses to establish support systems of peers with whom to share experiences and problems, identify aspects of similarity, identify areas of clinical research, and gain support. The purposes of a peer group are: (1) to provide a safe and supportive environment to discuss feelings related to the professional role; (2) to provide a confidential opportunity to explore, understand, and receive feedback on clinical issues; (3) to identify researchable areas of practice; and (4) to promote professional identity, development, and collegiality (Lewis & Levy, 1982). Peer support groups can be helpful for CNS consultants regardless of clinical specialty (see Chapter 14).

## Supervision

Lewis and Levy (1982) define psychiatric clinical supervision and describe formal and informal methods of supervision. Supervision as used in this context does not refer to administrative supervision. Clinical supervision is a supportive, stimulating, educational process whereby various clinical practice issues are presented to a more experienced and expert clinician. The goals of supervision are enhancing knowledge, increasing clinical skill, and developing professional autonomy and self-esteem. In formal psychiatric supervision, a contractual relationship is established, and the less experienced clinician regularly presents clinical work to the more experienced clinician, who may assume clinical accountability for the work. In informal supervision, an experienced practitioner is considered a resource, a formal contract is not negotiated, and the supervisee determines the need for consultation. Nursing peer groups, workshops, patient care rounds, and case conferences are also sources of informal supervision. While supervision is discussed by Lewis and Levy within the context of psychiatric practice, the models (particularly informal supervision), methods, and goals of supervision can have relevance for all CNS consultants. Consultants may use these concepts to promote their own growth and development as well as that of the staff with whom they work. This concept of supervision may be used regardless of a CNS's organizational placement.

## Evaluation

Evaluation is the final step of the consultation process, as it is the final step of the nursing process. The consultant and consultee consider several questions together. Were the goals of the consultation met? If not, why not? Were any revisions necessary in the plan of care? Were the recommendations of the consultant carried out? If not, why not? Was the consultant helpful? Was the consultant-consultee relationship strengthened? More case-specific questions may be appropriately considered by the consultant and consultee during the evaluation. The process of evaluating the overall effectiveness and helpfulness of the consultation and bringing the process to closure is the important final phase of each consultation.

In addition to evaluating individual consultations, CNSs evaluate the effectiveness of the role or consultant subrole. In these rigorous economic times, evaluation of all aspects of the CNS role is essential for the role to survive (Hamric, 1983). As CNSs consider their work as consultants, they may want to incorporate feedback from three sources: themselves, nursing administrators, and staff with whom they consult. Girouard and Spross (1983) and Hamric, Gresham, and Eccard (1978) cite the importance of nursing leaders seeking feedback from the staff with whom they work and describe the tools they designed to elicit and document staff evaluation. The evaluative criteria they developed were based on job descriptions, role models described in the nursing literature, and the CNSs' ideas about what the role ought to be. The feedback from staff offered important information, and the process of involving the staff was viewed as positive for both CNS and staff. CNSs who are not unit-based (as most consultants are not) may wish to involve units where they are particularly active in the evaluation process. This method of evaluation is described in Hamric, Gresham, and Eccard (1978).

Lewis and Levy suggest that liaison nurse consultants be evaluated in the areas of the actual consultations, interpersonal skills, leadership and professionalism, teaching skills, and academic advancements. Nursing administrators can assist with the implementation and analysis of staff feedback and can also evaluate the CNS in relation to other criteria such as those described by Lewis and Levy (1982), those specified in the job description, and the annual goals for the CNS position.

The records that consultants keep can also yield important evaluative data. Lewis and Levy (1982) suggest several questions to consider as consultants examine their practices over time. Is the consultant recontacted by staff after initial consultations? Are units that were initially reluctant to utilize consultation services becoming more open? Are consultation requests becoming more sophisticated over time? In addition, the author considered the following questions as she periodically examined the records of her consultation activities. Was the consultant able to respond to all requests? Is there evidence that glaring needs or issues are going unrecognized and unmet? Are there patterns developing in terms of theme and location of the consultations? Answers to these questions can also help to identify needs for educational programs for the staff.

Finally, consideration of the subjective experiences of the consultant, though impossible to quantify and measure, can offer important data in terms of evaluation. For example, sensing staff openness and enthusiasm toward consultation can be exhilarating and reinforcing, while staff resistance and lack of interest can have the opposite effect. Feelings consultants have about situations and relationships can help to identify problem areas and successful areas of practice. One would not want to rely solely on subjective experience for evaluation, but consideration of those experiences can be a rich part of the evaluation process.

## SUMMARY

Consultation is an important aspect of CNS practice. It is a complex and highly professional activity that can be both challenging and rewarding. The mutual and creative problem-solving that occurs during a consultation can be a catalyst for the ongoing professional development of both consultee and consultant and can profoundly influence nursing practice.

### *References*

Barron, A. M.: The clinical nurse specialist as consultant. *In* Hamric, A., and Spross, J. (eds): The Clinical Nurse Specialist in Theory and Practice. New York, Grune and Stratton, 1983.

Benner, P.: From Novice to Expert: Excellence and Power in Clinical Nursing Practice. Menlo Park, CA, Addison-Wesley, 1984.

Blake, P.: The clinical specialist as nurse consultant. J Nurs Admin 7:33–36, 1977.

Brown, S. J.: Administrative support. *In* Hamric, A., and Spross, J. (eds): The Clinical Nurse Specialist in Theory and Practice. New York, Grune and Stratton, 1983.

Caplan, G.: The Theory and Practice of Mental Health Consultation. New York, Basic Books, 1970.

Davis, D., et al.: Evaluating advance practice nurses. Nurs Management 15:44–47, 1984.

Fenton, M.: Identifying competencies of clinical nurse specialists. J Nurs Admin 15:31–37, 1985.

Flynn, G.: The romance of consultation. *In* Busman J., and Davidson, D. (eds): Practical Aspects of Mental Health Consultation. Springfield, IL, Charles C Thomas, 1972.

Girouard S., & Spross, J.: Evaluation of the clinical nurse specialist: Using an evaluation tool. *In* Hamric, A., and Spross, J. (eds): The Clinical Nurse Specialist in Theory and Practice. New York, Grune and Stratton, 1983.

Hamric, A.: A model for developing evaluation strategies. *In* Hamric, A., and Spross, J. (eds): The Clinical Nurse Specialist in Theory and Practice. New York, Grune and Stratton, 1983.

Hamric, A.: Role development and functions. *In* Hamric, A., and Spross, J. (eds): The Clinical Nurse Specialist in Theory and Practice. New York, Grune and Stratton, 1983.

Hamric, A., Gresham, M. L., and Eccard, M.: Staff evaluation of clinical leaders. J Nurs Admin 8:18–26, 1978.

Hitchens, E.: Mental health nursing consultations: Some distinctions. J Psychiatr Nurs *15*:13–16, 1973.

Lehman, F.: Liaison nursing: A model for nursing practice. *In* Stuart, G., and Sundeen, S. (eds): Principles and Practice of Psychiatric Nursing. St. Louis, C. V. Mosby Company, 1979.

Lewis, A., & Levy, J.: Psychiatric Liaison Nursing: The Theory and Clinical Practice. Reston, VA, Reston Publishing Co., Inc., 1982.

Lipowski, Z. J.: Consultation-liaison psychiatry: An overview. Am J Psych *131*:623–630, 1974.

Lipowski, Z. J.: Liaison psychiatry. Liaison nursing and behavioral medicine. Compr Psychiatry *22*:554–561, 1981.

Lipowski, Z. J.: Current trends in consultation psychiatry. Can J Psychiatry *28*:329–338, 1983.

Nelson, J., & Schilke, D.: Evolution of psychiatric liaison nursing. Perspect Psychiatr Care *14*:60–65, 1976.

O'Connor, P., & Malone, B.: A consultation model for nurse specialist practice. Nurs Econ *1*:107–111, 1983.

Prouty, M.: Contributions and organizational role of the clinical nurse specialist: An administrator's viewpoint. *In* Hamric, A., and Spross, J. (eds): The Clinical Nurse Specialist in Theory and Practice. New York, Grune and Stratton, 1983.

Polk G.: The socialization and utilization of nurse consultants. J Psychiatr Nurs *18*:33–36, 1980.

Robinson, L.: Liaison Nursing Psychological Approach to Patient Care. Philadelphia, F. A. Davis Company, 1974.

Roy, S. C., & Martinez, C.: A conceptual framework for clinical nurse specialist practice. *In* Hamric, A., and Spross, J. (eds): The Clinical Nurse Specialist in Theory and Practice. New York, Grune and Stratton, 1983.

Sedgwick R.: The role of the process consultant. Nurs Outlook *21*:773–775, 1973.

Simmons, M. K.: Psychiatric consultation and liaison. *In* Critchley, D., and Maurin, J. (eds): The Clinical Specialist in Psychiatric—Mental Health Nursing. New York, John Wiley & Sons, 1985.

Tarsitano, B., Brophy, E., and Snyder, D.: Demystification of the clinical nurse specialist role: Perceptions of clinical nurse specialists and nurse administrators. J Nurs Educ *25*:4–9, 1986.

# The CNS as Educator

*Ann-Reid Priest*

## INTRODUCTION

Educational responsibilities are a traditional part of the CNS role. To understand the educational component of the CNS role, it is helpful and important to compare and contrast it with other educator roles in nursing—specifically, those of nurse faculty and staff developers. While all three nurse roles use similar educational processes, the differences between CNSs and either nurse faculty or staff educators can be conceptualized in terms of base of practice and access to and control over the clinical environment. *Education* is the practice base, the raison d'etre, for faculty and staff development instructors. *Patient care* is the practice base, the raison d'être, for CNSs. Because of their involvement in a nursing unit and/or with a patient population, CNSs have more access to and control over the clinical environment. For example, the CNS should have close working relationships with head nurses, physicians, and staff nurses, which arise from (or are inherent in) the clinical immersion of the CNS in a practice setting. Such relationships facilitate the educator subrole of the CNS. Nurse faculty and staff developers would find such relationships hard to build because their encounters with these health care providers are intermittent and are usually structured rather than spontaneous. The lack of such relationships can be an obstacle to their education roles.

While there is a considerable body of literature on nursing education addressing such topics as staff development, continuing education, and education of graduate and undergraduate students, little is available on the educator component of the CNS role. Although the CNS can use the other literature to an advantage, it is important that CNSs have a grasp of their educator subrole in order to offer strategies for implementation, identify constraints, and discuss approaches to evaluating this subrole.

## EDUCATOR ROLES IN NURSING

Stafford commented in an account of the CNS in a faculty appointment that, "Every nurse is a teacher; not to teach is not to nurse" (1985, p. 102). The educator roles that exist in nursing include patient educator, staff developer, and student educator. The task of educator has also been identified as a distinct function of the CNS (Blount, et al., 1981; Georgopoulous & Christman, 1970; Menard, 1987; Perry, 1985; Stafford, 1985). It is necessary to compare the educator functions of the CNS with those of other nurse educators because the educator subrole, although distinct, is only one in a myriad of CNS functions. Another reason in support of such a comparison is that in some institutions, attempts may be made to place the CNS in solely educator roles. The following discussion compares and contrasts the education subrole in relation to the focus and purpose of each role.

STAFF NURSE. The education focus of the staff nurse is primarily on the patient and family.* Experienced staff nurses also assume preceptor relationships with new and/or inexperienced staff. Nurses involved in direct patient care are expected to balance competing roles including those of direct care provider, patient care planner, and supervisor of professional and nonprofessional staff. Staff nurses utilize informal and formal opportunities to provide information to patients and families. Assessment of patient knowledge deficits and dissemination of information often occur while other forms of care such as medication administration, AM care, wound care, and the like are provided. These informal teaching strategies are sometimes augmented by the development of structured educational resources such as patient education pamphlets and unit-based classes. Staff nurses often participate in the development of such resources.

Staff nurses may also participate in the education of other nurses through preceptorship programs and supervision of undergraduate student clinical experiences. In this way, staff nurses share clinical knowledge and skills developed from day-to-day bedside practice.

STAFF EDUCATOR. The work of the staff educator focuses on the general educational needs of staff nurses. Staff educators may function within staff development departments or they may be unit-based and work collaboratively with staff development personnel.

Staff development departments are traditional providers of formal education opportunities. Services provided include orientation of new employees, inservice training involving new procedures and equipment,

---

*It is understood that the educational process of patients includes family members and significant others. A reference to patient implies the inclusion of these other parties.

and certification of basic competencies such as Basic Life Support. Continuing education programs on advanced nursing topics for the experienced nurse may also be offered. Unit-based staff educators provide similar services but tailor orientation and skill development to the particular needs of the unit.

FACULTY. Nurses in faculty positions have as their primary focus the preparation of students for basic and advanced clinical nursing practice. Faculty prepare students for beginning or advanced nursing roles through lectures, seminars, skills labs, and clinical practicums. While patients and staff may benefit from faculty resources in the clinical setting, the emphasis is on the education of students. Unless faculty have joint appointments in the clinical setting, they and their students are not immersed in the culture of the unit or organization. This is a major difference between the CNS and faculty educator roles. Nursing faculty may find they have to explain or accept a disparity between practice and academic learning because they have little power to influence the system. Faculty have said they often feel like guests in the agencies where students have their practical experience. The CNS is not a guest. A collaborative practice model between schools of nursing and practice settings is one mechanism to share clinical expertise and educate students using the best that both education and practice have to offer (see Chapter 16). Ideally, this approach can strengthen educator roles of faculty and staff practitioners, with improved patient care and student education as outcomes.

CLINICAL NURSE SPECIALIST. The focus of practice for the educator subrole of the CNS is the patient and family. In this respect, the educator subrole of the CNS overlaps with the functions of staff nurses. However, the CNS also participates in programs designed to meet continuing education needs. The CNS functions as a preceptor, resource person, program planner, and lecturer in the education of undergraduate and graduate students. One characteristic that separates the CNS from other educators is the CNS's ability to perform in several subroles requiring multiple skills and competencies, often teaching patients, staff, and students simultaneously. The CNS may act as a consultant to determine patient teaching needs and then provide the teaching while acting as a role model for staff nurses and nursing students.

## ORGANIZATIONAL SUPPORTS FOR EDUCATOR SUBROLE OF CNS

CNS position descriptions usually include responsibilities associated with education. In order to implement these responsibilities, the CNS should be aware of resources within the setting. The CNS should assess the organizational resources and determine what other departments or individuals are responsible for educating staff, patients, and students.

CNS orientation should include meetings with appropriate individuals in staff development departments to determine the following: resources for program planning and development of educational materials; CEU application process; audiovisual equipment and borrowing procedures; conference room booking procedures; available educational materials; individuals responsible for arranging contracts for student placement; existing patient education program/support groups in the specialty area; budgeting for program/resource development and CNS access to such funds; and the best means for establishing relationships and developing initial plans for collaborating with appropriate individuals in mutual educational endeavors. The CNS should determine the extent of secretarial support for such services as typing, ordering equipment, and so forth. Another aspect of assessing the organization is to identify existing policies that govern participation in CE (honoraria, use of compensatory time, and the like).

CNSs have varying levels of knowledge and skill regarding educational theory and technology; the novice should find out if there are programs and other resources for assisting CNSs to develop particular skills. Often resources for the educator subrole may be found in the agency's training and development department, public relations department, medical arts department, faculty and learning resource labs of affiliated schools, and with audiovisual technicians associated with other departments, such as the surgical divisions of large institutions. In addition, CNSs should identify sources of materials and funding for educational programs and booklets, such as voluntary agencies (American Heart Association, National Cancer Institute) and speakers' bureaus (company pays speaker honoraria) of companies that manufacture drugs and other health care products. These companies often have excellent patient and professional educational materials. Some units or programs have special funds established by patients or their families which may be used to support educational endeavors.

## THE CNS AS STAFF EDUCATOR

The CNS participates in the education and development of nursing staff. The subrole of staff educator is expressed, in part, by participation in selected aspects of orientation, inservice education, continuing education, needs assessments, program planning, and speaker services.

However, as an expert practitioner, the influence and expertise of the CNS extends far beyond traditional education models. By definition the CNS is committed to furthering excellence in clinical practice and seeks innovative ways to share knowledge with other practitioners. One means to this end is developing a relationship with the staff development department.

Models for interfacing with various other departments are described in the literature. Schwartz-Fulton (1985) described how a CNS within a hospital consultation department provided hospital-based and community consultative services. Blount (1981) described CNS interface with the staff development department as including workshop planning, orientation, and unit-based instruction. This collaboration is one mechanism for extending the CNS's influence and improving the quality of nursing care. These descriptions support the intent of the educator subrole as one in a constellation of subroles.

In contrast, Everson proposed the placement of the CNS in the staff development department. Everson cited lack of successful integration of the CNS role in tertiary care settings as a reason for such organizational placement. She reasoned that placement of the CNS in staff development would obviate the problems of role implementation and utilization and focus on a consultation/liaison structure for the role. Clinical specialists functioning in the role of staff developers know that their accountability is not "to improve the care of any one patient or even a group of patients through direct patient contact, but to build a strong, collegial nursing staff so that all care is improved" (Everson, 1981, p. 19).

This idea may have some initial appeal but is fraught with potential and real problems. While CNSs interface frequently with staff development programs, their influence and expertise should extend beyond traditional education models. Furthermore, the consultation/liaison model limits the expression of the four CNS subroles and potentially emphasizes the educator subrole. As originally conceived, the CNS role is patient-centered; a shift in focus compromises both the spirit and purpose of the role. Placement of the CNS in staff development threatens not only to erode the patient/family focus of practice but also to skew the balance of the four subroles. It would also interfere with the ongoing development of the CNS's practice expertise. The time demands of orientation and continuing education can be burdensome to the practitioner with a patient-centered focus.

How then does the CNS find appropriate expression of the educator subrole and still balance the remaining roles of consultant, clinical expert, and researcher? Participation in selected formal educational offerings utilizing the clinical expertise of the CNS is one approach.

Assessment of formal and informal learning needs often occurs as the CNS practices in a consultant or direct patient care role.

Another way to utilize CNS expertise in the educator subrole is to address learning and developmental needs of experienced staff nurses. This would enable the CNS to contribute to the institution's effort to retain and satisfy experienced clinicians. Benner's work (1984) provides insight into the identification and acquisition of clinical knowledge by nurses. She described five levels of competency in clinical practice and some of the ways nurses acquire clinical knowledge. The passage through these levels from novice to expert practitioner depends upon the accrual of knowledge and development of expertise, which are acquired over time with experience in clinical situations.

Dolan (1984) addressed the retention issue by charging staff development departments with the task of identifying professional development needs of the experienced nurse. Using Benner's work with clinical knowledge acquisition, Dolan described a program that included preceptor orientation, clinical judgment programs for nurses to discuss their practices, and seminars to educate nursing administrators in the practical application of Benner's work. Dolan's emphasis on career development serves as both a retention strategy as well as a forum to advance nursing practice.

> Staff development departments should provide a forum for discussion of clinical practice in which nursing knowledge is carefully charted and explored. . . . Teaching rounds by expert nurses open vistas to the advanced beginner and the competent nurse while recognizing the value of expertise and its importance in the transmitting of wisdom and judgment (Dolan, 1984, p. 283).

While refinement of advanced practice using Dolan's ideas is one approach, other strategies can enhance the professional growth of staff. These include assisting staff to submit abstracts, developing presentations or posters for intramural/extramural conferences, and writing for publication. These strategies benefit staff as well as enable CNSs to overcome staff jealousy, which is sometimes expressed overtly or covertly over the CNS's job flexibility and variety.

Participation in the education and development of all levels of staff is an appropriate function of the CNS. Clinical expertise, analytic skills, and an understanding of advanced practice issues are particular assets the CNS brings to the effort of staff development. The CNS must be aware of the need to balance all subroles over time and to remain true to a patient-centered practice.

## Vignette

The development of the Intensive Care Unit (ICU) component of a liver transplant program serves as a paradigm case for the CNS as staff educator. A major university teaching center with an established clinical transplant program expanded to include liver transplantation. One ICU was designated to provide care for adult patients in the immediate postoperative period. A CNS was hired to coordinate the multidisciplinary team and assist in development of nursing staff. The staff already possessed knowledge and expertise in caring for patients with multisystem failure and were eager to learn more about the particular needs of transplant patients.

Initially, past experiences with other complex, critically ill patients were used to guide nursing care. The CNS contributed her knowledge of liver disease and transplant issues, such as intraoperative complications, immunology, and rejection, while experienced nursing staff developed sets of instructions about the technical care of the patient. Gradually, an understanding of the range of physiological, psychological, and spiritual responses emerged.

With each new transplant patient, the CNS and nursing staff exchanged informal observations and data about the patient's physiological and psychological responses to transplant and of subsequent nursing and medical interventions. The CNS shared current data from the literature and other transplant programs which improved patient care. This was done in conversations with individual staff nurses during transplant and multidisciplinary rounds, in patient care conferences, and in periodic day-long workshops for nursing staff. A set of clinical guidelines for the care of liver transplant patients was developed by nursing staff and the CNS, and a computerized critical care order set was available for housestaff use.

The CNS facilitated the formation of relationships between the ICU, OR, and anesthesia staffs to exchange information about the perioperative needs of the patient. Initially, ICU nurses assigned to care for transplant patients were taken to the OR by the CNS to observe the surgery and learn about intraoperative routines and problems. Informal communications with the anesthesia staff developed into a formal reporting process by the patient's anesthetist to the nurses preparing to care for the patient. While the CNS remained in contact with the OR team at the time of transplant for overall coordination of transplant activities, the OR nursing staff contacted the ICU as the transplant neared completion. The ICU staff came to the OR and received reports from the OR team and assisted with the transport of the patient to the ICU.

A cadre of nurses experienced in the immediate postoperative care of liver transplant patients prepared other nurses through a preceptorship program. Explicit guidelines for nursing responsibilities were delineated by the CNS and ICU administrative team, but refinement of these guidelines continued to occur as clinical experience revealed new information about caring for patients with their individual responses to the illness experience.

Preoperative teaching needs of patients and families have been identified, and a preoperative visit program has been implemented. Nurses experienced in the care of transplant patients visited the patient and family, assessed their needs, and provided information. The CNS identified the appropriate time for a patient and family to obtain further information about the immediate postoperative period and communicated particular concerns and needs to the visiting ICU staff nurse. The ICU nurse visited the patient and family and performed her own needs assessment. Written guidelines to assist the nurse were available. The ICU nurse brought the patient and family to the ICU, conducted a tour, and provided information on isolation, ventilators, lines and drains, psychological issues, visiting policies, and nursing routines. A written summary of this interaction was returned to the CNS with any questions or issues requiring CNS follow-up. A copy of this form was on file at the unit and was retrieved by the nurse caring for the patient at the time of transplant. The CNS provided updated information and shared particular problems or concerns that emerged during the waiting period. The ICU visit summary was placed on the bedside chart as a reference for family members, with phone numbers and particular nursing concerns.

This vignette illustrates two points. The first is that the care of liver transplant patients is planned and that needs are identified and documented at critical periods in the transplant process. Second, the responsibility for developing expertise in the care of these patients is ongoing, growing out of a rich interchange between the CNS and experienced staff and including both structured and unstructured teaching situations. Each party takes responsibility for evaluating the care delivered and for looking at ways to improve perioperative care. Finally, the task of providing high-quality care requires identification and development of clinical knowledge and the commitment to finding new and better ways to communicate that knowledge.

## Constraints to the Staff Educator Subrole

As mentioned previously, a measure of successful practice in this subrole is the CNS's ability to balance its expression with that of other CNS subroles. Institutional goals, assessments of learning needs, and staff development programs can easily and often subtly demand time of the CNS, creating imbalance in the practice of the various subroles.

Staff shortages place a constraint on the CNS's practice, and they are of increasing concern. The shrinking supply of staff nurses creates a stress on the teaching-learning situation and provides daily staffing concerns. The CNS can share expertise and assist in the development of staff only if staff are available and receptive. Keys to success in the current climate of shortage will involve principles of economy of effort. Possible strategies include teaching staff while teaching patients, clarifying and maximizing staff's role in patient education, and preparing audiovisual tapes for teaching small groups of staff. Collaborating with other CNSs to meet needs that cut across services (e.g., nursing diagnosis, ethics) will promote effective time management for the CNS.

Other constraints to successful implementation of the staff educator subrole include lack of institutional resources (e.g., financial and human resources), lack of support from unit administrative staff, and lack of staff motivation to learn. The latter may be related to existing staff shortages and increasing burdens and responsibilities on staff. Creative problem-solving, flexibility, and perseverance will be essential skills for the CNS in dealing with these long-term, complex constraints.

Periodic review of time utilization, administrative understanding, and support of the CNS role, and individual goals and objectives can assist the CNS in directing energies to balance all the subroles. The CNS will likely experience periodic high demands for educational services because of specific unit or departmental needs. These needs require flexibility on the part of the CNS to respond appropriately and vision to remember that, while temporary needs may be served, long-term commitment to patient-centered practice must be preserved.

## THE CNS AS PATIENT EDUCATOR

With expert knowledge and skills in a specialty, the CNS is in a strategic position for patient and family education. Benner commented, "Nurses provide benchmarks and time tables to the hospitalized patient who does not know what to expect . . . nurses become experts in coaching a patient through illness" (1984, p. 77). Benner further stated that expert nurses become effective coaches because they possess clinical expertise "characterized by an in-depth knowledge of a particular clinical population so that the nurse knows in theory and practice the illness trajectory of that patient population" (1985, p. 41). The CNS as clinical expert actively coaches patients through the illness experience and guides other nurses to perform selected aspects of the coaching function.

The contributions of the CNS to patient education may focus on individual or group education. For the individual patient, the CNS may assess a patient's understanding of the illness and implications during hospitalization and after discharge, formulate a teaching plan, implement all or part of that plan, assist nursing staff in the assessment and implementation of a teaching plan, and evaluate effectiveness of teaching through patient follow-up. For groups of patients, the CNS may be involved in planning unit-based education programs such as cardiac or postpartum classes as well as in designing the education component of more comprehensive programs, such as a home ventilator program or pulmonary rehabilitation. Other examples of appropriate use of CNS expertise is the development of patient education materials and protocols for staff use. The CNS uses an in-depth understanding of the particular illness experience to anticipate the needs of groups of patients in planning such programs. Knowledge of adult learning theory and strategies promotes program development. These topics are addressed in detail by Echols (1984), Knowles (1980), Menard (1987), and Smith (1978). Knowledge of growth and development assist the pediatric CNS to tailor teaching strategies to an age-appropriate level.

Possession of knowledge and clinical expertise, however, does not ensure successful patient education. All levels of professional nursing claim responsibility for patient teaching, so the CNS must carefully assess each opportunity before intervening to determine if patient teaching needs are being met by unit staff and other health care providers, such as the dietitian and physical therapist. More than one CNS has reported an ambitious attempt to educate a patient or family member, only to find a subsequent wellspring of anger and resentment on the part of unit staff for the perceived overstepping of boundaries.

The CNS is often used as a consultant to determine learning needs of a complex patient. In this context, the CNS may also act as a role model for staff in problem-solving and addressing certain learning needs. This process demonstrates the overlapping nature of CNS subroles in actual practice. CNSs must decide which aspect of patient education for their patient population will be handled by themselves and which will be delegated. Ideally, the patient education process is a collaborative effort. The CNS uses expert knowledge to identify learning needs, address complex problems, and coordinate teaching, especially in the case of multidisciplinary problems and needs.

As a clinical expert and manager of often complex patient situations, the CNS is in an ideal position to assume the role of expert coach in certain circumstances. Benner (1984) defined the coaching function as the process of taking what is "foreign and fearful to the patient and making it familiar and less frightening" (p. 77). Oftentimes, there is a population of patients with complex or unusual learning needs who are seen infrequently by staff nurses but are known to the CNS. This population may include patients with rare diseases, patients undergoing radical and/or new surgical procedures, patients treated with new therapies and modalities, and patients on research protocols or non-standard therapies.

These patients need an expert coach to help them navigate through the experience, since the illness trajectory may not be known or may be known to only a few. Benner contended that the expert coach learns what the illness means to the individual and what resources, skills, and demands are required of the patient at each stage of the illness (1985). The CNS can accomplish this task by assuming direct care and educator roles. The CNS learns the trajectory as it unfolds and uses knowledge from past experiences to coach the patient through the illness. This knowledge can be shared with the staff, and certain aspects of patient education may be delegated to staff nurses. For example, a patient is admitted to an oncology unit for epidural catheter placement for management of chronic pain. This treatment modality is seen infrequently by the nursing staff but is familiar to the CNS. The CNS provides much of the direct care in the first few days after catheter placement and offers information about the catheter to the patient, family, and staff. As staff familiarity increases through formal and informal learning experiences provided by the CNS, designated staff begin to provide care and selected teaching to the patient. It is unrealistic, however, to expect a staff nurse to independently coach patients through complex or uncommon illness trajectories. Staff nurses often lack the clinical expertise needed to provide such care.

As expert coach, CNSs can also use their assessment of patient readiness to guide the teaching efforts of other disciplines. For example, a child with chronic renal failure and developmental delay is placed on a diet with sodium, potassium, and fluid restrictions. The CNS assesses the patient and family readiness to learn and prioritizes learning needs. The CNS advises the dietitian and occupational and physical therapists regarding the optimum time for teaching. This coordinated effort lessens the likelihood of information overload, optimizes each interaction, and guides the patient through the illness experience.

Clinical expertise and knowledge of the illness trajectory enable the CNS to impart cognitive information and to assist the patient in developing judgment about the illness experience. For example, patients need to know not only the name, dose, and side effects of their medication but also what to do when they suspect adverse drug interactions or what exactly to do when they just do not "feel right." Lifestyle changes related to illness are frequently overlooked by less experienced staff, but the expert coach can help patients anticipate changes and provide a framework for decision-making about issues that arise after discharge. Development of this kind of judgment usually occurs over time and is a hallmark of the CNS as expert coach.

The CNS often provides continuity of care to a particular population and is in a position to evaluate the effectiveness of the teaching process. This feedback can be given to the staff to improve the quality of teaching for subsequent patients. The CNS must be sensitive to the nursing staff's need to be involved in the education process, and negotiation for specific tasks must take place according to patient needs and time constraints of staff. Encouragement of staff motivated to learn and teach is essential to CNS success in the patient educator subrole.

### Vignette

L.P. is a 40-year-old Oriental man accepted for kidney transplant at a United States transplant center. He is married, has children, and emigrated to the United States several years prior to needing a transplant. He is a deeply religious man as a result of his conversion to a major western religion and has remained active in his church throughout his illness. During the initial evaluation for transplant, it became clear that all information about transplant would be given to the patient and his minister, and L.P. would decide the information to be shared with his wife and children. Furthermore, the decision in favor of transplant would be made only if God gave him a sign. Attempts to educate the patient of the urgency of the decision were seemingly disregarded until the sign from God was received. The CNS became aware of the patient when he refused to discuss his feelings and concerns with the transplant psychologist and social worker. He also refused psychological testing. The CNS spent time with L.P. and his minister to determine the extent of cultural and religious influences on his decision-making. It was learned that information flowed into the family via the father, and it was believed unnecessary and ill-advised to include the wife in decision-making. The CNS also learned that L.P. could speak limited English but was even further limited in the reading of English. He wrote in his native language characters.

The informed consent process initially involved a line-by-line discussion of the two-page consent form with the CNS and one of the transplant physicians. The CNS later learned that L.P. could not read the consent form, and upon further inquiry, it was questionable if he gleaned much from the first discussion of transplantation. The CNS asked a transplant surgeon speaking L.P.'s native language to visit the patient and review the consent form. This interchange proved to be successful because L.P. began asking the CNS many questions and indicated his pleasure in speaking with the doctor concerning his transplant. Further assessment by the CNS revealed that L.P. believed physicians were divinely inspired, and that the recent visit by the transplant surgeon was a sign from God to proceed with transplant.

The CNS continued to visit L.P. during his in-hospital wait for transplant to further assess his religious and cultural perceptions of his illness and impending surgery. It was learned that continued respect and support was sought from his congregation and that he would probably not develop strong trusting bonds with hospital staff. He began to selectively confide in the CNS but remained distant with other staff. He declined the invitation to conduct a preop visit to the ICU because he believed God would take care of him and show him the way after transplant. The CNS reviewed very basic information about the ICU experience and did not insist on the tour. The data collected on L.P.'s cultural attitudes and religious convictions were shared with the staff through patient care conferences, and the planning of his care during the perioperative phase began.

At the time of transplant, L.P. revealed that only God could sign his consent form since it was His will that the transplant be performed. The CNS convinced the patient that the location of a suitable donor organ could be seen as a sign from God to proceed. This idea was supported by the minister and L.P. agreed to sign the consent. It was also during this time that the CNS met L.P.'s wife. She was attended by the minister, and all information about the patient's progress during the procedure was communicated to the minister, who explained the details to Mrs. L.P. The patient was successfully transplanted with an uneventful postoperative course. Information about L.P.'s religious and cultural views assisted the ICU staff in planning his care, understanding his demeanor, and respecting his deep religious convictions. For example, the staff did not call the hospital chaplain when L.P. seemed depressed but waited for L.P.'s minister to come to discuss their concerns. The staff did not take offense or question their own abilities when a warm therapeutic bond between patient and nurse did not form. They discovered that L.P. respected their competency but showed gratitude in very subtle ways.

Following the ICU stay, L.P. returned to the same general care area for convalescence and discharge teaching. He confided in the CNS that he felt God had healed him during the transplant such that lifetime immunosuppression would be unnecessary. The CNS used the patient's strong appeal to physician authority to deal with this question. Another visit by the Oriental transplant surgeon was arranged, and the importance of immunosuppression was discussed. L.P. believed that, since the physician strongly believed in the value of the medication, it was a sign from God to continue the medication regimen.

The CNS continued to provide short discharge teaching sessions that were well-received by the patient. The CNS arranged for written instructions to be translated into his native language, and L.P. agreed to share these with his wife and minister. L.P. was discharged and found to be highly compliant with diet, medications, exercise, and other instructions given at the time of discharge.

### Constraints to the Patient Educator Subrole

Resources are the major constraint to the implementation of the patient educator subrole. There are many patients with complex problems in need of expert coaching, and there are also fewer nurses available to care for and teach these patients. CNSs must make decisions that reflect the best use of expert resources. The need to balance all subroles requires careful assessment of learning needs, since direct patient education is a time-intensive enterprise.

Another resource constraint is the declining number of staff nurses available to provide patient education. The staff nurse may value patient education, but other demands on time may preclude its operation. The CNS must negotiate with staff to ensure that patient education needs are met in a time of diminishing resources. Flexibility and creativity on the part of the CNS and the staff nurse will be keys to the success and quality of patient education.

Administrative support for this subrole is essential. Nursing administrators need to understand and value all four CNS subroles. Patient education, like staff development, is a pressing need, but it cannot monopolize CNS time. Administrators can assist CNSs to develop strategies that best utilize their talents while meeting the needs of patients and staff.

## THE CNS AS STUDENT EDUCATOR

The clinical practice base of the CNS provides a compelling reason for the CNS to participate in the education of nursing students particularly at the graduate level. The CNS's practice is fertile ground on which education and practice can meet to serve the needs of students. It is here that students not only apply knowledge learned in the classroom but also experience the rich complexities of human responses to health and illness. The practice setting is used by undergraduate students to develop beginning skills in nursing practice. One way CNSs participate in education of undergraduate nursing students is through the consultative subrole. The CNS acts as consultant by providing insight into complex patient care situations and dilemmas faced by patients as well as staff. These activities and others, such as patient care conferences and inservices, enrich the clinical experience of undergraduate students while demonstrating the CNS's leadership in the clinical setting.

However, CNSs have the greatest impact on educating advanced practitioners. With the preceptor relationship as the foundation for learning, the student contracts with an advanced practitioner in a specialty to exchange knowledge about clinical issues. This relationship presupposes basic understanding of the content area by the student and a strong mutual commitment to learning. The clinical experience enables graduate students to have experiences in which they can apply theoretical knowledge and gain practical knowledge in a specialty area.

A second prerequisite to a successful preceptor relationship is clear identification of goals and objectives for the clinical experience. As a negotiated relationship, the goals of the student and expectations of the CNS must be clearly articulated. Glass (1983) proposed student and preceptor guidelines to facilitate this communication. These guidelines also describe the CNS role in evaluation of the clinical experience. A third prerequisite is that student and CNS must share a fundamental commitment to clinical practice; furthermore, they must share a common interest in the designated patient population. They must respect individual needs and appreciate the constraints of institutional, professional, and personal obligations such as committee work, research activities, and CNS-imposed time constraints. The richness of the clinical experience depends upon the willingness of the CNS and student to discuss, describe, and analyze complex clinical practice issues. In essence, there must be a "good fit" between the student and CNS.

The exchange of clinical knowledge occurs in several formats and settings. Directed readings can increase students' content expertise and sensitize them to clinical issues. However, student observation and participation in specific CNS activities effectively communicates the complex nature of CNS practice (e.g., allowing the student to respond to a consultation). Perry (1985) used Benner's model (1984) to describe a goal of graduate student clinical experience. Benner described seven domains of nursing practice and competencies within each domain. Perry used the domain of Teaching-Coaching to focus on one of her goals as a preceptor.

> Through structural sessions or bedside chats, I will model the teaching ability that can sense the "question behind the question" and relate from experience how to assess what the patient wants to know from the way the patient phrases the question . . . . The newly admitted patient may be a rookie in the patient role but a "seasoned veteran" in the experiences of life. Knowing how to encourage the patient in a way that acknowledges these two roles is a skill . . . that can be learned . . . by the graduate student (Perry, 1985, p. 83).

Other examples of the Teaching-Coaching domain are seen in CNS interaction with nursing staff. In a study by Fenton (1985) of CNS competencies, it was found that part of the consultative role included identification of issues that created discomfort for patients, families, and staff. Fenton concluded that the CNS is in a pivotal role to sense issues that have been avoided and determine strategies for addressing them. In the context of a preceptor relationship, the CNS can role model complex decision-making using avoided issues.

## Vignette

A CNS experienced in the care of AIDS patients was asked to consult on a patient in the terminal stage of the disease. The patient was attributed with many behavioral problems including angry outbursts toward his family and staff and noncompliance with isolation techniques. He also made threatening and inaccurate remarks to other patients regarding the contagious nature of his disease. The staff, in turn, expressed anger about the patient's manipulative and alienating behavior and began to withdraw. Patient care assignments were rotated, and the primary nurse wished to relinquish her role. It was unlikely that the patient would leave the hospital, and staff felt trapped, frustrated, and unable to meet the patient's needs.

The CNS and graduate student listened to the concerns of staff and discussed identified problems. The CNS reflected on past experiences with difficult patients and, with the assistance of the graduate student, sought additional information from the staff. The student observed these interactions including an assessment of the patient by the CNS. The CNS discovered that the patient was desperately angry at his sexual partner for violating their monogamous relationship and contracting the disease. The patient had not had recent contact with his partner and felt abandoned by his partner and his family. The patient's level of frustration and powerlessness was thought to be the source of the previously described behaviors. The CNS and student listened to his concerns and discussed ways the patient might re-establish contact with his partner. They provided support to the patient and began to reframe the staff's perception of the patient by providing additional information about the issues and needs of AIDS patients. The student convened a patient care conference to share the insights gained and allow staff to express their concerns. The CNS and student suggested some possible interventions and encouraged the staff to identify other strategies for renegotiating their relationship with the patient. Out of new sense of support and encouragement, the patient initiated contact with his partner and had an opportunity to discuss his feelings. The staff continued to renegotiate their relationship, and contracting around acceptable behaviors was initiated. The CNS provided a successful consultation to a troubled patient and staff, and the student had a learning experience while participating in the interaction.

## Constraints and Supports to Student Educator Role

Relationships between practice and education are described in several ways. Joint appointment, shared appointment, adjunct faculty, dual role, and faculty associate are just a few terms that describe a relationship between the CNS and the academic environment. Schwartz-Fulton (1985), Donovan (1985), Cox (1985), and Stafford (1985) described their experiences in this role, and similar constraints were found. Commonly identified problems include insufficient clinical practice time, lack of support networks in the practice and academic setting, and lack of financial reward. The primary threat to this dual role is that excessive time demands from competing agencies may erode the clinical practice base of the CNS. Without conscious effort to preserve the practice base, outside forces will dictate other priorities. Cox stated, "To be successful, the shared appointment must be designed and executed with the finely honed skills and determination of all the principal participants" (1985, p. 138).

Cox (1985) also determined that a good fit between school and hospital must exist. She found that success is contingent on consistency of goals and values among the CNS, the hospital, and the educational institution.

The potential for a successful relationship between student and CNS exists. The relationship between the practice and academic environment must be harmonious and must support the work of the CNS and student. Conflict between the two agencies regarding the education of students diminishes the quality of experience. The individual relationship negotiated between CNS and student is of equal importance. Goals and objectives must be clear and a commitment to clinical practice should be a priority. Given these criteria, it is possible that a relationship between CNS and student can be fruitful. It is an opportunity to examine practice, develop clinical experts, and continue to find meaning in a practice discipline. Schwartz-Fulton (1985) commented, "Students bring new perspectives, ask questions and cause reflection. . . . Reflection is a healthy balance point for a job that has no end" (p. 96).

## IMPLEMENTATION OF THE EDUCATOR SUBROLE

The real challenge for the CNS extends beyond just an understanding of the dimensions of the educator subrole. The CNS must find appropriate expression of the educator subrole and still balance the remaining roles of consultant, clinical expert, and researcher. The CNS may act as a consultant to determine patient teaching needs and provide patient teaching, while acting as a role model for staff nurses and nursing students. The following scenario illustrates the synthesis of the many teaching roles of the CNS.

The staff on a busy oncology unit were preparing a patient for discharge with a new central venous access for chemotherapy. A CNS with expertise in venous access placement was asked to see the patient to assist in identifying learning needs. The CNS and primary nurse drafted initial discharge teaching guidelines and arranged a discharge teaching process. The patient, family, and student nurse were present for the first meeting. The CNS presented the information, and other staff observed both the process of patient teaching as well as the content delivered. The primary nurse presented information to the same group during a second session and was critiqued by the CNS.

In the above scenario, the CNS functioned as a consultant to determine complex learning needs, as a role model for staff and students, as a patient and family educator, as a clinical leader, and as a staff developer. The simultaneous practice of several subroles is a trademark of advanced nursing practice and the ultimate challenge for the CNS.

## EVALUATION OF THE EDUCATOR SUBROLE

A thorough discussion of evaluation used in CNS practice is presented in Chapter 4. The following comments are limited to practical ways to assist with structure, process, and outcome evaluation.

Structure evaluation is a basic level of evaluation and provides useful data about the activities of the CNS. Structure evaluation of the educator subrole could include the following: content outlines of courses/classes/programs, a listing of education activities of the CNS, time documentation, and membership on committees (intramural and extramural) with an educational focus. Clinical guidelines, teaching protocols, and development of patient or professional educational resources are further examples of structures within CNS practice that can assist in evaluation.

In Chapter 4, Hamric states that, although structural evaluation is valuable, it cannot be used as a single method. She describes process evaluation as examination of caregiver's functions. Process evaluation yields data regarding the CNS's ability to perform in each subrole. This form of evaluation is especially useful in evaluating CNS effectiveness, because some measure of quality rather than just quantity of activity is desired. Examples of process evaluation include peer review conducted while the CNS is involved in some aspect of teaching; staff, student, and patient evaluations aimed at the effectiveness of the teaching interventions; and self evaluations and documentation of paradigm coaching examples kept in a CNS log.

Outcome evaluation examines the impact of CNS educational activities on patients. This is a more difficult indicator to measure, since changes in patient health status could be multifactorial in origin. An example of outcome evaluation might be demonstrating that a patient education program shortened the length of stay for a particular population. There are obvious problems with this example of outcome evaluation because there are other factors affecting length of stay. Cognitive and psychosocial outcomes can be another method for meas uring effectiveness of patient teaching. An example of an outcome measure is testing the extent of a patient's knowledge before and after an education program. Identification of coping strategies and monitoring of anxiety postdischarge may also be used as an indicator of effectiveness of discharge teaching.

The CNS operating in a program-based practice such as a transplant program may have greater opportunity to utilize outcome evaluation. Continuity of care provides the CNS with an opportunity to observe patients as they integrate discharge teaching into daily living. The CNS can observe behavioral outcome changes manifested by an appropriate use of resources and the adherence to routine regimens such as blood pressure monitoring, exercise programs, and laboratory testing. The patient's ability to judge illness and wellness may be valuable in measuring outcome. Patient's ability to initiate appropriate calls to CNS or physician, self-assessment of signs and symptoms of illness, and integration of healthy lifestyle behaviors are outcomes that reflect development of good judgment and adaptation to illness and wellness. A long-term relationship with patients may create an opportunity for the CNS to evaluate, both formally and informally, the effectiveness of teaching patients good health behaviors.

## SUMMARY

The purpose of this chapter was to describe the CNS role of staff, patient, and student educator. This role was compared with other educator roles in nursing; the elements of advanced clinical knowledge and a patient-centered practice make CNS contributions to education unique. Threats to the CNS role included the concern that excessive educational demands may erode the practice base and prevent appropriate expression of the other CNS subroles. Strategies for addressing this concern were described.

The coaching of staff and patients was described but needs further study to determine the elements of that function which are most effective in the teaching-learning process. Finally, implementation and evaluation strategies were discussed. Outcome evaluation may be possible and beneficial to CNS practice, which strives for continuity of care.

*References*

Benner, P.: From Novice to Expert: Excellence and Power in Clinical Practice. Menlo Park, CA, Addison-Wesley, 1984.
Benner, P.: The oncology clinical nurse specialist: An expert coach. Oncol Nurs Forum *12*:40–44, 1985.
Blount, M., Burgo, S., Crigler, L., et al.: Extending the influence of the clinical nurse specialist. Nurs Admin Q *6*:53–63, 1981.
Cox, C.L.: Nursing practice in action: Diary of a casualty. *In* Barnard, K.E., and Smith, G.R. (eds): Faculty Practice in Action: Second Annual Symposium of Nursing Faculty Practice. Kansas City, American Academy of Nursing, 1985.
Dolan, K.: Building bridges between education and practice. *In* Benner, P.: From Novice to Expert: Excellence of Power in Clinical Practice. Menlo Park, CA, Addison-Wesley, 1984.
Donovan, C.T.: Clinical nurse specialist practice in an acute care setting. *In* Barnard, K.E., and Smith, G.R. (eds): Faculty Practice in Action: Second Annual Symposium of Nursing Faculty Practice. Kansas City, American Academy of Nursing, 1985.
Echols, J.L.: The teacher-facilitator role of clinical nursing leaders. Topics Clin Nurs *6*:28–40, 1984.
Everson, S.L.: Integration of the role of clinical nurse specialist. J Cont Ed Nurs *12*:16–19, 1981.
Fenton, M.V.: Identifying competencies of clinical nurse specialists. J Nurs Admin *15*:31–37, 1985.
Georgopoulous, B.S., & Christman, L.: The clinical nurse specialist: A role model. Am J Nurs *70*:1030–1039, 1970.
Glass, E.C.: The clinical nurse specialist as graduate student preceptor. Momentum *1*:3,5,8, 1983.

Knowles, M.S.: The Modern Practice of Adult Education. Chicago, Association Press, 1980.

Menard, S.W.: The CNS as teacher. *In* Menard, S.W. (ed): The Clinical Nurse Specialist: Perspectives on Practice. New York, John Wiley & Sons, 1987.

Perry, K.M.: Clinical preceptors: Communicating knowledge in clinical practice. *In* Barnard, K.E., and Smith, G.R. (eds): Faculty Practice in Action: Second Annual Symposium of Nursing Faculty Practice. Kansas City, American Academy of Nursing, 1985.

Schwartz-Fulton, J.: The clinical nurse specialist: Where the rubber meets the road. *In* Barnard, K.E., and Smith, G.R. (eds): Faculty Practice in Action: Second Annual Symposium of Nursing Faculty Practice. Kansas City, American Academy of Nursing, 1985.

Smith, C.E.: Principles and implications for continuing education in nursing. J Cont Ed Nurs 9:25–28, 1978.

Stafford, M.J.: The clinical nurse specialist's faculty role. *In* Barnard, K.E., and Smith, G.R. (eds): Faculty Practice in Action: Second Annual Symposium of Nursing Faculty Practice. Kansas City, American Academy of Nursing, 1985.

# The CNS as Researcher

Deborah B. McGuire
Kerry V. Harwood

## INTRODUCTION

Involvement in research is generally accepted as one of the major components of the clinical nurse specialist (CNS) role and, indeed, is mandated by our major national professional organization (American Nurses' Association [ANA], 1980a; 1981; 1985). The specifics of such involvement have been debated over the years, ranging from the actual conduct of research to its application in the clinical setting (Hodgman, 1983). As a result, expectations of administrators, CNSs themselves, and others with respect to the research role have varied widely, creating role confusion and even conflict (Harrell & McCulloch, 1986; Sisson, 1987; Tarsitano, et al., 1986). It is clear that a more specific and useful conceptualization of this role needs to be developed.

The involvement of clinicians in nursing research is viewed as critical to the profession (ANA, 1980b, 1985; Colton, 1980; McClure, 1981; Werley, 1972). In this chapter, literature that contributed to this view is explored. The conceptual framework for the research role of the CNS is explicated and expanded into a model consisting of levels of research involvement which are both reasonable and realistic. Factors essential for involvement at the different levels, and methods to acquire them, are described. Obstacles to research involvement are delineated along with strategies for overcoming them. Finally, some ideas for evaluation of the research role are presented.

## REVIEW OF THE LITERATURE

Research in clinical nursing practice has been urged for more than three decades, beginning with Henderson (1956), Werley (1962; 1972),

**169**

Ellis (1970), and Lindeman (1973), and continuing through the present (Gortner, 1975; Mercer, 1984; Moore, 1980; McClure, 1981; Pollock, 1987). Clinical research priorities have been described for critical care, oncology, and general nursing by many authors (ANA, 1980b; 1985; Lewandowski & Kositsky, 1983; Lindeman, 1975; Oberst, 1978). The need for clinicians to participate in careful, scholarly documentation of their clinical knowledge and the impact of such documentation on practice so that a research base might evolve have been noted by Diers (1983a; 1983b) and Benner (1983; 1985).

This section covers literature discussing research participation by "clinicians," that is, nurses with direct patient contact regardless of academic preparation. In 1973, the ANA defined the integration of nursing research as a responsibility of nursing service organizations. Schlotfeldt (1974) described the greatest hope for enhancing nursing's research activities as being the commitment to inquiry on the part of *all* nurses. In 1979, Padilla acknowledged that "the gap between introduction of the written standard and its operationalization has been difficult to bridge" (p. 49). She recommended incorporation of nursing research into the institutional nursing audit process based on Lewin's change theory (1958), which suggested that the most efficient and economical means of implementing and maintaining change was through an existing institutional mechanism. For similar reasons, Whitney and Roncoli (1986) recommended a model for developing research projects which used the problem-solving methods of the nursing process.

Several authors have discussed specific research responsibilities of clinicians. Bowie (1980) described a hierarchy of participation which the clinical nurse could move up as skills developed, starting with being a research subject, providing supportive care to research subjects, and providing technical assistance to researchers. The next three steps were being a consumer of research, providing consultation about specific clinical areas to researchers, and functioning in an investigative role. The first three activities are consistent with Stetler's (1983) belief that a basic research expectation of *all* nurses is understanding the importance of and facilitating nursing research.

The incorporation of nursing research activities into practice has been recommended through research teams or committees. Loomis (1982) described collaborative efforts between clinician and academic members of the Conduct and Utilization of Research in Nursing (CURN) Project. The American Hospital Association (1985) proposed a hospital-based research committee as a viable method, advocating nurse representation from all levels within the department. Hoare and Earenfight (1986) presented a model for unit-based nursing research teams supported by a research consultant. All participants were volunteers, and this model encouraged participation in the research process by a significant number of staff (22 per cent) who might not otherwise have become involved.

Despite this focus on clinical research and the various models and recommendations for accomplishing it, there is still little clinical research to support or direct most nursing practices. Additionally, several investigators have documented that even when well-replicated research findings exist, nurses rarely are aware of or utilize them in daily clinical practice (Ketefian, 1975; Kirchhoff, 1982; Stokes, 1981), nor do they appear to value research (Stokes, 1981). Kirchhoff (1983), however, questioned whether staff nurses should even be expected to use research findings and recommended that nurses with more preparation in research assume more responsibility for implementing research findings into practice. Although specific academic preparation or research skills were not prerequisites for participation in the research models just described, the majority of participants had master's degrees, were acquiring them, or had done additional coursework or independent study in research methods and statistics. This evidence, along with Kirchhoff's (1983) suggestions, has direct import for the research role of the CNS.

## CONCEPTUAL FRAMEWORK

This section is confined to literature that specifically addresses the research role of the CNS and forms the basic conceptual framework for such a role. Georgopoulous and Christman (1970) initially proposed research performance expectations in their historical paper on the role of the CNS. Two of the 14 core functions and activities in their model involved research: communication and interpretation of research findings to nursing staff and translation of scientific findings into practice, and investigation of specific problems of nursing practice. In a paper discussing problems inherent in doing clinical research, Jacox (1974) clearly implied that actual conduct of research was the role of the CNS.

In 1979, at a conference on the role of CNS, Hodgman presented her vision of specific research expectations for the CNS, which then formed the basis of her chapter in the first edition of this book (Hamric & Spross, 1983). She stated that each CNS's individual characteristics influenced whether, and how, a research component was operationalized. These characteristics include particular values and beliefs about nursing research; values about research techniques and methodology; preparation for engaging in research; and individual interests, motivation, and natural abilities. As a result, Hodgman believed that CNSs participated in a variety of research activities, which she classified empirically into three separate levels.

At the first and most basic level, CNSs should be able to interpret, evaluate, and communicate to nursing staff research findings pertinent to their own areas of specialization. Inherent in these steps is keeping up with current literature, judging reliability and validity of findings, identifying conceptual difficulties in the research, and drawing implications for patient care. Thus, this expectation requires the CNS to engage in research utilization and serve as a "communicator of nursing research" (Hodgman, 1983, p. 78).

In the second level of research activity, the CNS should be able to test and apply the findings of research produced by others. Hodgman envisioned this activity to include translation of research findings into protocols for innovations in nursing care. Because utilization projects are complex, the CNS would simultaneously function as a research collaborator (with other staff), research coordinator (in assuming leadership and administrative responsibilities), and research generator (of evaluation research). She considered this an advanced level of activity that also falls into the area of research utilization along with the basic level.

The third level of research activity included a variety of approaches depending upon the individual CNS's motivation, interests, abilities, and amount of knowledge about research. These approaches consisted of replicating the research of others, precepting students in research projects, generating original studies at all levels of inquiry, and collaborating with other nurses and physicians. Girouard (1983) described her experiences with research at this level.

Hodgman emphasized that research and research utilization were two different processes—a fact only recognized by nursing within the past 15 years—and proposed that the differences between the two were in part responsible for confusion about the research role of the CNS. She also declared that evaluation, communication, and utilization of new knowledge to improve patient care, rather than the actual discovery of new knowledge, should be the focus of both the CNS's education and practice, as this would ". . . allow the greatest number of clinical specialists to have the greatest impact on clinical practice through research activities" (Hodgman, 1983, p. 81).

In 1981, the American Nurses' Association published *Guidelines for the Investigative Functions of Nurses*. Of importance to the research component of the CNS role are the investigative functions for the nurse with a master's degree in nursing (Table 8–1). These go beyond research utilization at the basic level to include identification of researchable

**TABLE 8–1.  American Nurses' Association Guidelines
for the Investigative Functions of Nurses\***

*Master's Degree in Nursing*
Analyzes and reformulates nursing practice problems so that scientific knowledge and
scientific methods can be used to find solutions.

Enhances the quality and clinical relevance of nursing research by providing expertise
in clinical problems and by providing knowledge about the way in which these clinical
services are delivered.

Facilitates investigations of problems in clinical settings through such activities as
contributing to a climate supportive of investigative activities, collaborating with others
in investigations, and enhancing nursing's access to clients and data.

Conducts investigations for the purpose of monitoring the quality of the practice of
nursing in a clinical setting.

Assists others to apply scientific knowledge in nursing practice.

\*Adapted from the American Nurses' Association *Guidelines for the Investigative
Functions of Nurses,* 1981.

clinical problems, provision of consultation in the clinical site to researchers, facilitation of and collaboration in research activities, and
conduct of quality assurance investigations. Independent research or
generation of new knowledge for nursing practice were not recommended.

Fawcett (1985), however, suggested that nurses with master's degrees should generate clinical research, as well as disseminate and utilize
research findings. Oberst (1985) contended that the nursing profession
could not depend solely on generation of research by the still-small
cadre of doctorally prepared researchers but must enlist the participation of the CNS. The extent to which qualified CNSs became involved
in the research aspects of their role would ". . .directly affect the level
of research productivity in nursing" (Oberst, 1985, p. 46). Thus, she
recommended integration of the research and clinical practice roles for
the CNS; implicit in her view was the conduct of research.

Cronenwett (1986a) reported that, although many CNSs had research expectations built into their job descriptions, few felt successful
in achieving these expectations. She attributed the problem to general
confusion about the research role and what CNSs should or could be
held accountable for. Before the actual conduct of research was assumed
as an appropriate activity, she recommended that an assessment be
made of the organization's readiness for and commitment to research,
as well as of the research competence and commitment of the CNS. If
the organization and/or particular CNS were not ready to conduct
research, efforts aimed at research facilitation, dissemination, or utilization might be more appropriate as well as attainable (Cronenwett,

1986b). In this way, realistic expectations for the research role of the CNS could be set and evaluated.

A realistic formulation of the CNS's research role today must take into account individual attitudes and values about research, interest in and commitment to research, educational preparation, job description, clinical setting, and administrative support for research. It is naive and unfair to expect that all CNSs will be interested *and* involved in research at the *same* level. Expanding upon the conceptual framework for the CNS research role just described, the authors propose three levels of involvement in research (Table 8–2). Each level is composed of specific research expectations and functions; at least one level will be commensurate with an individual CNS's personal and institutional characteristics. The first level should be the *minimum* expectation for the CNS's research involvement; however, for many CNSs it will be the only level at which they are involved in research, and this is both appropriate and sufficient. The second level involves activities that some CNSs might pursue after substantial post-master's experience in the clinical area, while the third level includes more advanced research functions. The different expectations and activities of each level represent more or less sophisticated use of the research and research utilization processes, but it is not necessary, and indeed not appropriate, for all CNSs to strive

**TABLE 8–2.  Levels of Research Involvement
for the Clinical Nurse Specialist**

**LEVEL 1**
1. Identifies nursing practice problems and translates them into research questions.
2. Enhances the clinical relevance and quality of research through collaboration with researchers.
3. Facilitates the research of nurses and others in the clinical setting.
4. Assists others to apply scientific knowledge in practice.

**LEVEL 2**
1. Conducts investigations to monitor or assess the quality of nursing practice in the clinical setting.
2. Conducts virtual replication studies of others' research.
3. Tests the research findings of others in the clinical setting and applies the findings when appropriate.
4. Participates in collaborative research, assuming responsibility for minor aspects of the research process.
5. Conducts single subject (case study) research.
6. Conducts research using secondary analysis.

**LEVEL 3**
1. Conducts independent nursing research.
2. Conducts constructive replication research.
3. Participates in collaborative research, assuming responsibility for major aspects of the research process.
4. Serves as a research preceptor or advisor for student or other researchers.
5. Seeks out sources of financial support for research and writes grant applications for such funds.

for the second or third levels. Additionally, the levels are not mutually exclusive; a CNS can be involved in one or more of them simultaneously.

## LEVELS OF RESEARCH INVOLVEMENT

### Level 1

A minimal research expectation of the CNS involves identification of nursing practice problems and formulation of research questions from these problems. Through practitioner and consultant roles, the CNS is in an ideal position to identify practice problems. Although problem identification leads to problem-solving behaviors, a routine activity of nurses, problem-solving is not synonymous with research. While similarities exist between the research and problem-solving processes, there are some key differences. Most importantly, problem-solving is specific to the situation in which it occurs; the results cannot be generalized because "neither the sampling methods used nor the theoretical basis reflect the universal nature of the problem being studied" (Phillips, 1986, p. 22).

Of all the clinical problems encountered by the CNS, which should be pursued with research? Fuller (1982) identified four characteristics of clinical problems that lead to good research studies:

> Each occurs frequently in a definable population of patients; the current way that the problem is being dealt with is unsatisfactory to patients and the professional staff; an index of the problem can be reliably measured and the proposed solution alters the patient care (Fuller, 1982, p. 60).

The CNS could engage in multiple activities to identify clinical problems appropriate for research. A log of consultations and clinical problems seen in patient interactions may be kept. Alternatively or additionally, staff nurses working with the clinical specialist's patient population could be asked about patient management problems. Assessments may be validated by reports of the same problem in the literature. When a specific problem is identified, current nursing actions and patient outcomes should be identified. This assumes that nursing actions have been uniform and that some measurable outcome exists. If these actions are unsatisfactory, alternative nursing actions may be identified on the basis of either theoretical rationale alone or in combination with some limited clinical experience described in the literature.

The next step is to transform the clinical problem into a research question. Fleming (1984) cited four characteristics of an appropriate research question. First, it is phrased in the form of a question showing a relationship between two or more variables. Second, the research question must be empirical and based on observable phenomena. Third, the research question must be free of value judgments; and finally, it clearly attempts to fill a gap in the knowledge of the topic under study. While many research questions may be generated by the CNS, assistance may be required depending upon the complexity of the problem identified. Sometimes formulation of a research question may indicate a need for further descriptive study of the area or for tool development in order to measure the outcomes of the nursing actions in question.

A second minimal expectation of the CNS, consistent with the ANA guidelines (1981), is to "enhance the quality and clinical relevance of nursing research." This involves collaboration between nurse clinicians and nurse researchers. Hinshaw and colleagues (1981) identified the complementary roles of these two groups in research:

> Clinicians will be vigilant about the usefulness of the question being researched and the relevancy of the data being collected. The researcher will make sure that the study is systematic and the data usable from a research point of view (Hinshaw, et al., 1981, p. 34).

The relevance of research conducted by faculty or nurse researchers with little patient contact is highly dependent upon their communication with CNSs or other expert clinicians (McClure, 1981). Traditionally, communication between researcher and clinician flows in only one direction—from researcher to clinician in the form of a written research report at the conclusion of a study (Phillips, 1986). The clinical relevance of nursing research is enhanced by two-way communication, when the CNS:

> . . . share(s) information with researchers about new nursing procedures, lab tests, disease conditions, or societal changes that are affecting health care and producing new dilemmas. Thus, they could inform their research colleagues about aspects of nursing care that are currently creating problems or suggest questions worthy of research (Bishop, 1981, p. 110).

This two-way communication can avoid what Mahoney (1978) has referred to as Type III error—the problem of having conducted the wrong experiment.

The most obvious sources for this collaboration are nurse researchers based in the CNS's own institution or faculty in an associated school of nursing. If these resources are not available, the CNS may solicit collaboration more creatively, looking to nurse and other researchers at outside institutions (based on geographic proximity and related research interests), or membership in either an institutional consortium or cooperative research group. Insecurity about one's research experience should not discourage this initiative as faculty discomfort with the clinical area and their need for clinical exposure have been well described (McClure, 1981).

A third basic expectation of the CNS research role is facilitation of nurses' and others' research in clinical settings, which may be accomplished through both participatory and collaborative roles. Shiplacoff (1981) defined participation as "taking part in the implementation of a research study" (p. 337), whereas collaboration denotes not only the quantitative effort but also a qualitative contribution, "sharing in the identification of a research problem, in the formulation of a research question, and in designing the study" (p. 337). The importance of the CNS's participation should not be negated. "Gatekeepers," or those who "grant" access to patients, are usually thought to be physicians and administrators. Nurses at many levels, however, may be equally or more important in granting such access (Kirchhoff & McGuire, 1985).

The CNS can facilitate clinical nursing research by verbally supporting nursing research to staff nurses, administrators, and physicians'; translating the research question into language understandable to the staff nurse and relevant to physicians and administrators; assisting the researcher(s) with entry into the clinical environment in a manner least disruptive to patient care routines; and assisting in data collection through either individual efforts or knowledge of routine nursing data collection, which could be utilized for research purposes.

The final basic expectation in fulfilling the research role is that the CNS assist others to apply scientific knowledge in nursing practice. While the research process was previously considered to be complete at the time of publication of findings, it now includes efforts aimed at use of results in practice (Kirchhoff, 1983), a concept called research utilization (Stetler, 1985). In order to effect the utilization of research findings in day-to-day nursing practice, the CNS must be able to "find the findings, find the good findings, and implement the good findings" (Diers, 1972).

To "find the findings," CNSs must be current in literature related to their specialty, including publications from both nursing and other disciplines. The periodic, systematic review of well-defined topics from the area of specialization may be facilitated by computer searches, which in many libraries can be generated on a regular basis and mailed to the practitioner. In order to "find the good findings," the CNS must be able to critically evaluate pertinent research studies, considering conceptual framework, study design, instrumentation and procedures, data analysis, and the applicability of the findings.

Following critical evaluation of research findings, implementation involves both dissemination of information and application of findings to practice. While the application of findings is designated a Level 2 activity, a basic expectation of Level 1 includes communication of findings. This may be accomplished within the CNS's institution through journal club participation, use of a newsletter, special or routine inservice programs, or by sharing research articles informally with other staff. The CNS can also disseminate research findings to a much broader audience by writing and publishing review articles in his or her area of expertise, as exemplified in Sheidler's (1987) paper describing new methods in analgesic delivery.

## Level 2

The second level of research activity involves both qualitative and quantitative participation in clinical nursing research, without primary responsibility for the entire research process. This level of involvement necessitates additional knowledge and skills beyond those required for Level 1 participation and is likely to require a larger time commitment. Concurrently, the potential impact of Level 2 activities on development of a scientific basis for nursing practice is greater than that of Level 1. Several different activities constitute Level 2 research involvement.

First, the CNS can conduct investigations to monitor the quality of nursing practices in a clinical setting, an activity identified by the ANA (1981) as appropriate for nurses with master's degrees. Such evaluation research is integrally linked to the CNS's role in research problem identification, since problems are derived from assessment of unsatisfactory outcomes resulting from current practice. Formulation of a research question depends upon the ability to measure outcomes; thus, the logical focus for evaluation research is on outcomes of nursing actions prescribed by the nursing policy and procedure manual. Since few nursing practice actions are based on well-designed (let alone replicated) clinical studies, the policy and procedure manual offers a plethora of evaluation research opportunities.

A related activity is the evaluation of products for patient care. This evaluation involves assessment of patient outcomes when the product is used (similar in methodology to evaluation research) and also assessment of potential risks of the product, nursing time involved in its usage, and comparative cost with other alternative products.

A second way in which the CNS may be involved in research is through replication of previously conducted studies. Among several types of replication studies (Haller & Reynolds, 1986), virtual replication is most appropriate for the CNS at this level. Also known as approximate or operational replication, virtual replication attempts to repeat the original study under similar conditions, following the methods as closely as possible. This strategy precludes the need for the CNS to determine the study design, measurement methods, and statistical procedures to be used. Mayer's (1987) replication study of cancer patients' and oncology nurses' perceptions of nurse caring behaviors is an example of virtual replication.

A third area of research involvement is through testing and application of others' research, a logical progression from Level 1 activities of finding and critically evaluating research studies in one's area of specialization. When evaluation of both original and replication research supports the need for changes in nursing practice, the CNS can initiate and direct this process. In introducing planned change, the CNS should use outcome evaluation measures after the application of findings to practice. Because research findings are never definitive or completely generalizable, the application of research findings should be approached as "research in action" (Stetler & Marram, 1976) or as "an innovation trial" (Horsley, et al., 1978).

A fourth avenue for participation in research is as a participant in a collaborative research effort. This activity may be classified as a Level 2 or 3 function, depending upon the level of participation. At Level 2, the CNS is involved in some, but not all, of the steps of the research process. Most commonly, the CNS will provide qualitative input into problem identification, development of the research question, and design of the study; quantitative input is provided through the collection of data. Other collaborators will be responsible for determining appropriate outcome measures, data analysis, interpretation, and publication (Lindeman, 1973; Krone & Loomis, 1982).

Two additional activities, although rarely used in nursing, are appropriate for Level 2 research involvement. The first is single subject or case study research (Holm, 1983; Meier & Pugh, 1986). Two approaches may be taken (Holm, 1983). The descriptive approach involves description and/or quantification of an individual's response to nonexperimental situations over time. Using this approach, the CNS may note unique or previously undescribed phenomena and generate questions for further study. An example is the initial identification of local toxicity caused by a specific chemotherapeutic agent at a prior venipuncture site (Johnston-Early & Cohen, 1981). The experimental approach may also be employed—baseline measures of a dependent variable are recorded, an experimental intervention is introduced, and the dependent variable is again measured. Single subject research may generate both valuable information and questions for further study.

Secondary data analysis has also rarely been used in nursing, although the potential for its use is increasing with the greater availability of secondary data bases through computer technology (McArt &

McDougal, 1985) and other venues. Secondary data analysis "makes use of data gathered for the purposes of a primary research analysis (original research) but looks at questions not addressed by the original investigator, or addresses the same questions using different methods of analysis" (McArt & McDougal, 1985, p. 54). A recent example of this type of secondary analysis is Barbour and colleagues' (1986) paper on nonanalgesic methods of pain control used by cancer outpatients, which utilized data from a larger study of analgesic scheduling in cancer outpatients (McGuire, et al., 1987). If there is a good fit between available data and the new research question, then the time-consuming data collection process becomes unnecessary, and a cost-efficient method of research is the result.

The research activities described for Level 2 generally do not necessitate competitive grant-writing for funding. This further supports the appropriateness of these activities since inexperienced nurse researchers, particularly those without doctoral degrees, may have difficulty obtaining large grants (Stetler, 1983). The limited resources necessary for the types of studies described above may be available through the CNS's department, the hospital, in-hospital volunteer service groups, and perhaps a few outside organizations. Some studies may involve a parallel multidisciplinary approach in which the physician's grant may provide support for related nursing activities. For example, a physician who had a contract with a pharmaceutical company to study the effects of interferon in cancer patients was willing to purchase various instruments for a CNS's use in concurrently evaluating neurologic side effects of interferon (K. Harwood, personal communication, 1987).

## Level 3

The third level of research involvement can be viewed as the most advanced and deals primarily with the actual conduct of research in the clinical setting. Although the ANA (1981) did not recommend that master's-prepared nurses conduct research, it did state that "some nurses may have the capacities to perform investigative activities beyond their preparation." A small number of CNSs have been, are, or will be involved in the actual conduct of research; several different activities or functions can fulfill this Level 3 expectation.

First, the CNS can independently formulate a research question, then design, implement, and analyze a study to answer the question. An example of original research conducted by a CNS is Foltz's (1985) study of weight gain among patients with stage II breast cancer. Although the study was a doctoral dissertation, the research question emanated from her clinical practice and was conducted while she was employed as an oncology CNS.

An interesting variant of this approach can be original clinical nursing research conducted in tandem with medical cooperative clinical trials. Oberst (1980) described this as multidisciplinary research, in which several disciplines conduct parallel studies of a related topic. Hubbard and Donehower (1980) discussed the various opportunities open to nurses using such an approach in the cancer research setting. Harwood (personal communication, 1987), for example, is conducting a study within the Eastern Cooperative Oncology Group to examine the effects of duration of cooling on extravasation of a parenterally administered and locally toxic chemotherapy. The parallel medical studies are examining the responses of various tumors to the chemotherapy. Harwood's research question, design, and implementation are original; the patients, however, are obtained through the medical clinical trials. It should be noted that, although Harwood's research is a collaborative venture with other nurse colleagues, this type of study can be done by the CNS alone. The key point is that the CNS is responsible for conceiving and carrying out the study, although consultation with methodologists, statisticians, clinicians, and others is appropriate and most likely necessary.

A second way in which the CNS may be involved in the conduct of research is through replication of research previously performed by others. In this third level of involvement, however, the CNS does not conduct a virtual replication as in Level 2 but rather modifies the research to fit the setting, thus requiring some original contribution. Haller and Reynolds (1986) described various strategies for replicating the studies of others, including constructive methods that use new methodologic and measurement approaches to the same research question. Replication research has been neglected in nursing for a variety of reasons (Reynolds & Haller, 1986), and this neglect is a significant obstacle to research utilization. In a review of 145 research articles published in nursing research journals over an 18-month period, Fawcett (1982) reported that only five replication studies were found. Thus, the conduct of all types of replication studies is an important and valuable mode of research involvement for the CNS.

The third major way the CNS can conduct research is to function as a member of a collaborative research group. Such groups can be nursing or interdisciplinary (Oberst, 1980). In this approach, the research question and design, implementation, and analysis are undertaken by the entire group. Individual members may participate in all or in selected steps of the research process; the key difference between this level and Level 2 is that the CNS participates in several *major* aspects of the process, such as formulation of the research question, overall design, data analysis and interpretation, or writing up the findings. The literature abounds with papers describing various forms of collaborative research, including CNSs, other clinicians, a graduate student, and a pharmacist (Hagle, et al., 1987); clinicians, faculty, and non-nurse researchers (Bergstrom, et al., 1984); clinicians within a medical cooperative clinical trial group (Scogna, 1981); clinicians and outside researchers (Bishop, 1981; Krone & Loomis, 1982; Loomis & Krone, 1980); and clinicians, administrators, and researchers within one institution (Hinshaw, et al., 1981). Advantages and disadvantages of collaborative research are also discussed; the CNS who is interested in a collaborative endeavor would be well-advised to read the pertinent papers.

The fourth way in which a CNS can be involved in the conduct of research is as an advisor or preceptor to someone who is designing or actually conducting research. For example, a CNS who is both a faculty member at a school of nursing and a clinician in an agency may be responsible for helping a graduate student design and carry out a research project to meet graduate program requirements. In another situation, a CNS in an agency may advise an outside researcher or doctoral student who wishes to carry out a study in that agency. Finally, a CNS who is already engaged in a research endeavor might include a graduate student in various aspects of the study, functioning as a preceptor by guiding the student through selected components of the research process.

Finally, a fifth function of the CNS conducting research is seeking out, applying for, and obtaining funding. This function was discussed in the second level of research involvement; the difference at the third level, however, is that the CNS is seeking funds for original, formal research rather than for tandem, quality assurance, or virtual replication research. The function may be carried out in individual or collaborative research efforts, both directly (as a principal investigator or co-investigator) and indirectly (as an advisor or consultant). There are many sources of funding for research, including private and public organizations (Lawson, 1986). Writing an application for such awards can range from a simple one-page abstract to a lengthy and complex document with extensive budget justifications. Several authors have described this process (DeBakey, 1976; Eaves, 1973; Gortner & Kayser-Jones, 1984).

In summary, it is obvious from the preceding discussion of Levels 1 through 3 that many viable alternatives exist for the CNS to become involved in research, thus fulfilling the research component of the overall CNS role. As alluded to earlier, each CNS has a different configuration of characteristics that will contribute to research interest, commitment, and involvement. These many factors are addressed below.

# FACTORS CONTRIBUTING TO RESEARCH INVOLVEMENT

A number of characteristics, or factors, are absolutely essential for involvement in research, while others are helpful but certainly not essential. All of these may be present in greater or lesser quantities; some may not be present at all. These factors can be dichotomized into two general categories—*internal* (personal) factors such as attitudes, beliefs, values, knowledge, and skills; and *external* (environmental) factors such as administrative and organizational support, financial support, and professional affiliations.

## Internal Factors

Essential internal factors fall into the two broad categories of values, attitudes, and beliefs; and knowledge and skills (Table 8–3). How these internal characteristics manifest themselves in the individual CNS will influence the level of research involvement exhibited. Self-assessment in these areas will guide the CNS in determining an appropriate level of research involvement as well as areas in which further development is needed.

**TABLE 8–3.   Internal Factors Necessary for Research Involvement**

*Values, Attitudes, and Beliefs*
• Personal commitment to research involvement based on value of nursing research.
• Intellectual curiosity, creativity, independence, tolerance for error and uncertainty, minimal discomfort with not knowing everything.
• Personal belief that research involvement is an expected and legitimate role for the CNS.

*Knowledge and Skills*
• Clinical expertise.
• Knowledge of basic research designs, measurement techniques, and statistical methods.
• Knowledge of research utilization models.
• Ability to identify and secure appropriate consultants.
• Interpersonal skills.
• Critical thinking skills and conceptual ability to deal with abstractions and theoretical formulations.
• Writing skills.
• Knowledge of ethical issues and guidelines and regulations for clinical research activity.

### Values, Attitudes, and Beliefs

With several functions competing for time in the overall CNS role, freeing up time for research activities requires a strong personal commitment to clinical nursing research. Eisz (1984) recommended that the CNS examine personal values regarding a role in research and assess current activities as they relate to those expressed values. When activity level does not represent a commitment consistent with expressed values, Eisz (1985) recommended activities to strengthen one's individual commitment, such as spending time with research role models and others with positive research attitudes, strengthening one's knowledge and skills to avoid fear-related procrastination, and considering and recording how one's research activities might help meet personal career goals.

Several of the requisites cited in the literature for successful research contribution relate to attitude. Schlotfeldt (1974) described intellectual curiosity and creativity as essential for research involvement. The necessity of this type of attitude has also been recognized by Larson (1978) who described the "inquisitive nurse" and Oberst (1985) who listed as essential to research productivity the characteristics of creativity and a lively curiosity. Oberst (1985) also described other essential attitudes such as independence, tolerance for error and uncertainty, and minimal discomfort with not knowing everything.

Finally, what the individual CNS believes are the institution's research expectations will influence the level of research involvement. Girouard (1983) said, "We CNS's believe that we are expected to do research. How could we possibly believe otherwise?" (p. 83). However, in evaluating coworkers' perceptions of the CNS role, Sisson (1987) discovered that the research role of the CNS in an institution with 16 CNSs was not identified by nursing directors, head nurses, staff nurses, or physicians (N = 120). Alternatively, Tarsitano and colleagues (1986) found that nurse administrators placed a higher value on research than did CNSs. The CNS's belief that research involvement is a legitimate and expected role (in addition to the nurse administrator's beliefs) is a basic requirement to operationalizing that role amidst many competing CNS activities.

### Knowledge and Skills

Absolutely essential to the CNS research role at any level is clinical expertise (Girouard, 1983; Hamric & Spross, 1983; Schlotfeldt, 1974; Oberst, 1985). The knowledge level of research and statistics, however, is highly variable among CNSs and will help determine the CNS's level of research involvement. Some research and statistics background is necessary for the CNS to fulfill Level 1 expectations and should also be an expectation of graduate programs. Problem identification will evolve from the CNS's clinical expertise, but transformation of the problem into a research question will necessitate that the CNS be familiar with and able to appropriately select from alternative research designs, measurement techniques, and basic statistical methods. A good resource to review appropriate usage of these areas is the text *Reading Statistics and Research* (Huck, et al., 1974). Other research texts (Abdellah & Levine, 1986; Polit & Hungler, 1987) are helpful in this regard, especially for Level 2 and 3 activities. Critique of others' research (Level 1) requires a similar level of knowledge and an ability to determine a study's relevance for practice (Fleming & Hayter, 1974; Jacox & Prescott, 1978).

The application portion (Level 2) of the research utilization process requires additional knowledge. Nurses advocating a change in practice based on research findings assume a professional responsibility to be knowledgeable not only about the practice area and research process but also about criteria for applying research findings to practice (Stetler, 1983). The reader is referred to the following models for evaluating and applying nursing research findings to practice: Haller, et al., 1979; Horsley, et al., 1983; Phillips, 1986; Stetler & Marram, 1976; and Tanner, 1987. By reviewing this material in depth, the CNS will gain both expertise and confidence in the application of research findings.

While Level 1 research involvement requires basic, textbook knowledge of the research process and statistical procedures, Levels 2 and 3 require some practical knowledge and skills generally acquired through experience. It is not until one has actually been involved in clinical research that one can estimate the time involved in data collection, both for investigators and patients, or how long it will take to gather the needed number of subjects. The novice cannot anticipate and plan for the multiplicity of problems and complications that can arise in the course of clinical research. The CNS who conducted thesis research during the master's program will have fundamental experience with these issues. Alternatively, CNSs who have implemented medical research or collaborative nursing research may have gained experience and expertise that would enhance more independent research activities (Hubbard & Donehower, 1980).

In considering the knowledge and skills necessary for the CNS's research involvement, the frequent lack of congruency between education at the master's level and subsequent role expectations must be addressed. Although research utilization is considered an appropriate activity for master's-prepared nurses, an informal survey of several such nurses (K. Harwood, personal communication, 1987) revealed that neither formal critiquing methods nor models of research utilization were included in their curricula. The absence of this content did not indicate inattention to research, however, as their curricula focused on preparing them to perform all the steps of a controlled experiment.

Ackerman (1976) questioned the legitimacy of teaching research in master's degree programs for the purposes of preparing graduates to conduct research for theses, doctoral dissertations, or postgraduate work. She declared that the only legitimate expectation was to prepare the nurse as a research consumer. Hodgman (1983) seconded this opinion when she wrote ". . . the emphasis in both the research training and research practice of clinical specialists needs to be on the evaluation, communication, and utilization of new knowledge to improve practice rather than the discovery of new knowledge . . ." (p. 81). Since the ANA (1981) did not cite the conduct of original research as a research function of the master's-prepared nurse, the authors agree that, with rare exceptions, research curricula in graduate programs should focus on the evaluation and utilization of research. Congruency between the academic and service environments regarding research preparation and expectations of the CNS would help relieve conflict in this area and provide direction for research curricula in master's degree programs. In the interim, the nurse administrator's expectations for the CNS's research activities must be considered in the context of the CNS's educational preparation and postgraduate training and experience.

The actual implementation of a clinical study, whether evaluation research, product evaluation, replication, or original research, requires knowledge and skills beyond those needed for Levels 1 and 2, including some related to research design and statistical analysis. Just as important for the CNS as pursuing higher level knowledge is the ability to identify and secure appropriate consultants (Todd & Gortner, 1982; Oberst, 1985) who may be experts in research design, measurement, and/or statistics. Gaining access to these consultants has been described through collaborative efforts with academic researchers (Bishop, 1981; Hinshaw, et al., 1981) or through medical cooperative research groups (Scogna, 1981).

Because clinical nursing research is generally conducted in the "real world" as opposed to an isolated laboratory setting, interpersonal skills are critical to the success of the CNS-researcher. Resistance to study approval and patient access may come from administrators, physicians, staff nurses, and others (Brooten, 1984; Girouard, 1983; Kirchhoff & McGuire, 1985; Lasoff, 1986; Oberst, 1980; Todd & Gortner, 1982). Brooten (1984) detailed "stumbling through" approval of her first clinical research study with the subsequent recommendation to the nurse-researcher to pay close attention to possible resisters, in both medicine and nursing, who may limit access to the patient population and to solicit their suggestions and comments. Staff assistance with data collection may be enhanced by sensitivity to the routines of the nursing unit and the impact of the research study on these routines. In addition to nursing and medical staff, the research may also have an impact on the workload of medical records staff, laboratory staff, secretarial staff, and others. Sensitivity to their routines and other job requirements is essential, as are acknowledgement and appreciation of their involvement. A basket of fruit or box of doughnuts has also been described to facilitate the conduct of clinical research (Brooten, 1984)!

Critical thinking skills and problem-solving ability, while not specific to the research process, are requisites for research activities (Oberst, 1985). Beyond the problem-solving skills needed for the advanced practice role, the CNS must possess conceptual ability to deal with not only the concrete evidence but also the abstractions and theoretical formulations associated with research (Schlotfeldt, 1984).

Another skill that will influence the CNS's research involvement is the ability to write both clearly and concisely. Following the development of a research question, a written research proposal must be generated. In most cases, a clinical nursing research proposal would be reviewed by nursing administrators and/or a nursing research committee, as well as by the institutional review board. Approval is dependent not only upon the merit of the study but also upon the ability of the investigator to convey that merit using a clear, scientific approach without the use of meaningless nursing jargon.

Furthermore, when one examines the norms of researchers and practitioners regarding writing for publication, there is a major difference between the two (Batey, 1977). The norm in the research world is that a study is not completed until it is published, a norm not generally shared by practitioners. To function at Level 2 or 3, the CNS must possess the ability and willingness to summarize the study in publishable form. Many helpful resources exist to aid the CNS in improving writing skills and selecting a journal (DeBakey, 1972, 1976; Johnson, 1982; Kolin & Kolin, 1980). Additionally, some institutions and organizations such as Sigma Theta Tau may sponsor inservice programs or courses on the writing process.

Finally, to function at any level of research involvement, the CNS must understand the need for protection of human subjects, the federal regulations designed to ensure this protection, and the potential conflict between researcher and caregiver roles (Kaempfer, 1982). Ethical considerations are inherent in every clinical research study. Research arises from the "need to solve a problem, answer a question, or resolve a conflict" (Larson, 1978, p. 10), but this need must be balanced with those of the specific individual participating in the study. When preparing for involvement in clinical research, the CNS should review the ANA guidelines for nurses in research (ANA, 1986). If the CNS is responsible for obtaining consent from research subjects, familiarity with the federal regulations for informed consent by research subjects is essential (Levine, 1981; United States Department of Health and Human Services, 1983). The CNS must also recognize the essentially different responsibilities of the clinical and investigative roles (Batey, 1977), a potential conflict discussed later in the obstacles section. The patient may not understand the research role of the nurse, and if he has entrusted himself to the nurse for care and not for research, autonomy and self-determination may be at risk (Todd & Gortner, 1982). Additionally, the patient may expect that data collected for research purposes will be used immediately for patient care purposes. In some study designs, this would preclude evaluation of outcomes. Finally, patients may also fear that refusal to participate in research may adversely affect their care (Davis, 1982). It is incumbent upon the CNS to provide the patient with a clear explanation of what is involved in the research.

## External Factors

External factors fall into the broad categories of administrative support, organizational (institutional) support, financial support, and professional affiliations (Table 8–4). Multiple types of support exist within these broad categories of which varying amounts are needed depending upon the levels of research involvement.

### Administrative Support

Administrative support is required for any level of research involvement. There are many types of administrative support, most of which should emanate from the institution's goals and philosophy. The first requisite is that the importance of nursing research to both quality and cost of patient care must be recognized by the overall organization and the nursing department (Baker, 1978; Conway, 1978; Dean, 1982; Fagin, 1982; Moore, 1980). The role of nurse administrators in, and various strategies for, the implemention of nursing research in the clinical setting have been described (AHA, 1985; American Society for Nursing Service Administrators, 1982; Davis, 1981; Padilla, 1979). Clear, unequivocal administrative support for nursing research activities within the department sends the message to all staff that research is

**TABLE 8–4.   External Factors Necessary for Research Involvement**

*Administrative Support*
Departmental support of research through goals and philosophy
Integration of research role in position description
Release or compensatory time
Physical/technical resources (office, duplication, secretarial and technical,
   supplies and equipment)
Reward system
Books and journals
Formal nursing research program

*Organizational Support*
Incorporation of research into institutional goals and philosophy
Comprehensive library
Computer facilities
Consultants

*Financial Support*
Departmental
Institutional
Private funding
Public funding
Industry funding

*Professional Affiliations*
Networking (internal/external, formal/informal, nursing/other)
Professional organizations (publications, access to research)

valued as an essential part of nursing practice and is a valid activity. Some nursing administrators may not yet value or support research activity by CNSs or other staff. In such cases, the CNS must use change agent skills to help facilitate awareness of the need for research-based nursing practice and research activities within the department.

With respect to integrating research into practice, the next important factor is that the CNS's position description include the research component of the role (Donoghue & Spross, 1985). The specific research functions or activities can be mutually determined by the CNS and nurse administrator using as guides the levels of research involvement, available institutional resources, departmental goals, and the CNS's interests, skills, and commitment. For example, one position description for a Veterans Administration CNS included identifying researchable clinical problems; initiating or participating in nursing research activities; identifying, interpreting, and implementing research findings; and maintaining current knowledge of research in nursing and health care (Norby, 1986). The inclusion of the research role in the position description legitimizes research activities, makes them an expectation, and theoretically provides a basis for evaluating this aspect of the CNS's role. Whether these activities are actually engaged in depends upon other important administrative factors.

Time is the third important factor related to research involvement, as release time from clinical activities or designated research time is essential (Davis, 1981; Eisz, 1986; Larson, 1981; Oberst, 1980; Varricchio & Mikos, 1987). If research is an expectation in the CNS's position description, then time should be designated for related activities. A minimal amount could be 4 hours a week, or 10 per cent of the CNS's time (M. Hagle, personal communication, 1987) for Level 1 activities. Time required for Level 2 and 3 activities could be greater, perhaps 20 to 30 per cent respectively, but obviously would depend upon specific research activities of the individual CNS. Research time should be discussed when the CNS and nurse administrator write the position description. Whether the research time is "release" time, compensatory time, or some other arrangement is not as important as the fact that formal research time is negotiated and agreed upon in advance.

A fourth important factor involves a variety of physical and technical resources that are needed for all levels of research involvement (Dean, 1982; Varricchio & Mikos, 1987). Personal office space is important to the CNS for many reasons, including research activity. It is unrealistic to expect any research involvement when the basics of a desk and chair are not available for regular use. Duplication services are necessary as CNSs seek out and obtain research reports in their specialty, conduct literature reviews, and prepare materials for dissemination to nursing colleagues. Secretarial and other forms of technical assistance are needed for development of bibliographies; general correspondence; preparation of materials for inservice programs, outside presentations, or other methods of disseminating research findings; preparation of research proposals; and preparation of abstracts, manuscripts, or other written materials. Finally, supplies and equipment such as paper, stationery, stamps, audiovisual materials, computers, typewriters, and overhead and slide projectors are needed. All of these resources may not be available in the nursing department, but various arrangements can be made with other departments for their provision in exchange for fees or services such as inservice programs or consultation (O'Connor & Malone, 1983; see also Chapter 19).

A fifth important factor that facilitates research involvement is a reward system within the nursing department. Even when such involvement is an expectation and in theory should occur automatically, provision of a variety of rewards for research activities enhances participation. Dean (1982) recommended that rewards be actual, overt, and recognized. Publicity about CNSs' research involvement (at whatever level) in departmental or institutional newsletters is one form of recognition. Additionally, this method informs other health disciplines about nursing research, an important goal in enhancing the image of nurses. Other departmental mechanisms such as nursing grand rounds, poster sessions during Nurses' Week, or annual research conferences provide additional showcases for CNSs who have been involved in research. Presentations at these affairs do not have to be reports of completed or even ongoing research but can be reviews of the literature, clinical papers, or other means to disseminate research findings to nursing staff.

Paid leave and partial or full travel funding to attend research or clinical conferences demonstrate the department's commitment to research (Davis, 1981), both internally as well as externally. Such support is critical when the CNS attends a meeting to present a research-related paper, but it is also quite important when attendance will allow oral presentations in other aspects of the conference program (i.e., instructional sessions, symposia) or will provide opportunities for continuing education and professional networking. In many institutions, a reward system may be in place; if it is not, the CNS may again need to use change agent skills to help develop such a system.

A sixth way in which nursing administration can support research involvement is by providing journals and books that facilitate the expected research activities of the CNS. For example, books on the utilization of research findings in clinical practice (Horsley, et al., 1983; Lieske, 1986; Phillips, 1986) would be helpful for Level 1 activities, while books on the conduct of evaluation studies (Rezler & Stevens, 1978; Weiss, 1972), the research process (Abdellah & Levine, 1986; Polit & Hungler, 1987), and the instruments for use in clinical research (Frank-Stromborg, 1988) would help with Level 2 and 3 activities. Similarly, subscriptions to *Nursing Research, Research in Nursing and Health, Western Journal of Nursing Research, Journal of Nursing Administration, Research Review, Journal of Professional Nursing,* and *Clinical Nurse Specialist,* among others, would be valuable. The availability of such publications is important in the absence of a readily accessible library, especially since lack of access to research findings can interfere with applying them to practice (Miller & Messenger, 1978).

A seventh and final way in which nursing administration can support CNSs' research involvement is through the development of a formal nursing research program. Many such programs have been instituted in hospitals throughout the country, with varying goals and organizational structures. There are clearly many research-related roles the CNS can play in formal nursing research programs. Space limitations preclude any discussion of these programs, but the interested reader is referred to the extensive literature on the subject (AHA, 1985; Chance & Hinshaw, 1980; Davis, 1981; Hoare & Earenfight, 1986; Lieske, 1986; Lindeman, 1973; Marchette, 1985; Padilla, 1979; Stetler, 1984; Zalar, et al., 1985).

### Organization Support

As stated earlier, organizational support for research in terms of the institution's goals and philosophy is required in order for nursing administrative support to be available. The inclusion of a nurse on an institution's human subjects review board also indicates support for nursing research (Cronenwett, 1986b). However, additional organization factors must be present for meaningful research involvement to be a reality.

Access to a library with a comprehensive and current collection of books and journals is critical to any level of research involvement. Through the library, the CNS can also gain access to extensive computer data bases from the National Library of Medicine (Sparks, 1984) or other organizations or to unavailable documents through interlibrary loan.

Computer facilities are invaluable aids to CNSs engaged in all levels of research involvement, particularly Levels 2 and 3. Beyond simple word processing, computers are useful and, in many circumstances, necessary for entering, storing, and analyzing data from all sorts of nursing studies. Competent consultation and/or instruction is essential for users of computer hardware and software.

A third important organizational factor that is particularly germane to research involvement at Levels 2 and 3 is availability of and access to consultants for design, methodologic, and statistical aspects of a proposed nursing study. It is unrealistic to expect that an individual can design, implement, and complete a study without such consultation.

If these three types of organizational support are lacking, various solutions may be available depending upon the nature of the CNS's institution. In a university setting, there may be schools of nursing, public health, or medicine with computer facilities, as well as faculty who are willing to consult with clinical staff. Similarly, institutions that affiliate with universities may have access to these resources. In smaller organizations, reciprocal arrangements might be worked out with local universities in exchange for use of the institution as a clinical practice site for nursing or medical students. Additionally, access to computers might be obtained through contractual arrangements. Finally, in some areas, independent consultants or computer facilities might be available on a fee-for-service basis.

### Financial Support

The administrative and organizational resources discussed above obviously represent substantial although indirect financial support for

CNS's involvement in research at all three levels. In Levels 2 and 3, however, there can be a need for direct financial support.

Research of any kind can rarely be performed without some costs, and a careful analysis must be made of the potential expenses before starting (Lawson, 1986). For some studies, necessary supplies, equipment, or personnel needs may go beyond what the institution already has available or can reasonably support. The use of institutional or departmental "seed" monies to fund some of these expenditures is a possible solution. In other circumstances, equipment or supplies may be borrowed from other departments, or exchanged for certain services. When departmental or institutional resources have been exhausted, the CNS may have to seek funding from outside sources (Hagle, et al., 1987).

A myriad of funding sources, both private and public, are available for research. Lawson (1986) discussed these sources and how to identify them in a comprehensive review of funding for research. Many such organizations encourage research applications from master's-prepared nurses, for example, the American Heart Association (D. Becker, personal communication, 1987) or the Competitive Extramural Grants Program of the American Nurses' Foundation. Nursing specialty groups such as the Oncology Nursing Society or the Association of Critical Care Nurses have competitive funding mechanisms for members who wish to conduct research. Additionally, many local chapters of Sigma Theta Tau, the international nursing honor society, have funds earmarked for research which are awarded on a competitive and usually annual basis.

Additional sources of funding for research only recently explored by nurses are pharmaceutical and hospital supply corporations. Studies of specific products, bactericidal soaps or sterile dressings for example, might be supported by the manufacturers. Some firms might commit monies to a study of a treatment technique or intervention related to their products. For example, a manufacturer of a narcotic analgesic may fund a study of several analgesics (V. Sheidler, personal communication, 1987).

The sources of funding cited here represent only a smattering of those potentially available. Since a discussion of the grant writing process is beyond the scope of the chapter, the interested reader is referred elsewhere (DeBakey, 1976; Gortner & Kayser-Jones, 1984).

## Professional Affiliations

Affiliation with nurses, members of other health care disciplines, and research experts is extremely important in research involvement.

The purposes of networking include sharing resources, clarifying practice standards and professional roles, enhancing professional growth and development, and ensuring a forum for creativity (Hunt, 1986). Additionally, the benefits of networking are access to information and opportunities and establishment of mechanisms for feedback and referral.

Networking can be internal or external to the work setting (Hunt, 1986). Additionally, networking can be informal or formal, depending upon circumstances and goals. Informal networking is often used to exchange ideas and information and is the sort that frequently occurs at professional conferences. Formal networking involves a structured group that convenes to accomplish a definite goal. Some informal networking efforts may result in collaborative research among clinicians (Hagle, et al., 1987), thus fostering research involvement for CNSs and others.

While networking with individuals within the institution is essential to the CNS at all levels of research involvement, membership in various professional organizations offers many benefits to the CNS as well, including some with direct applicability to the research role. The opportunities for formal and informal networking are perhaps one of the most important benefits. This benefit is accrued through attendance at local, regional, and national meetings or conferences of organizations, and the friendships, professional contacts, colleagial relationships, and collaborative writing or research efforts that may develop.

Most organizations include a publication with membership, for example, the ANA Council of Nurse Researchers' *CNR*, the ANA Council of Clinical Nurse Specialists' *Momentum*, the Oncology Nursing Society's *Oncology Nursing Forum*, or the American Association of Critical Care Nurses' *Heart and Lung*. These publications serve a variety of functions related to research involvement, including sharing activities of members of the organization, announcing funding sources, discussing strategies for involvement in research activities, presenting review articles of a specific clinical area, and reporting the results of research.

The CNS may seek affiliations with a variety of health professionals outside the institution through external networking efforts. Some of the possibilities have been discussed previously, including identification of individuals who can collaborate in research, offer consultation for various aspects of the process, or provide access to libraries or other facilities.

Finally, a most important benefit of professional affiliations, whether obtained through membership in organizations or through internal or external networking, is access to current information in a particular research or clinical area. In this way, the CNS is exposed to a variety of sources that make keeping abreast of recent developments and research findings in the specialty area far easier, thus facilitating involvement in research at the chosen level.

## OBSTACLES TO RESEARCH INVOLVEMENT

Despite the presence of necessary internal and external factors for research involvement, there are several obstacles that can inhibit this process. These include lack of inter- and intraprofessional support, conflict between the clinician and researcher components of the CNS role, and difficulty balancing one's workload.

Lack of inter- and intraprofessional support refers to either absent or minimal support for research activities from colleagues outside of and within nursing, respectively. Forms of support include verbal and behavioral validation of the importance of research activities and provision of an environment conducive to such activities. Factors such as failure to recognize research as important or as part of the CNS role, insufficient understanding of or preparation for research, lack of visibility or accessibility of the researcher, language barriers between clinicians and researchers or between disciplines, and differing values and roles of researchers and clinicians have been offered as reasons for this problem (Batey, 1977; Davis, 1968, 1981; Kirchhoff, 1987; Sisson, 1987; Todd & Gortner, 1982; Varricchio & Mikos, 1987).

There are many ways to increase cooperation and support from colleagues. In some instances, educational efforts related to the purpose of and need for research involvement can be directed at those who have difficulty understanding or condoning it (Girouard, 1983). For research efforts at Levels 2 and 3, the establishment of credibility as a researcher (Girouard, 1983) and the development of a "research posture" (Davis, 1981) are extremely important. These goals can be achieved through a willingness to publicly present and defend one's activities at a variety of multidisciplinary meetings such as departmental physician committees, institutional review boards, and so on. Within the nursing department, it is helpful to study problems relevant to clinicians at all levels, to communicate all pertinent aspects of research activities including the findings, to encourage involvement wherever possible, to praise any efforts made to help, and to share information about the research process and amount of work involved in its successful completion (Bowie, 1980; Davis, 1981; Girouard, 1983; Lasoff, 1986).

Related to support for research involvement from professional colleagues is the second major obstacle—conflict between the clinician and researcher roles. This area has not been addressed at any length in the literature, although problems such as reluctance to approach patients for participation in studies (sometimes resulting in small samples), fear of imposing on colleagues by asking for help with workload, reluctance to make needs known to colleagues, and difficulty with objectivity can be found in a few reports (Davis, 1968, 1981; Hagle, et al., 1987; Larson, 1981; McHugh & Johnson, 1980). Batey (1977) attributed this role conflict to the very different role performance expectations, methods, knowledge, values, and norms held by researchers and practitioners.

Several avenues of action can help CNSs resolve this conflict. Strong administrative support and individual internalization of the research aspect of the CNS role are essential. If CNSs are committed to research, they will be better able to deal with individuals who demand time and do not recognize the value of their research activities. Additionally, Hagle, et al. (1987) recommended that clinicians involved in the actual conduct of research have some latitude and flexibility in scheduling both their time and their workload, thus decreasing conflicts related to patient care issues. McHugh and Johnson (1980) advised nurse researchers who are tempted to give patient care while conducting research to "exercise careful judgment and act so as to protect the client and at the same time not jeopardize the research unduly" (p. 356). Finally, Batey (1977) commented that nurses (as well as others) have created a mystique surrounding research that is "dysfunctional" to the profession. She urged better communication between researchers and clinicians, improved dissemination of findings, and more conscious consideration of the implications for practice.

The last area that can present an obstacle to research involvement is balancing one's workload in order to make time for research activities. Even when time is allotted for research in the CNS's position description, and despite the best intentions of the CNS, conflicting role responsibilities and unexpected clinical crises can intervene. Because research involvement is usually not viewed as immediate, it is often relegated to "tomorrow" or to one's private time (M. Hagle, personal communication, 1987).

To solve this persistent and insidious problem, the individual CNS will have to devise strategies to *make* time. Eisz (1986) offered six actions to help achieve this goal—create a research activity plan, publicize it, eliminate time wasters, evaluate competing job priorities, control procrastination, and practice time-effectiveness strategies daily. Similarly, Girouard (1983) wrote of the importance of setting priorities and scheduling activities in order to "remain goal-, rather than task-directed" (p. 86). She also recommended combining efforts to overcome time constraints. For example, a CNS who wanted to study patients' reactions to gastroscopy could work with staff nurses who wanted to develop an educational program to prepare patients for the procedure. Using this strategy, standards for care could be developed, helping the CNS meet the role expectation of expert clinician responsible for setting practice expectations. Additionally, the CNS could help the staff learn more about research and appreciate its usefulness, while enlisting their help as research assistants. Last, but not least, the staff could achieve their goals as well.

Careful appraisal of these obstacles and their potential impact on the research activities will help the individual CNS devise strategies for eliminating or minimizing them. This effort, in combination with the variety of internal and external factors necessary for research involvement, can result in the chosen level of involvement and fulfillment of the research aspect of the role.

## EVALUATION

Evaluation of the overall CNS role was discussed at length in the first edition of this book (Girouard & Spross, 1983; Hamric, 1983; Leibold, 1983) and is covered elsewhere in the present volume. Thus, there is no need to review or discuss the various conceptual frameworks for evaluation which could be applied to the research component of the CNS's role. Rather, a few very general ideas for application of these classic evaluative strategies to research involvement are offered below.

As mentioned previously, the CNS's position description should include a research component, with specific activities and functions. Given the conflicting role expectations of the CNS identified by Cronenwett (1986a), Harrell and McCulloch (1986), Sisson (1987), and Tarsitano, et al. (1986), it is imperative that the CNS and nurse administrator agree with what constitutes the research component of the role. Evaluation should then emanate from the specific research activities delineated in the CNS's position description.

Depending upon the level of the CNS's research involvement or combination of levels, different evaluation goals and methods can be devised. For example, in an institution that has many organizational barriers to research and in which even Level 1 activities would be difficult, structural evaluation could be used. The CNS could carry out some of the activities described by Cronenwett (1986b), such as serving on an institutional review board (IRB), developing or refining a process for screening research proposals, designing and developing proposals for commitment of resources to research, or building and maintaining contacts with local nurse researchers. These activities could then be examined for their impact on the institution. Does the institution support a nurse member on the IRB? Is a workable process for reviewing and approving research proposals now in place? Can the department commit resources to research, and if so, what are they and how will they be accomplished? Structural evaluation is a helpful starting point for any CNS wishing to begin research activity, as it evaluates whether needed supports are in place. An additional structural evaluation method suggested by Hamric (1985) relates to the CNS's use of time. Records of time spent on research activity in relation to the time allotted in the position description could be kept, with adjustments made as needed.

Process evaluation could be applied to the CNS's performance of various activities within the research role. Level 1 research involvement, for example, consists of identifying nursing practice problems and translating them into research questions, collaborating with researchers, facilitating the research of others, and applying research findings to clinical practice. These activities could be evaluated through peer review of appropriateness of the research question, feedback from team members regarding the CNS's facilitation skills, or CNS self-evaluation and concomitant staff evaluation of success with application of findings. These same methods, which focus on the processes used by the CNS to accomplish research, could also be used to evaluate Level 2 and 3 research involvement.

Finally, the evaluation of outcomes related to research activities is a possibility, although probably more difficult than structural or process evaluation. As an example, a CNS could conduct a quality assurance study of a particular nursing practice and evaluate selected patient care outcomes, including cost data in this time of shrinking resources. The nurse administrator could then, in turn, evaluate the impact the study has had on costs of patient care or other parameters. In another example, patients' responses to a specific innovation in nursing care initiated by the CNS could be evaluated.

In summary, deliberate and well-planned evaluation of the research component of the CNS role is extremely important. The research role that is proposed in this chapter is multifaceted yet realistic and should lend itself well to evaluation. Participation at any level of research involvement will enable the CNS to contribute substantially to the exciting and continually expanding body of knowledge which underlies nursing practice, while fulfilling one of the critical components of the role of clinical nurse specialist.

### Acknowledgments

The authors thank Mary E. Hagle, R.N., M.S., for her thoughtful comments on the research role of the CNS; and Linda M. Arenth, R.N., M.S., and Constance Ziegfeld, R.N., M.S., for their review of the manuscript.

## References

Abdellah, F.G., & Levine, E.: Better Patient Care Through Nursing Research (3rd ed). New York, Macmillan, 1986.

Ackerman, W.B.: The place of research in the master's program. Nurs Outlook 24(12):754–758, 1976.

American Hospital Association: Strategies: Integration of nursing research into the practice setting. In: Nurse Executive Management Strategies. Chicago, author, 1985.

American Nurses' Association: 111. Specialization in nursing practice. In: Nursing: A Social Policy Statement. Kansas City, author, 1980a, pp. 21–30.

American Nurses' Association: Standards for Nursing Services. Kansas City, author, 1973.

American Nurses' Association Cabinet on Nursing Research. Directions for Nursing Research: Toward the Twenty-First Century. Kansas City, American Nurses' Association, 1985.

American Nurses' Association Commission on Nursing Research: Generating a scientific basis for nursing practice: Research priorities for the 1980s. Nurs Res 29(4):219, 1980b.

American Nurses' Association Commission on Nursing Research: Guidelines for the Investigative Function of Nurses. Kansas City, American Nurses' Association, 1981.

American Nurses' Association Commission on Nursing Research: Human Rights Guidelines for Nurses in Clinical and Other Research. Kansas City, American Nurses' Association, 1986.

American Nurses' Association Council of Clinical Nurse Specialists: The Role of the Clinical Nurse Specialist. Kansas City, American Nurses' Association, 1986.

American Society for Nursing Service Administrators: The Role of the Nursing Service Administrator in Nursing Research. Informational bulletin. Chicago, American Hospital Association, 1982.

Baker, V.E.: Nursing administration and research. Nurs Leadership 1(1):5–9, 1978.

Barbour, L.A., McGuire, D.B., and Kirchhoff, K.T.: Nonanalgesic methods of pain control used by cancer outpatients. Oncol Nurs Forum 13(6):56–60, 1986.

Batey, M.V.: Nursing research: Conflict or congruence with nursing service goals? In: Conflict Management: Flight, Fight, Negotiate? New York, National League for Nursing, 1977, pp. 7–13.

Benner, P.: Uncovering the knowledge embedded in clinical practice. Image 15(2):36–41, 1983

Benner, P.: The oncology clinical nursing specialist: An expert coach. Oncol Nurs Forum 12(2):40–44, 1985.

Bergstrom, N., Hansen, B.C., Grant, M., et al.: Collaborative nursing research: Anatomy of a successful consortium. Nurs Res 33(1):20–25, 1984.

Bishop, B.E.: A case for collaboration. Nurs Outlook 29(2):110–111, 1981.

Bowie, R.B.: Research responsibilities of the clinical nurse. AORN J 31(2):238–241, 1980.

Brooten, D.E.: Making it in paradise. Nurs Res 33(6):318, 1984 (editorial).

Chance, H.C., & Hinshaw, A.S.: Strategies for initiating a research program. J Nurs Admin 10(3):32–39, 1980.

Colton, M.R.: Research: Will it help us come to age as a profession? Supervisor Nurse 11(12):12–14, 1980.

Conway, M.E.: Clinical research: Instrument for change. J Nurs Admin 8(12):25–32, 1978.

Cronenwett, L.R.: The research role of the clinical nurse specialist. J Nurs Admin 16(4):10–11, 1986a.

Cronenwett, L.R.: Research contributions of clinical nurse specialists. J Nurs Admin 16(6):6–7, 1986b.

Davis, A.J.: Ethical issues in nursing research. West J Nurs Res 4(1):111–112, 1982.

Davis, M.Z.: Some problems to identify in becoming a nurse researcher. Nurs Res 17(2):166–168, 1968.

Davis, M.Z.: Promoting nursing research in the clinical setting. J Nurs Admin 11(3):22–27, 1981.

DeBakey, S.: Basic principles of good writing. AORN J 15(6):69–72, 1972.

DeBakey, S.: The persuasive proposal. J Tech Writ Commun 6(1):5–25, 1976.

Dean, P.G.: Facilitating research. Nurs Management 13(5):23–24, 1982.

Diers, D.: Clinical scholarship. Image 15(1):3, 1983a (editorial).

Diers, D.: Clinical scholarship II. Image 15(2):35, 1983b (editorial).

Diers, D.: Application of research to nursing practice. Image 5:7–11, 1972.

Donoghue, M., & Spross, J. (eds): Recommendations for administrative support of the oncology clinical nurse specialist. Oncol Nurs Forum 12(2):71–73, 1985.

Eaves, G.N.: The project-grant application of the National Institutes of Health. Fed Proc 32(5):1542–1550, 1973.

Eisz, M.K.: Freeing up time for nursing research. Part I: Making the commitment. Momentum 2(4):1–4, 1984.

Eisz, M.K.: Freeing up time for nursing research. Part II: Translating commitment to action. Momentum 3(1):1–4, 1985.

Eisz, M.K.: Freeing up time for nursing research. Part III: Time-effectiveness strategies. Momentum 4(1):2–3, 1986.

Ellis, R.: The nurse as investigator and member of the research team. Ann NY Acad Sci 169(2):435–441, 1970.

Fagin, C.M.: Nursing as an alternative to high-cost care. Am J Nurs 82(1):56–60, 1982.

Fawcett, J.: Utilization of nursing research findings. Image 14(2):57–59, 1982.

Fawcett, J.: A typology of nursing research activities according to educational preparation. J Prof Nurs 1(2):75–78, 1985.

Fleming, J.W.: Selecting a clinical nursing problem for research. Image 16(2):62–64, 1984.

Fleming, J.W., & Hayter, J.: Reading research reports critically. Nurs Outlook 22(3):172–175, 1974.

Foltz, A.T.: Weight gain among stage II breast cancer patients: A study of five factors. Oncol Nurs Forum 12(3):21–26, 1985.

Frank-Stromborg, M. (ed): Instruments for Clinical Nursing Research. East Norwalk, CT, Appleton & Lange, 1988.

Fuhs, M.F., & Moore, K.: Research program development in a tertiary care setting. Nurs Res 30(1):24–27, 1981.

Fuller, E.O.: Selecting a clinical nursing problem for research. Image 14(2):60–61, 1982.

Georgopoulous, B.S., & Christman, L.: The clinical nurse specialist: A role model. Am J Nurs 70(5):1030–1039, 1970.

Girouard, S.: Implementing the research role. In Hamric, A.B., and Spross, J. (eds): The Clinical Nurse Specialist in Theory and Practice. New York, Grune and Stratton, 1983, pp. 83–89.

Girouard, S., & Spross, J.: Evaluation of the CNS: Using an evaluation tool. In Hamric, A.B., and Spross, J. (eds): The Clinical Nurse Specialist in Theory and Practice. New York, Grune and Stratton, 1983. pp. 207–218.

Gortner, S.R.: Research for a practice profession. Nurs Res 24(3):193–197, 1975.

Gortner, S.R., & Kayser-Jones, J.: Research grant applications: What they should be. West J Nurs Res 6(4):459–462, 1984.

Hagle, M.E., Barbour, L., Flynn, B., et al.: Research collaboration among nurse clinicians. Oncol Nurs Forum 14(6):55–59, 1987.

Haller, K.B., & Reynolds, M.A.: Using research in practice. A case for replication—Part two. West J Nurs Res 8(2):249–252, 1986.

Haller, K.B., Reynolds, M.A., and Horsley, J.A.: Developing research-based innovation protocols: Process, criteria, and issues. Res Nurs Health 2:45–51, 1979.

Hamric, A.B.: A model for developing evaluation strategies. In Hamric, A.B., and Spross, J. (eds): The Clinical Nurse Specialist in Theory and Practice. New York, Grune and Stratton, 1983, pp. 187–206.

Hamric, A.B.: Clinical nurse specialist role evaluation. Oncol Nurs Forum 12(2):62–66, 1985.

Hamric, A.B., & Spross, J. (eds): The Clinical Nurse Specialist in Theory and Practice. New York, Grune and Stratton, 1983.

Harrell, J.S., & McCulloch, S.D.: The role of the clinical nurse specialist. J Nurs Admin 16(10):44–48, 1986.

Henderson, V.: Research in nursing practice—When? Nurs Res 4(3):99, 1956 (editorial).

Hinshaw, A.S., Chance, H.C., and Atwood, J.: Research in practice: A process of collaboration and negotiation. J Nurs Admin 11(2):33–38, 1981.

Hoare, K., & Earenfight, J.: Unit-based research in a service setting. J Nurs Admin 16(4):35–39, 1986.

Hodgman, E.C.: The CNS as researcher. In Hamric, A.B., and Spross, J. (eds): The Clinical Nurse Specialist in Theory and Practice. New York, Grune and Stratton, 1983, pp. 73–82.

Holm, K.: Single subject research. Nurs Res 32(4):253–255, 1983.

Horsley, J., Crane, J., and Bingle, J.: Research utilization as an organizational process. J Nurs Admin 8(7):4–6, 1978.

Horsley, J., Crane, J., Crabtree, M.K., et al.: Using Research to Improve Nursing Practice: A Guide (CURN Project). New York, Grune and Stratton, 1983.

Hubbard, S.M., & Donehower, M.G.: The nurse in a cancer research setting. Semin Oncol 7(1):9–17, 1980.

Huck, S., Cormier, W., and Bounds, W., Jr.: Reading Statistics and Research. New York, Harper & Row, 1974.

Hunt, V.: Networking for nursing research development. In Lieske, A.M. (ed): Clinical Nursing Research: A Guide to Undertaking and Using Research in Nursing Practice. Rockville, MD: Aspen, 1986, pp. 161–174.

Jacox, A.: Nursing research and the clinician. Nurs Outlook 22(6):382–385, 1974.

Jacox, A., & Prescott, P.: Determining a study's relevance for clinical practice. Am J Nurs 78(11):1882–1889, 1978.

Johnson, S.H.: Selecting a journal for your manuscript. Nurs Health Care 3(5):258–263, 1982.

Johnston-Early, A., & Cohen, M.H.: Mitomycin C-induced skin ulceration remote from infusion site. Cancer Treat Rep 65(5–6):529, 1981.

Kaempfer, S.H.: A care orientation to clinical nursing research. Oncol Nurs Forum 9(4):36–38, 1982.

Ketefian, S.: Application of selected nursing research findings into nursing practice: A pilot study. Nurs Res 24(2):89–92, 1975.

Kirchhoff, K.T.: A diffusion survey of coronary precautions. Nurs Res 31(4):196–201, 1982.

Kirchhoff, K.T.: Using research in practice: Should staff nurses be expected to use research? West J Nurs Res 5(3):245–247, 1983.

Kirchhoff, K.T.: Nurses and physicians must interact for valid clinical research. Res Nurs Health 10(3):149–154, 1987.

Kirchhoff, K.T., & McGuire, D.B.: Gaining access to a clinical setting for research. Nurse Educ 10(5):24–26, 1985.

Kolin, P.C., & Kolin, J.L.: Professional Writing for Nurses in Education, Practice, and Research. St. Louis, CV Mosby Company, 1980.

Krone, K.P., & Loomis, M.F.: Developing practice-relevant research: A model that worked. J Nurs Admin 12(4):38–41, 1982.

Lasoff, E.M.: Improving nurses' cooperation with clinical research. J Nurs Admin 16(9):6–7, 1986.

Larson, E.: The inquisitive nurse: Bringing research to the bedside. Nurs Admin Q 2(4):9–12, 1978.

Larson, E.: Nursing research outside academia: A panel presentation. Image 13(3):75–77, 1981.

Lawson, L.: Funding for research In Lieske, A.M. (ed): Clinical Nursing Research: A Guide to Undertaking and Using Research in Nursing Practice. Rockville, MD, Aspen, 1986, pp. 211–228.

Leibold, S.: Peer review. In Hamric, A.B., and Spross, J. (eds): Clinical Nurse Specialist in Theory and Practice. New York, Grune and Stratton, 1983, pp. 219–233.

Levine, R.L.: Ethics and Regulation of Clinical Research. Baltimore, Urban & Schwarzenberg, 1981.

Lewandowski, L.A., & Kositsky, A.M.: Research priorities for critical care nursing: A study by the American Association of Critical-Care Nurses. Heart Lung 12(1):35–44, 1983.

Lewin, K.: Resolving Social Conflicts: Selected Papers on Group Dynamics. New York, Harper, 1958.

Lieske, A.M. (ed): Clinical Nursing Research: A Guide to Undertaking and Using Research in Nursing Practice. Rockville, MD, Aspen, 1986.

Lindeman, C.A.: Nursing research: A visible, viable component of nursing practice. J Nurs Admin 3(2):18–21, 1973.

Lindeman, C.A.: Priorities in clinical nursing research. Nurs Outlook 23(11):693–698, 1975.

Loomis, M.E.: Resources for collaborative research. West J Nurs Res 4(1):65–74, 1982.

Loomis, M.E., & Krone, K.P.: Collaborative research development. J Nurs Admin 10(2):32–35, 1980.

Mahoney, M.J.: Experimental methods and outcome evaluation. J Consult Clin Psych 46(4):660–672, 1978.

Marchette, L.: Developing a productive nursing research program in a clinical institution. J Nurs Admin 15(3):25–30, 1985.

Mayer, D.K.: Oncology nurses' versus cancer patients' perceptions of nurse caring behaviors: A replication study. Oncol Nurs Forum 14(3):48–52, 1987.

McArt, E.W., & McDougal, L.W.: Secondary data analysis—A new approach to nursing research. Image 17(2):54–57, 1985.

McClure, M.L.: Promoting practice-based research: A critical need. J Nurs Admin 11(11–12):66–70, 1981.

McGuire, D.B., Barbour, L., Boxler, J., et al.: Fixed-interval versus as-needed analgesics in cancer outpatients. J Pain Symp Management, 2:199–205, 1987.

McHugh, J.G., & Johnson, J.E.: Clinical nursing research: Beyond the methods books. Nurs Outlook 28(3):352–356, 1980.

Meier, P., & Pugh, E.J.: The case study: A viable approach to clinical research. Res Nurs Health 9(3):195–202, 1986.

Mercer, R.T.: Nursing research: The bridge to excellence in practice. Image 16(2):47–51, 1984.

Miller, J.R., & Messenger, S.R.: Obstacles to applying nursing research findings. Am J Nurs 78(4):632–634, 1978.

Moore, F.: Research in a clinical setting: Promises & potential. Supervisor Nurse 11(6):35–38, 1980.

Norby, R.B.: Collaborative relationships among nursing service, education, and research. In Lieske, A.M. (ed): Clinical Nursing Research: A Guide to Undertaking and Using Research in Nursing Practice. Rockville, MD, Aspen, 1986, pp. 121–140.

Oberst, M.T.: Priorities in cancer nursing research. Cancer Nurs 1(4):281–290, 1978.

Oberst, M.T.: Nursing research: New definitions, collegial approaches. Cancer Nurs 3(6):459, 1980.

Oberst, M.T.: Integrating research and clinical practice roles. Topics Clin Nurs 7(2):45–53, 1985.

O'Connor, P., & Malone, B.: A consultation model for nurse specialist practice. Nurs Econ 1(2):107–111, 1983.

Padilla, G.V.: Incorporating research in a service setting. J Nurs Admin 9(1):44–49, 1979.

Phillips, L.R.F.: A Clinician's Guide to the Critique and Utilization of Research. Norwalk, CT, Appleton-Century-Crofts, 1986.

Polit, D.F., & Hungler, B.P.: Nursing Research: Principles and Methods (3rd ed). Philadelphia, J.B. Lippincott Company, 1987.

Pollick, S.E.: Clinical nursing research: The needed link for unifying professional nursing. Clinical Nurse Specialist 1(1):8–12, 1987.

Reynolds, M.A., & Haller, K.B.: Using research in practice. A case for replication—Part I. West J Nurs Res 8(1):113–116, 1986.

Rezler, A.G., & Stevens, B.J.: The Nurse Evaluator in Education and Service. New York, McGraw-Hill, 1978.

Scogna, D.M.: Nursing Research in a cancer cooperative group setting. Cancer Nurs 4(4):277–280, 1981.

Schlotfeldt, R.M.: Cooperative nursing investigations: A role for everyone. Nurs Res 23(6):452–456, 1974.

Sheidler, V.R.: New methods in analgesic delivery. In McGuire, D.B., and Yarbro, C.H. (eds): Cancer Pain Management. New York, Grune and Stratton, 1987, pp. 203–222.

Shiplacoff, J.A.G.: The oncology nurse: Clinical oncology team research. In Vredevoe, D.L., et al. (eds): Concepts of Oncology Nursing. Englewood Cliffs, NJ, Prentice-Hall, 1981.

Sisson, R.: Co-worker's perceptions of the clinical nurse specialist role. Clinical Nurse Specialist 1(1):13–17, 1987.

Sparks, S.M.: The National Library of Medicine's bibliographic databases: Tools for nursing research. Image 16(1):24–25, 1984.

Stetler, C.B.: Nurses and research: Responsibility and involvement. NITA: The Official Journal of the National Intravenous Therapy Association 6(3):207–212, 1983.

Stetler, C.B.: Nursing Research in a Service Setting. Reston, VA, Reston, 1984.

Stetler, C.B.: Research utilization: Defining the concept. Image 17(2):40–44, 1985.

Stetler, C.B., & Marram, G.: Evaluating research findings for applicability in practice. Nurs Outlook 24(9):559–563, 1976.

Stokes, J.E.: Utilization of research findings by staff nurses. In Krampitz, S.V., and Pavlovich, N. (eds): Readings for Nursing Research. St. Louis, C.V. Mosby Company, 1981, pp. 227–234.

Tanner, C.A.: Evaluating research for use in practice: Guidelines for the clinician. Heart & Lung 16(4):424–431, 1987.

Tarsitano, B.J., Brophy, E.B., and Snyder, D.J.: A demystification of the clinical-nurse specialist role: Perceptions of clinical nurse specialists and nurse administrators. J Nurs Educ 25(1):4–9, 1986.

Todd, A.H., & Gortner, S.R.: Researchmanship: Removing obstacles to research in the clinical setting. West J Nurs Res 4(3):329–333, 1982.

United States Department of Health and Human Services, National Institutes of Health, Office for Protection from Research Risks. Protection of human subjects. Code of Federal Regulations Title 45, Part 46, 1983.

Varricchio, C., & Mikos, K.: Research: Determining feasibility in a clinical setting. Oncol Nurs Forum 14(1):89–90, 1987.

Weiss, C.H.: Evaluation Research: Methods for Assessing Program Effectiveness. Englewood Cliffs, NJ, Prentice-Hall, 1972.

Werley, H.: Promoting the research dimension in the practice of nursing through the establishment and development of a department of nursing in an institute of research. Milit Med 127(3):219–231, 1962.

Werley, H.: This I believe—about clinical nursing research. Nurs Outlook 20(11):718–722, 1972.

Whitney, F.W., & Roncoli, M.: Turning clinical problems into research. Heart & Lung 15(1):57–59, 1986.

Zalar, M.K., Welches, L.J., and Walker, D.D.: Nursing consortium approach to increase research in service settings. J Nurs Admin 15(7–8):36–41, 1985.

# The CNS as Collaborator

*Judith A. Spross*

## OVERVIEW AND HISTORICAL ASPECTS

Collaboration and interdisciplinary teamwork are words often used to describe health care as it is or as it should be. Through previous clinical experience and during graduate education, CNSs usually learn to value interdisciplinary work, at least as an ideal or goal toward which to work if it does not exist in practice. Part of the reality shock CNSs experience may result from settings in which collaboration and inter-disciplinary work are not valued. Lip service may be given to the concept, but structural, administrative, and professional support may be lacking.

The descriptions of interdisciplinary teams that function well are mainly anecdotal. The results of a study on the evaluation of intensive care suggest that interdisciplinary processes influence patient outcome (Knaus, et al., 1986). Much of the literature on collaboration describes the joint practice of nurse practitioners and physicians (Steel, 1986). In the early 1970s, the American Nurses' Association (ANA) and the American Medical Association (AMA) collaborated to form the National Joint Practice Commission (NJPC). The NJPC funded several demon-stration projects of joint practice in hospitals. One participant in the demonstration project described the collaborative practice that evolved in an acute care setting (Devereux, 1981). In the literature, joint practice consistently refers to nurse-physician collaboration. The demonstration projects were successful but have not led to widespread implementation of the NJPC's recommendations.

CNSs must be leaders in developing, promoting, and maintaining interdisciplinary collaboration and teamwork. Most CNS position de-scriptions contain expectations related to collaboration. CNSs not only collaborate but also teach and model collaborative behaviors to nursing staff with whom they work. In the author's experience, three particular collaborative situations offer the most challenge and promise for the growth and development of collaborative relationships within the health care professions: CNS participation on interdisciplinary teams, CNS collaboration with individual head nurses, and collaboration with physicians.

This chapter will discuss the imperatives and obstacles to collaboration, the elements of collaboration, and selected specific situations of collaboration. Strategies to promote collaboration will be discussed in the context of specific situations. Methods of evaluating this leadership function will also be presented.

## IMPERATIVES FOR COLLABORATION

CNSs and other nurse leaders have both social and professional obligations to promote collaboration. Professional, organizational, and social imperatives require CNSs to examine the concept of collaboration and to identify what CNSs can do to promote collaborative practice.

Baird discussed the concepts of communication, cooperation, and collaboration and stated that collaboration was the least developed in nursing and believed it should "command our attention." "Collaborative efforts are increasingly important as we look at new ways to maximize resources" (1985, p. 89).

The establishment of practice standards and certification processes by the ANA and other specialty organizations is imperative for collaboration. Standards of practice give nurses goals for care which need to be incorporated into the goals of interdisciplinary teams. CNSs can articulate these standards and apply them to the care of particular patients. Certification is a public statement of each individual's expertise and a public commitment to meeting the standards of care. Standards and certification in a specialty are public evidence of professionalism and of a commitment to excellence. Implementation of practice standards and certification processes can promote collegiality among nurses, CNSs, and other professionals.

Technology transfer, i.e., the transfer of scientific advances into the clinical setting, is an imperative. To plan for technology transfer requires analyzing and implementing needed role and practice changes. The orderly transfer of technology from laboratory to practice requires anticipatory planning and collaboration among nurses, physicians, and administrators. Nurses should not be in the untenable position of having to care for patients using invasive diagnostic or therapeutic interventions for which they have had no preparation.

Ethical dilemmas are another aspect of practice requiring exquisite collaboration. If health care providers do not communicate and collab-orate, either they may not be identifying ethical issues or they may not be grappling with them. Lack of provider collaboration on ethical problems threatens patient autonomy and inhibits team growth.

Some insightful studies of nurses and nursing give important reasons as to why collaboration must be given priority. In a study of why nurses leave nursing, factors related to collaboration which were ranked highly included lack of an environment that provides a sense of worth as a member of the health care team and a lack of positive professional interactions with physicians (Aiken, 1981). The National Commission on Nursing Study found that a "lack of recognition and understanding of the nurses' role in health care delivery—by the public, other health professionals, and by nurses themselves—was considered by many to be a key contributor to current nursing-related problems" (1983, p. 9). These studies suggest that a lack of collaboration among nurses and the people with whom they work influences job satisfaction and affects a nurse's decision to remain in the profession.

Benner, in her landmark study of advanced nursing practice, found that one of the seven functions expert nurses perform is making the system work to meet the needs of the patient (1984). This particular function is rarely taught, and its value is rarely acknowledged or recognized. Fenton's work, which applied Benner's results to CNSs, found that an important role of CNSs was "massaging the system" both for nurses and patients (1985). "Massaging the system" suggests the use of indirect techniques (perhaps because direct efforts to collaborate have failed). In addition, interpersonal role modeling was identified as an important means of supporting staff. These studies suggest that collaboration is an important component of advanced practice and that the CNS plays a major role in promoting collaboration.

Some studies, such as those of the NJPC (1981) and Knaus, et al. (1986), demonstrate that when collaboration exists, patient care im-proves. In an NJPC report, nurses and physicians reported improved communication and clinical collaboration. Physicians initiated commu-nication with nurses more frequently than they had prior to the demonstration project. Expanded statements on the scope of nursing practice were developed, giving nurses more decision-making authority. Patients interviewed expressed a high degree of satisfaction with the care from nurses and physicians participating in the project. Knaus, et al. (1986) found that the hospital with the best outcome of intensive care had systems that ensured excellent nurse-physician communication and a comprehensive nursing education support system. CNSs had primary responsibility for orientation and development of staff.

Cost containment and consumerism encourage competition, which can be either a driving or a restraining force for collaboration. As a driving force, competition may encourage professionals from different disciplines to ally with one another. One study demonstrated that collaboration may cut costs (Koerner & Armstrong, 1984). Alliances may increase efficiency and cost-effectiveness. As a restraining force, competition may compel individuals to protect their territories, hoard information, and otherwise obstruct collaboration. CNSs, with their clinical, interpersonal, and organizational skills, may be able to shift the balance so that cost containment becomes a driving force.

## ELEMENTS OF COLLABORATION

Collaboration means to work together, especially in a joint intellectual effort. Collaboration is essential to effective inter- and intradisciplinary work. If one reviews the literature on collaboration, interdisciplinary teams, and joint practice (Given & Simmons, 1977; Challela, 1979; Ryan, Edwards, and Rickles, 1980; Devereux, 1981; MacElveen-Hoehn, 1983; Burchell, Thomas, and Smith, 1983; Steel, 1986; Riegel & Murrell, 1987; Crowley & Wollner, 1987), three elements essential to collaboration emerge. The first element is that of a common purpose or mission; the second is that collaborators have diverse and sometimes complementary skills and contributions to apply to clinical decision-making; the third is effective communication processes. These elements are vital for both intra- and interdisciplinary collaboration. Further analysis of these elements will help CNSs understand the state of collaborative practice in their own settings.

### Common Purpose

The development of a common purpose as a prerequisite to collaboration may seem straightforward. The purpose may be as broad as to improve patient care or as specific as to ensure that a particular patient is discharged with the appropriate resources for home care.

When a common purpose is not understood by the parties involved, conflict may arise or an important need of a patient or staff member may go unmet. In one example, a CNS was consulted to evaluate and teach a cancer patient relaxation exercises to decrease anxiety. During the evaluation, the CNS determined that the patient was not anxious, as the primary nurse had assessed, but was suffering from chronic, unrelieved cancer pain. The CNS reviewed her proposed plan, which included a need for medication adjustment, with the primary nurse. The CNS and primary nurse approached the resident physician. The physician was surprised to learn that the patient had pain and asked the CNS for her recommendations. When the CNS suggested an increase in narcotic dosage, the physician said he did not want the patient to become constipated. The CNS replied that constipation was a reasonable concern to raise but that it was preventable and identified the steps that would be taken to avert the side effects. The physician ended the interaction by walking away. The goal of the CNS and primary nurse had been to relieve the patient's pain; the physician did not have the same goal. One could speculate on the reasons—he did not know the patient had pain (nor did the primary nurse); he did not know the CNS and nurse well enough to trust their information; or he truly believed the risk of constipation outweighed the benefit of pain relief in a patient with advanced cancer. The conflict illustrates the absence of a common purpose and its potential impact on patient care.

An example of shared leadership between a CNS and a head nurse shows the value of a common purpose. Based on staff input and their own observations, the CNS and head nurse recognized a need to promote professional growth among the staff and decided the unit should be represented at the annual national oncology conference. Priority would be given to staff who were presenting or exhibiting. The CNS helped three staff members prepare abstracts and posters for the meeting. The head nurse arranged the staff's schedules to allow for some professional time to devote to these activities. One staff member indicated that this activity influenced her to stay in her staff nurse position—she had been looking for another job. The head nurse and CNS had a common goal and worked together to achieve it.

These examples illustrate that the development of a common purpose presupposes certain values and characteristics of collaborators. Collaborators want to work together. They believe that their combined efforts are synergistic—that the sum of their combined efforts is greater than independent efforts. They trust each other and acknowledge interdependence (Given & Simmons, 1977; MacElveen-Hoehn, 1983). These elements may not be present in a particular situation, and the CNS may have to focus on helping coworkers develop trust and value collaboration—a resocialization process (Given & Simmons, 1977; Challela, 1979). Until these values and characteristics develop, a collaborative environment is unlikely to exist.

## Diverse Professional Skills and Contributions

The second element of collaboration is the existence and recognition of divergent and complementary skills and contributions. In the first example cited, divergent and complementary skills of two professionals were available (the CNS's expertise in pain assessment and intervention and the doctor's ability to prescribe drugs). The absence of a common purpose rendered these contributions useless. In the second example, the CNS's clinical and coaching skills were complemented by the head nurse's administrative authority to assign and schedule staff.

Like the first element, the second presumes that certain values and processes exist. In order to appreciate what each professional can contribute to solving a particular problem, collaborators must know what knowledge and skills each colleague has to offer. Health care providers often presume they know this; their professional education may give them some knowledge of which disciplines offer particular services. However, unless professionals collaborate and talk together about the talents they can offer to solve problems, it is probable that no one could articulate another colleague's skills. Discussion and clarification of roles assist individuals to recognize and accept the areas where one discipline's practice overlaps another's.

In addition to knowing what services colleagues can offer, it is important for colleagues to value that service. Not valuing the divergent, often complementary skills of fellow team members has been cited as a reason for ineffective teamwork (Hamric, 1977; Gilliss, 1983). Undervaluing the contributions of colleagues can lead to costly and inefficient use of resources and may be an underlying reason for conflict. It contributes to power imbalances, which can ultimately affect patient care. There is also personal cost in terms of diminished self-esteem.

## Coordinating and Communicating Processes

The third element critical to collaboration is effective coordination and communication. Structures and processes for communication must be identified and implemented. Individuals working together must articulate these structures and processes. Examples of structure include regular meetings and documentation of guidelines for collaborative decision-making. Processes that must be addressed include issues of power, leadership, decision-making, and conflict resolution.

Collaboration that incorporates all three elements is rare, yet effective collaboration requires them. Absence of conflict is not necessarily a sign of collaboration. CNSs should analyze their settings to determine whether the elements of collaboration exist. For some, it may be necessary to foster the elements that promote collaboration in order to be able to collaborate effectively with other providers.

# OBSTACLES TO COLLABORATION

Obstacles to collaboration have been reviewed by a number of authors (Mount, 1985; Wise, et al., 1974; Given & Simmon, 1977; Challela, 1979; Goren & Ottaway, 1985). Observations made by some of these authors pertain to both the affective and interactive difficulties encountered when attempting to build a successful team. One author wrote of the "team as stressor," a source of burnout for health care professionals (Mount, 1985). To care for a patient holistically "demands the input of an interdisciplinary team. Such teams are in vogue!. . . Teams don't just happen. They slowly and painfully evolve." "It is naive to bring together a highly diverse group of people and expect that, by calling them a team, they will, in fact, behave as a team. It is ironic indeed to realize that a football team spends 40 hours a week practicing teamwork for the two hours on Sunday afternoon when the teamwork really counts. Teams in organizations seldom spend two hours per week practicing when their ability to function as a team counts 40 hours per week" (Wise, et al., 1974, p. 73).

Obstacles to collaboration can be conceptualized as organizational and professional. Both types of obstacles are amenable to CNS intervention. A discussion of these obstacles will enable CNSs to analyze issues of collaboration in their settings and help target plans for promoting and enhancing collaborative work.

## Organizational Obstacles

Increased acuity in both inpatient and outpatient settings is an obstacle to collaboration. Providers move from one crisis to another; whether the crisis is a life-threatening emergency or an overbooked clinic, the time available to providers to sit down, communicate, analyze the data they have collected, and make decisions is minimal. In addition to being one-minute managers, health care providers are now one-minute nurses, doctors, social workers, and chaplains.

If team members change every month (i.e., house staff) or every year (i.e., staff nurses), it is difficult to engage in team *building* activities. Shift changes, assignment changes, and models of care delivery such as team nursing can interfere with continuity of care; in these situations, caregivers often have insufficient information about patients, thus making them unable to communicate about and coordinate care. If the turnover of nurses is high, there may never be the right mix of experienced and novice nurses capable of working (or learning to work) with those in other disciplines to solve complex clinical problems. A shortage of nurses may mean that the processes essential to interdisciplinary communication and collaboration become subordinated to providing critical, lifesaving care.

A lack of planning can contribute to poor communication and collaboration. In most settings in which the author has worked, nurses have been the last to know that a new medical treatment is being introduced. Sometimes it is the patient who informs the nurse, or the investigator tells the head nurse shortly before the first patient to be treated is admitted. In certain cases, this lack of communication can threaten safe nursing care—for example, when the treatment is unlike those usually administered on the unit.

Specialization and subspecialization may be obstacles to collaboration, yet they are part of the development of health professions which have created a great need for collaboration. One patient may be seen by a half dozen consultants in nursing, medicine, and other professions. How can a staff nurse coordinate the nursing consultants along with the medical consultants? How can a staff nurse work with an attending physician who will not coordinate the input of the medical consultants brought in on a case?

Lack of administrative support may restrain collaboration—for example, if there is no system to ensure that nurses' patients will be cared for while they attend an interdisciplinary meeting. For CNSs, lack of administrative support for collaboration may be apparent in a number of ways. The administrator who holds the CNS responsible for collaborating with the head nurse but does not have similar expectations of the head nurse to collaborate with the CNS is not providing support for a vital collaborative relationship. The administrator who requires the CNS to get involved in many departmental projects may not be allowing time to establish collaborative relationships. When efforts to collaborate with physicians concerning important clinical issues meet with resistance, the CNS should expect support from the nursing administration.

Goren and Ottaway (1985) described the "chronicity" condition of health care teams and organizations—that is, rapid or successful response to team-building interventions is unlikely to occur. Intractable organizational problems often defy solution because of collusion. Problem behaviors are maintained by the unacknowledged support of the system and because solutions that are tried may be problematic. Collusion, in this case, refers to either a conscious or an unconscious commitment to maintain the status quo. While not referring specifically to CNSs, Goren and Ottaway's description of organizational obstacles is relevant to collaboration and may help CNSs understand systems that are unresponsive to interventions that promote collaboration. In efforts to promote collaboration, CNSs may find verbal support for "team efforts" but not the supportive behaviors. For example, the passive primary nurse or the physician who never attends the team conference has not made a "behavioral commitment" to team work/collaboration.

## Professional Obstacles

In specialty settings, in which both the CNS and the nursing staff possess expert knowledge, there may be a disparity between the knowledge of nurses and that of house physicians who are responsible for the daily care of patients. This disparity may be advantageous if the expertise of the CNS and staff is acknowledged and used as a resource by the house staff. In many cases, however, this disparity is a threat and gives rise to conflict, frustration, lack of collaboration, and suboptimal care. In these cases, it is unlikely that the caregivers can identify a common purpose toward which collaborative efforts could be directed.

Nurse clinicians and clinical specialists with fairly narrow specialties may have difficulty working with generalist house physicians who may not appreciate or accept the special expertise of these nurses. The author has encountered this problem in attempting to work with physicians to address chronic cancer pain, which requires both medical (e.g., medications) and noninvasive nursing methods to achieve good control. The CNS may have a good sense of the appropriate medication needed to control the pain, but the physician may be unwilling to prescribe the drug based on an irrational fear of causing addiction in a dying cancer patient. Specialists in nursing can sometimes be thwarted in their efforts to apply their specialty knowledge when it cuts across professional territorial lines.

Role overlap may be an obstacle or an advantage. It is an obstacle when there is role ambiguity. When members of the interdisciplinary team are not clear about their own range of talents or that of their colleagues, the team cannot be effective. Overlap can be advantageous when members understand what each has to offer—the team may not have to depend upon one person to provide a particular service, and leadership can be shared depending upon the nature of the problem and the skills of individual members.

Differing philosophies of the caregivers can restrain collaboration. These conflicts may occur among nurses or between nurses and other providers. In the oncology setting, the author has encountered an occasional staff nurse who believed a patient would become addicted from the administration of round-the-clock analgesics and would withhold a dose until the patient asked for it. In neurology, oncology, and intensive care settings, nurses and physicians may have very different philosophies about terminally ill patients which lead to conflicts over "do not resuscitate" prescriptions.

Another example of a situation in which differing philosophies inhibited collaboration occurred on a surgical unit on which the author worked as a CNS. The unit had a large number of nurses who viewed themselves as oncology nurses and believed their practice was specialized. By contrast, the surgical oncology fellows, who had daily responsibility for the medical care of patients, saw themselves as surgeons in a setting where they could learn unusual surgical techniques. These physicians had no long-term interest in oncology. This difference in perspective led to conflicts over pain and side effect management of cancer patients undergoing treatment.

Differing standards of care offer yet another obstacle to collaboration. An illustration would be a setting where both physicians and nurses administer chemotherapy intravenously. In this setting, the nurses are required to become certified in the procedure through a combination of study and clinical supervision. The physicians are not required to go through this process. Patients are subject to two different standards of care. (In this case, one standard is safer than the other.) Patients may observe this difference and may make comments to providers or constantly ask for one provider (often the nurse). Nurses may take it upon themselves to offer training to the physician to avoid errors (equivalent to supervising medical practice). And in some cases, nurses may feel responsible when an error occurs even though they did not administer the drug.

Another obstacle is that the nurse is often a "coordinator without portfolio" (Hamric, 1977). This stems from a lack of recognition of nurses' efforts to fulfill this collaborator role and from an unwillingness on the part of some nurses to assume this role.

### Other Obstacles

Some writers have identified other forces that restrain efforts to promote collaboration between nurses and other health professions (Hamric, 1977; Morgan & McCann, 1983; Gilliss, 1983). These include the hierarchical structures of many health care agencies, which place physicians in authoritative positions over other health professions; sexism; time conflicts; and lack of assertiveness and conflict resolution skills. CNSs attempting to promote collaboration should be aware of the variety of factors that can restrain team building efforts.

## STRATEGIES

After assessing the setting, the CNS should include collaborative efforts in work plans and annual goals. Such goals may reflect the need to develop a collaborative climate as well as particular collaborative endeavors with other providers. Thus, initial efforts may, of necessity, have an interpersonal focus—developing relationships with key people, planning inservices, and coaching individual staff to develop assertiveness and conflict resolution skills. At the same time, CNSs may develop and participate in specific programs requiring collaboration such as the neurology/rehabilitation CNS who, with a speech pathologist, developed a support group and standardized educational interventions for head-injured patients and their families.

The selection of specific strategies for promoting collaboration in one's setting depends upon the results of the CNS's analysis of the setting or organization. Such an analysis examines both intra- and interdisciplinary collaboration. Priorities for developing a plan of action for collaboration will depend upon the particular setting. A CNS may decide to try to improve relationships among nurses before trying to implement an interdisciplinary model of care. Well-established collaboration among nurses can enhance interdisciplinary collaboration, since such nurses would possess the attitudes, values, and behaviors essential to interdisciplinary team success.

Prior to discussing specific strategies, it seems worthwhile to identify, particularly for the novice CNS, an affective dimension of working to improve collaboration. This dimension seems to occur particularly in institutions and agencies where collaboration among disciplines is not well established. CNSs may feel as though they are the only ones interested in or committed to building a collaborative team. The CNS may not understand why the benefits of working together are not as clear to staff, a head nurse, or physicians. The CNS may feel alone in a struggle in which the primary purpose is to improve patient care. In the ideal situation, all parties are committed to a common purpose. In a "second best" situation, there is a laissez-faire attitude that allows CNSs to pursue efforts with little or no obstruction but with no active commitment to promoting collaboration. In this case, true collaboration may develop but will require considerable time and energy from the CNS, and results will probably take two or more years to evolve. One is less optimistic about settings in which there is active obstruction that continues unabated despite CNS efforts to build a team.

## Organizational Strategies

CNSs encouraging organizations to be supportive of collaboration should be aware of studies that examine nursing practice and trends in nursing. One such study was a demonstration project executed by the NJPC in 1981. From the project hospitals, strategies that fostered collaborative practice were identified. Although some of these strategies would be considered professional, they did require organizational commitment. Such strategies include a primary nursing model of practice, an integrated patient progress record (i.e., one in which all disciplines document in the same part of the chart), and joint quality review of records and explicit scope of practice statements for medicine and nursing. To do all of these at once in a setting where none exist is a major task. In implementing these suggestions, it would be logical to start with initiation of primary nursing, since that change would be under the control of nursing service. Implementation of joint review of records and scope of practice statements requires collaboration with medicine. The medical record may be the most difficult change to implement since such changes often involve long, drawn-out processes. For the CNS interested in promoting collaboration, the NJPC's recommendations suggest some possible directions for initiating the structures that may accomplish that objective.

The establishment of one or a few decision-making groups can provide the organizational structures needed to promote collaboration. One type of decision-making group would have regularly scheduled (monthly or bimonthly) planning meetings and would include the leaders in nursing, medicine, and hospital administration who have responsibility for the CNS's specialty unit(s). The agenda for these meetings should include problem-solving related to the clinical setting and discussion of major projected clinical initiatives and clinical programs that are going to be modified or cancelled. It was at this kind of meeting that the author and the head nurse with whom she worked learned that a bone marrow transplant program was to be initiated the following year. This information gave the nurse leaders time to plan required administrative changes (e.g., in staffing) and for staff education and procedure development. The newly employed CNS may find that these meetings already take place between the head nurse and chief physician, in which case the CNS needs to begin to participate. If such meetings do not take place, the CNS may need to provide the impetus to make them happen.

A second type of group that can promote successful collaboration is the interdisciplinary team whose purpose is to discuss, plan, implement, and review the ongoing care of particular patients. The team generally consists of nurses, physicians, social workers, chaplains, physical therapists, and other providers involved in the care of a group of patients. Such teams have been described in the literature (Challela, 1979).

A third type of group is a joint or collaborative practice committee similar to the one suggested by the NJPC (1981). This committee, generally composed of nurses and physicians (although other disciplines such as physical therapy may be involved), have several functions such as developing and promulgating scope of practice statements, developing and implementing standard protocols and standards of care, jointly reviewing and evaluating care, and taking other interdisciplinary actions that enhance patient care. Some of these activities deserve further discussion and will be viewed as professional strategies, since the actions themselves are professional strategies. Establishing such a group is often the most challenging part of developing a collaborative environment. If a joint practice committee does not exist, then it would probably be wise to initiate groups such as the first two described above, before attempting to start a joint practice committee.

In assessing the organization, the CNS should identify who makes clinical decisions (patient or program related) and determine if there is potential for such decisions to be made at interdisciplinary forums. Negotiating participation of the CNS in existing groups, such as meetings of specialty physician staff or grand rounds, and defining nursing participation in this group is one strategy. The author learned that decisions about initiating clinical trials were made in monthly hematology-oncology physician staff meetings. She successfully made a case for her participation in those meetings, specifying advantages to the physicians in terms of study implementation as well as advantages of having well-informed and prepared nursing staff. The CNS had the support of the nursing administrator who was prepared to intervene, but the intervention was not necessary.

## Professional Strategies

One CNS with whom the author worked believed that a way to elicit commitment to collaboration or to overcome obstruction was to make oneself indispensable to the parties involved. She did this by working effectively with patients whom the nursing staff, house staff, or attending physicians found difficult to manage, either because of personality problems, complex family problems, or other psychosocial issues or multiple clinical problems (e.g., the unstable diabetic with severe peripheral vascular disease).

The CNS may find it useful (and easier) to develop collaborative relationshps with those perceived as having good relationships (and influence) with key people. In one instance, the author recognized rapport between a head nurse (HN) and assistant head nurse (AHN); the HN was distant and authoritarian with others. Although the HN had advocated having a CNS for her unit, she did not seem as receptive to the CNS as did the AHN. Initial efforts on the part of the CNS were directed to both leaders; however, ultimately it was the trusting relationship that the CNS developed with the AHN (who was well-liked and trusted by the HN) which facilitated successful HN/CNS collaboration.

An important step toward promoting collaboration is developing scope of practice statements for institutions within which CNSs work. This recommendation of the NJPC originally focused on nurses and physicians. There may be enough overlap in clinical skills that the concept of scope of practice statements may need to include a range of providers, depending upon the specialty population served. For example, in a rehabilitation setting, the CNS and physical therapist may benefit from such a statement. The scope of practice statement identifies the discipline's authority for making clinical decisions. Such a statement would legitimize current nursing decisions that, either by tradition or law, are considered medical decisions. The kinds of clinical decisions nurses make have changed in the last 15 years; policies, nurse practice acts, and job descriptions should reflect these changes. CNSs are ideal nurses to identify the areas of clinical decision-making which should be examined and to develop scope of practice statements for nursing.

In addition to practice statements, joint practice committees should work together to develop clinical protocols. Paulen remarked on the irony that in critical care units, nurses and other therapists are guided by standing protocols for therapy, but on medical-surgical units nurses cannot even give an aspirin without a prescription (1985). Depending upon the specialty, the CNS should be instrumental in identifying situations that would benefit from standing clinical protocols. For example, units that have a high incidence of constipation could institute a protocol that includes nursing measures (such as activity, fluid intake), medical prescriptions (such as stool softeners), and dietary measures. With a protocol that has been reviewed and endorsed by a joint practice committee, the nurse can initiate both the nursing measures and medical prescriptions without having to contact the physician for a prescription for every patient who is at risk for constipation. In addition to protocols, systems would need to be in place to ensure that nurses (or other providers) would have the responsibility and the authority to activate the protocol. Such protocols could eliminate conflict in certain clinical situations and enhance patient care. A manual of protocols could be developed and distributed to new nurses and physicians.

Another strategy suggested by the NJPC is joint review of medical records. In the author's opinion, this should be a function of the joint practice committee. The focus of joint review of medical records is quality assurance, achieved by examining documentation and outcomes of care. The group would also be responsible for the regular evaluation of both standard protocols and practice standards. The committee would establish standards for the providers engaged in a particular activity. For example, all providers administering cancer chemotherapy would need to be certified in the practice and would be required to follow the same policies and procedures for administration and documentation.

The CNS must look for other opportunities to promote interdisciplinary collaboration and to model collaborative behaviors for other nurses. A strategy that several CNSs have used is to encourage staff nurses to participate in medical rounds (unit or "walk" rounds as well as conferences) during which patients known to the staff are discussed. Nurses are encouraged to share their knowledge of the patient(s) and to ask questions about the clinical problem(s) under discussion. CNS support of this behavior includes demonstrating participation as well as coaching staff prior to (or after) such rounds. The following situation illustrates the CNS coaching a staff nurse in collaborative behaviors.

On rounds, a patient with leukemia who was also septic was being discussed. The patient's sepsis had some puzzling features, and the usual triple antibiotic therapy had not been initiated. Due to the patient's fever and frustration over what he perceived to be the physicians' indecision regarding appropriate antibiotic therapy, the patient had become withdrawn and refused certain essential hygiene. The assistant head nurse's (AHN) contribution to the discussion was to urge them to begin antibiotics immediately. Her suggestion was ignored. After rounds, the CNS spoke to the AHN and explained that her suggestion was ignored probably because she had tried to tell the doctors how to practice medicine. The CNS suggested that the AHN approach the attending physician and explain that the physicians' indecision was clearly being picked up by the patient, and in fact, that the patient was experiencing anxiety that led him to refuse essential nursing and medical measures—in other words, the physicians' dilemma was making it difficult to nurse the patient. The AHN used this approach, which resulted in the attending physician having a meeting with the other doctors to urge them to be consistent with the patient. The attending would be responsible for communicating treatment decisions to the patient. The attending and the patient's intern went to talk to the patient, to listen to his concerns, and to explain why there was a dilemma over treatment and what was being done to make the final decision. The patient became less withdrawn and anxious and began to agree to the care he had been refusing. In this example, collaborative aspects included definition of the scope of practice of the two disciplines in a particular case, trust that allowed each provider to be open to information about how a patient's care was being hampered by certain behaviors, and a commitment to a common purpose (good patient care).

Over time, systematic efforts to promote collaboration pay off in terms of more interdisciplinary planning and consultation. Of more importance are the benefits to patient care, as well as professional satisfaction with a job well done and with professional growth and development.

## PREPARATION FOR COLLABORATION

In graduate programs, CNS students must be given opportunities to collaborate with other providers in clinical practica. One clinical project should focus on collaboration including analysis of the driving and restraining forces promoting or inhibiting collaboration within a particular setting as well as implementation strategies. Faculty should be aware of the stress elicited in students by these activities. Such projects often involve risk-taking, assertiveness, and use of conflict-resolution and group skills. "How can I be expected to do this (I am only a student)?" students ask. Depending upon the particular setting, the student may need more or less coaching by the faculty and/or preceptor.

The curriculum should include content on group dynamics, role theory, organizational theory, conflict resolution, and change in order to prepare students as well as possible for the role of collaborator and to address issues in collaboration. Learners should be asked to discuss examples of collaboration and noncollaboration from their own clinical experiences and identify what factors accounted for success or failure. Learners need to be aware of social, economic, and legislative forces that will influence collaborative efforts. Students should be able to articulate what nursing is so that they can explain the profession to both patients and non-nursing health providers. They also need to be aware of trends in specialization in other health professions which may affect CNS practice.

There should be ample opportunity for interdisciplinary interaction around clinical issues, particularly among students and physicians. Depending upon the specialty, it may be appropriate for the CNS student to practice with a physician. This happens more often in graduate programs that prepare CNSs with nurse practitioner skills; educators should examine this type of practicum for all CNS programs. In a review of literature on interdisciplinary education, several suggestions emerged for promoting interdisciplinary education around a shared knowledge base. These include real or simulated clinical experiences, presentation of complex and thought-provoking materials rather than a least-common-denominator approach, use of educators from many disciplines, interdisciplinary team experiences, and student peer teaching (e.g., graduate physical therapy student teaching graduate nursing student techniques for preventing pathologic fractures) (Shepard, Yeo, and McGann, 1985).

## EVALUATION OF THE COLLABORATIVE ROLE

Evaluation of the collaborative role will depend upon the nature of the collaborative activity. Evaluation strategies may be structure, process, or outcome oriented. Structure evaluation would consist of determining whether a forum for collaboration exists—i.e., are there regular meetings, do the appropriate people attend, and are decisions/minutes documented? This type of evaluation might also include data on staff retention before and after the introduction of a major collaborative initiative, documentation of time spent on collaborative work, and job satisfaction data.

Process evaluation would examine group functioning. Collaboration is a process and is probably best evaluated by process evaluation measures. In the case of an established interdisciplinary (ID) team or group, an evaluation of team processes may give the team clues as to areas of strength and weakness.

While an ID team exemplifies process evaluation, similar approaches can be used to evaluate collaboration among other individuals (HN/CNS, nursing staff). This could be done by inviting a consultant (with expertise in organization theory and group dynamics) to observe several meetings and engage the team in a discussion of strengths and weaknesses around communication and group dynamics. The team could periodically schedule time for a discussion of members' perceptions of group functioning and develop a plan for change (if needed) or for growth and development. Is leadership of the group shared depending upon the problem and the skills of the members or is a single leader emerging? Are the processes consistent with the goals of the group? Does the group continue to be bound by commitment to a common purpose? Have interpersonal issues emerged which interfere with team functioning? How do nurses and those in other disciplines who are involved in the care of the team's patients view collaboration—successful? Unsuccessful? Do they believe that they are able to make a contribution and that they can have a say in the decision-making? Are all disciplines represented at rounds and do these individuals speak up regarding patient issues? Rounds at which the physicians do the speaking and the representatives of other disciplines merely listen are not collaborative. Alternatively, one could undertake a pencil and paper survey of members to determine their views on group functioning such as communication evaluation, conflict resolution, accomplishments, and other aspects of group functioning. These data could be compiled and shared with the group, and decisions could be made about changes needed.

Other methods of process evaluation would include CNS documentation (in a log of some sort) of staff coaching around issues of collaboration; clinical ethnographies, which illustrate successes and failures of collaboration; administrative review with one's supervisor of the range of collaborative activities; peer review; and evaluation of the contribution made by the CNS to establishing/promoting collaboration by the staff, other providers, and consumers (Hamric, 1983). The CNS may ask a colleague to provide evaluative information regarding collaboration. For example, the speech pathologist cited in an earlier example might be asked to comment on the neuroscience/rehabilitation CNS's collaborative skills.

If standard protocols have been initiated by a joint practice committee, the CNS, as a member of the joint practice committee, should evaluate the impact of the protocols on nursing practice—through surveys of the staff nurses and physicians and through chart review. These evaluation measures can be done in tandem with other quality assurance activities as appropriate.

Outcome evaluation examines the impact of collaborative activities on patient care. Hamric pointed out the technical difficulties associated with trying to measure the impact of a CNS on patient outcome, given the numbers of providers often involved in delivering care to the same patient (1983). While evaluation of the impact of collaboration on patient outcome may not identify the unique contribution of the CNS, such data could be combined with data from structure and process evaluation to clarify the CNS's contribution. To measure effects on patient outcome, a CNS might collect data on length of stay, number of clinic visits, and readmissions for a population prior to initiation of an interdisciplinary team and use this as one measure of the impact of the team's efforts on patients. In a well-performed process-outcome study, one group found that mortality (patient outcome measure) was related to structures and processes that facilitated interdisciplinary communication and collaboration (Knaus, et al., 1986).

## COLLABORATION: SELECTED ISSUES

Two particular relationships warrant further discussion of collaboration—the HN/CNS relationships and the CNS/MD relationship.

## CNS/HN Relationship

Whether CNSs practice in inpatient or outpatient settings, they will have to relate to both head nurses and physicians. If the CNS is unit-based, the HN/CNS relationship is especially pivotal. If the CNS is a consultant, the HN can influence whether the CNS has access to the unit and patients and whether the CNS's recommendations are followed. CNSs who work in ambulatory settings may need to see their clients when they are hospitalized and even provide guidance or treatment to those patients. A good rapport with the HN and staff can affect how much the CNS can influence care.

During their orientation to a new CNS position, CNSs should become acquainted with head nurses with whom they will need to work closely. During this process, the CNS should elicit the goals of the HN for the unit, staff, and patient population. CNSs must explain their goals for the position (even if it is just to get oriented) as well as their background and skills. If the CNS is unit-based, the CNS must identify how to help accomplish some of the clinical goals the HN has established for the unit. Even CNSs who are not unit-based may find this approach helpful, especially if they will need to practice on the unit or follow patients (e.g., the CNS in joint practice with a physician). Providing a needed inservice may facilitate access to the unit and elicit the support of the unit staff for the CNS's interventions with clients.

If the CNS is in a nursing department, it is important that the HN/CNS relationship be articulated. If the administrator expects the CNS and HN to work together to provide joint (i.e., clinical and administrative) leadership for a unit, then the CNS and HN need to meet regularly and communicate exquisitely. The CNS and HN will have to work hard to articulate to the staff how this joint leadership functions (Gresham, 1976). This means that the CNS, for example, will refer problems of an administrative nature to the HN and will not get bogged down in discussions of time planning and the like. Likewise, the HN will refer staff to the CNS for clinical problems. The relationship is a delicate one and requires ongoing attention. The CNS who is the first for a unit and for a HN will find this particularly true. Even the HN who has dreamed of working with a CNS and has done the negotiation to have a position budgeted and filled may find the reality more dismaying or threatening than anticipated. Staff begin to take clinical problems to the CNS which they used to take to the HN. The HN may experience a sense of loss. This may be happening at the same time that nursing administration is giving HNs more and more administrative responsibilities. The HN who used to take pride in knowing all that was happening on the unit clinically may be unable to do this and may feel a sense of loss or inadequacy.

The author views the HN/CNS relationship as one providing mutual support—the CNS and HN may be the only two providers who have an intimate understanding of the daily ups and downs of the unit and can discuss unit issues that neither could discuss with staff. The CNS has access to clinical information that the HN may need to support budgetary requests for new clinical programs. The author has found that HN/CNS teamwork can effectively accomplish what neither professional could do alone. In two settings within which the author worked, the joint leadership concept was valued to the extent that the two leaders tried not to be on vacation at the same time. When the HN was on vacation, a staff nurse was placed in charge. The CNS was available to help support this person and assist with problem-solving.

The CNS/HN alliance is important, especially to unit-based CNSs, and deserves nurturing from the individuals themselves and their administrators. If CNS efforts to develop this alliance are not successful even after open discussion with the HN, CNSs should seek counsel from their administrators.

## CNS/MD Relationship

The CNS/MD relationship is another that deserves careful attention during the first few months of employment. In a discussion of collaborative practice in hospitals, Gilliss wrote that physicians continue to be unaware of nurse practice activities. She stated that it is essential for nurses to capture the attention of physicians and to demonstrate their finest practice skills (Gilliss, 1983). To meet the needs of nursing, one change that can promote joint practice in hospitals is to ensure that nurses "capable of advanced nursing practice must play a more central role in modeling expanded skills" (Gilliss, 1983, p. 40). Like Brown (1983) (see also Chapter 2), Gilliss proposed the idea of an attending nurse who works closely with both an attending physician and the hospital's nursing staff to provide excellent care. There are few documented descriptions of collaborative CNS/physician practice in hospitals. Crowley and Wollner described the implementation of collaborative practice in the hospital setting (1987). Nurse/physician collaboration in private practice is better documented primarily because of the nurse practitioner movement (Steel, 1986). However, some instances of collaborative private practices between CNSs and physicians have been reported (Ryan, Edwards, and Rickles, 1980; Littell, 1981; Riegel & Murrell, 1987).

Efforts to promote collaboration should begin early; CNSs should meet the physician chief of the CNS's specialty, preferably while interviewing and, if not, then during the first few weeks of employment.

CNSs should use this time to explain the role and their background and interest in working collaboratively. From physicians, the CNS can ascertain roles and research interests of those in the medical specialty. After a period of orientation and with the above information, the CNS can identify particular goals that would require nurse/physician collaboration and again meet with the appropriate physician to develop a plan for collaboration.

## SUMMARY

Establishing collaborative relationships with nurses and other professionals caring for a population of patients can be a demanding, frustrating, labor-intensive, but rewarding CNS activity, especially when there has been no tradition of collaboration. The investment of time and interpersonal energy is often significant. The rewards usually justify such an investment. The most tangible is that of better patient care. Other rewards include job satisfaction, improved communication and understanding among health professionals, and professional growth and development. The concept of collaboration has been described. Organizational and professional obstacles and strategies for promoting successful collaboration have been identified. CNSs play pivotal roles in fostering intra- and interdisciplinary communication, cooperation, and collaboration. To do this, graduate education must prepare CNSs by providing theoretical and experiential knowledge of collaboration, forces that drive and restrain collaboration, and strategies for fostering collaboration. The changing health care environment requires re-evaluating and reinventing the concepts of intra- and interdisciplinary collaboration. CNSs can provide leadership to ensure that nurses and nursing are clearly represented in collaborative clinical decision-making either about individual patients or clinical programs.

### References

Aiken, L. H.: Why nurses leave nursing. Am J Nurs *81*:73–77, 1981.
Baird, S. B.: Communication, cooperation, collaboration: Cornerstones for specialty achievement. Oncol Nurs Forum *11*(4):87–90, 1985.
Benner, P.: From Novice to Expert. Reading, MA, Addison-Wesley Publishing Company, 1984.
Brown, S. J.: The clinical nurse specialist in a multidisciplinary partnership. Nurs Admin Q *8*(1):36–46, 1983.
Burchell, R. C., Thomas, D. A., and Smith, H. L.: Some considerations for implementing collaborative practice. Am J Med *74*:9–13, 1983.
Challela, M. S.: The interdisciplinary team: A role definition for nursing. Image *11*:9–15, 1979.

Crowley, S. A., & Wollner, I. S.: Collaborative practice: A tool for change. Oncol Nurs Forum *14*(4):59–63, 1987.

Devereux, P.: Nurse/physician collaboration: Nursing practice considerations. J Nurs Admin *11*(9):37–39, 1981.

Fenton, M. V.: Identifying competencies of the clinical nurse specialist. J Nurs Admin *15*:31–37, 1985.

Gilliss, C. L.: Collaborative practice in the hospital: What's in it for nursing? Nurs Admin Q *7*(4):37–44, 1983.

Given, B., & Simmons, S.: The interdisciplinary health care team: Fact or fiction. Nurs Forum *16*:165–184, 1977.

Goren, S., & Ottaway, R.: Why health care teams don't change: Chronicity and collusion. J Nurs Admin *15*(7,8):9–16, 1985.

Gresham, M. L.: Conflict or collaboration: A head nurse's view. *In*: The Clinical Nurse Specialist. Indianapolis, IN, Sigma Theta Tau, 1976.

Hamric, A. B.: Deterrents to therapeutic care of the dying person. *In* Barton, D. (ed): Dying and Death—A Clinical Guide for Caregivers. Baltimore, Williams & Wilkins, 1977, pp. 183–199.

Hamric, A. B.: A model for developing evaluating strategies. *In* Hamric, A. B., and Spross, J. (eds): The Clinical Nurse Specialist in Theory and Practice. New York, Grune and Stratton, 1983.

Knaus, W. A., Draper, E. A., Wagner, D. P., and Zimmerman, J. E.: An evaluation of outcome from intensive care in major medical centers. Ann Intern Med *104*:410–418, 1986.

Koerner, B. L., & Armstrong, D.: Collaborative practice cuts costs of patient care: A study. Hospitals *58*(10):52–54, 1984.

Littell, S. C.: The clinical nurse specialist in a private medical practice. Nurse Admin Q *6*(1):77–85, 1981.

MacElveen-Hoehn, P.: The cooperation model for care in health and illness. *In* Chaska, N. L. (ed): The Nursing Profession: A Time to Speak. New York, McGraw Hill, 1983.

Morgan, A. P., & McCann, J. M.: Nurse-physician relationships: The ongoing conflict. Nurs Admin Q *7*(4):1–7, 1983.

Mount, B. M.: Dealing with our losses. J Clin Oncol *4*(7):1127–1134, 1985.

National Commission on Nursing Report. Chicago, The Hospital Research and Education Trust, 1983.

National Joint Practice Commission: Guidelines for establishing joint or collaborative practice in hospitals. Chicago, Neely Printing, 1981.

Paulen, A.: Practice issues for the oncology clinical nurse specialist. Oncol Nurs Forum *12*(2):37–39, 1985.

Riegel, B., & Murrell, T.: CNSs in collaborative practice. Clinical Nurse Specialist *1*:63–69, 1987.

Ryan, L. S., Edwards, R. L., and Rickles, F. R.: A joint practice approach to the care of persons with cancer. Oncol Nurs Forum *7*(1):8–11, 1980.

Shepard, K., Yeo, G., and McGann, L.: Successful components of interdisciplinary education. J Allied Health *14*:297–303, 1985.

Steel, J. E. (ed): Issues in Collaborative Practice. Orlando, New York, Grune and Stratton, 1986.

Wise, H., Beckhard, R., Rubin, I., et al.: Making Health Teams Work. Cambridge, MA, Ballinger, 1974.

# Clinical Leadership, Management, and the CNS

*Joyce L. Gournic*

## INTRODUCTION

Changes in financial reimbursement and consumer awareness have forced health care organizations—particularly hospitals—to re-examine their delivery of health care in terms of both quality and cost-effectiveness (Joel, 1985b). Health care programs and personnel are being re-evaluated as to their impact on the organization. Those programs and personnel that do not contribute to the viability of the organization are phased out, and additional responsibilities are assigned to those who remain. The author and other nursing leaders (Hoeffer & Murphy, 1984; Joel, 1985a; Malone, 1986) believe that a lack of understanding of the CNS role prompts administrators to specifically examine the contribution of CNSs to the organization and to quality, cost-effective patient care.

The cost-effectiveness and productivity of the CNS are often difficult to quantify and measure because of the inherent ambiguity of the CNS role. Lack of consistency by the CNS and the organization in defining the CNS's roles and responsibilities is a major factor contributing to this ambiguity (Farkas, 1982; Harrell & McCullough, 1986). Because of the lack of a role definition that is familiar to organizations and the shortage of valid and reliable objective measurements required to establish the effectiveness and contribution of the CNS, the CNS in a staff position is particularly vulnerable. The accomplishments of the CNS in a staff position are often not directly attributable to the actions of the CNS. This prevents identification of those behaviors that positively affect the organization and makes it difficult for the CNS to defend the role's value.

The possible administrative responses aimed at cost containment and revenue generation which may influence CNSs include eliminating the CNS position, restructuring the CNS role into a line position ( Joel, 1985a; Poulin, 1985), and restructuring the CNS role so that it remains a staff position but mainly generates revenue for the organization (see Chapter 19).

CNSs also respond to this changing environment in several ways. Those who no longer wish to be CNSs may choose to become nurse administrators or entrepreneurs. Other CNSs take on a line role hoping to maintain a practice and a CNS identity. Still others take a line position as a survival strategy and mourn the loss of the clinical CNS role. Some CNSs successfully merge clinical and management positions through careful and thorough planning.

In this competitive health care environment in which fiscal constraint is paramount, a clear delineation of CNS leadership and management behaviors and the critical mix of these behaviors may be one key to survival of the CNS role and CNSs' clinical contributions to patient care. Clinical leadership is a major component of the CNS role and is an expectation of administrators and staff. In addition, most CNSs would agree that management knowledge, skills, and processes enhance one's effectiveness as a clinical leader regardless of organizational placement. However, there is little information available in the literature to give the CNS needed guidance to make these leadership and management skills work to advantage. Consequently, there are CNSs in line positions who hope to maintain a clinical practice but who are unable to do so successfully.

Because of the leadership capabilities of the CNS, it is often assumed that the CNS is a natural for a management position, and the CNS may be placed in that position with little or no concern for the effect on direct patient care activities. For CNSs who wish to maintain a CNS identity, it is imperative that line positions for CNSs are structured carefully. Without such attention to line placement, a CNS runs the risk of losing the practice role and perhaps the ability to exercise *clinical* leadership.

This chapter will compare and contrast leadership and management skills as they pertain to the CNS role. It will also address how the CNS, regardless of organizational placement, acquires, integrates, and uses these skills. In addition, a leadership/management continuum will be described which will provide strategies for implementing leadership and management skills regardless of whether the CNS is in a line or staff position. Finally, the author will propose rationales and criteria for placing a CNS in a line management position as well as strategies for making it work to the advantage of both the CNS and the organization.

## LEADERSHIP AND MANAGEMENT

The terms leadership and management are often used interchangeably. Although similar in concept, they are not identical. Because leadership and management are interdependent, abstract concepts that continually evolve in a dynamic environment, no definition will ever accurately describe either term. It has been argued by experts that there are as many different definitions of leadership and management as there are leaders and managers (Drucker, 1974; Stodgill, 1974; Hershey & Blanchard, 1982).

Leadership has been defined by Stodgill (1974) as the process of influencing the activities of an individual or group toward goal setting and goal achievement. Leadership may exist on a formal or informal basis. Lundborg (1982) described the true leader as one who is a good communicator and morale builder and as one who accepts responsibility for the actions and results of the group.

In contrast to leadership, management can be defined as "working with and through individuals and groups to accomplish organizational goals" (Hershey & Blanchard, 1982, p. 3). Drucker (1974) delineated the work of the manager as setting objectives, organizing, motivating and communicating those objectives, measuring performance, and most importantly, developing the potential of people. The manager is the one who has legitimate authority to direct specific resources to accomplish organizational goals and who is expected to be the problem-solver of the organization (Zaleznik, 1981; Portnoy, 1986).

Contemporary management experts emphasize that, in our modern "fluid" society, the definition of management must expand to incorporate and encourage leadership behavior among managers if organizations are to flourish and retain leaders (Naisbitt, 1982; Drucker, 1985; Naisbitt & Aburdene, 1985). In addition, management principles and techniques must extend beyond the confines of administrative abilities and be internalized by all leaders regardless of organizational placement. Managers are responsible for developing the hidden potential of personnel by aligning personal goals with those of the organization. This results in an organization that fosters leadership behavior and that is rewarded by an innovative staff who embrace change and identify their own needs for personal and organizational goal attainment.

The shifting of management principles to include leadership behaviors further adds to the ambiguity between the two concepts. Since both leadership and management require interpersonal involvement for goal attainment, the major distinctions between these two concepts appear to be the authority of the person seeking the goal attainment and the goals themselves.

The authority bestowed on a manager is that which is attached to the position and not necessarily to the person who holds that position. The legitimate authority inherent in the manager position will exist regardless of the abilities of the individual manager. On the other hand, leaders enjoy expert authority that is earned as a result of their demonstrated ability to influence the behavior of others. Leaders may lose this authority if their followers fail to perceive them as influential.

The other major distinction between leadership and management is that of goal attainment. Managers work toward achievement of organizational goals, while leaders work toward personal goals that may or may not be the same as those of the organization. Hershey and Blanchard believed that the achievement of the organization's goals through leadership is itself management (1982). As management practices shift to encourage innovation, it becomes increasingly difficult to distinguish a leader's activities toward goal attainment from a manager's activities.

McFarland, Leonard, and Morris (1984) believed that not all managers are leaders and that not all leaders are found solely in management roles. By influencing the behavior of those in the organization to realize positive change and to accomplish both personal and professional goals, it is possible to be a successful leader without being a manager. However, it is nearly impossible to be a successful manager without being a leader. Without leadership ability, the issuance of orders does not guarantee successful implementation or completion of tasks or goals. Because leaders are not encumbered by the goals of the organization, they can dream of what could be while managers must face the reality of what is (Zaleznik, 1981). The best manager is one who can dream and then turn dreams into reality.

In the health care system, the CNS may be the ideal person for merging leader and manager roles. As the expert in a clinical practice area, the CNS can visualize what clinical practice *should* be. In addition, the combination of leadership and management skills inherent in any CNS role can serve as a complement to those managerial skills required in line positions. Placing CNSs in line positions without careful reflection on these ideas of leadership and management and on what a particular job requires may serve neither the CNS nor the organization well. In Chapter 11, Sample addresses organizational placement that can meet both the needs of the organization and of the CNS.

# CNS LEADERSHIP/MANAGEMENT CONTINUUM

The CNS leadership/management continuum is offered as a means for new and practicing CNSs to assess, implement, and evaluate leadership and management opportunities that may arise (Figure 10–1). Because of the leadership capabilities of the CNS, an administrator who needs to decrease personnel costs often sees a management position as the only option for CNSs if they are to remain in the system. This need not occur if the CNS has already considered all alternatives and knows what the needs of the oganization are and how to best meet them without compromising the CNS's clinical practice. The struggle to defend each component of the CNS role, especially that of clinical practice, lies with the CNS and requires the CNS to propose alternatives that integrate these components. It is only when the CNS has not done adequate preparation that the alternatives are limited and the choices are few. This evaluation process is important for the new or experienced CNS who is looking for a job and also for the CNS whose organization and position are being reorganized.

## Assumptions

The leadership/management continuum is based on the following assumptions that are critical to successful utilization of the CNS. The first assumption is that management principles are invaluable to leaders and managers alike. Regardless of organizational placement, CNSs need some familiarity with management language, skills, and processes. Knowledge of what an FTE (full-time equivalent) is and how a head nurse staffs a unit affords the CNS the opportunity to plan the optimum time for doing patient care conferences or offering continuing education (CE) opportunities. Management skills such as how to run a meeting can help the CNS accomplish goals more efficiently by delegating the

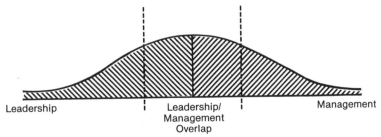

**Figure 10–1.** Leadership/management continuum with overlap of leadership and management knowledge, skills, and processes.

committee's activities to other participants. Time management skills prove useful to any CNS who feels the internal and external pressures of trying to accomplish so much in so little time. Survival and growth of patient care activities depend on the CNS's management knowledge of how to develop a clinical program or how to communicate both upward and downward in an organization.

Within the structure of the CNS role there are many leadership and management skills that need to be acquired, strengthened, and incorporated into practice, e.g., developing and implementing standards of care, introducing change successfully, and documenting effectiveness (Farkas, 1982; Hoeffer & Murphy, 1984; Fenton, 1985; Paulen, 1985). Poteet and Branyon (1986) believed that in order to be effective in their clinical practice CNSs, particularly those in staff positions, also need to have an understanding of communication networks, role relationships, and organizational behaviors.

The second set of assumptions relate to the leadership and practice aspects of the CNS role. Although it is not necesary that all CNSs be managers, it is imperative that all CNSs exhibit leadership behaviors in order to successfully influence patient care activities. However, if the CNS assumes a management position and wishes to retain a CNS identity, it is critical that each subrole, especially the clinical practice component, be maintained. If any component is lost, the CNS ceases to be a CNS.

The third assumption is that leadership and management behaviors are learned through various methods and utilized differently throughout CNS practice. As familiarization and confidence in the CNS role occur, the CNS is able to expand these behaviors and incorporate them more into practice.

## Description of Continuum

The leadership/management continuum consists of those leadership and management skills, knowledge, and processes that any CNS may need to use in practice depending upon the focus of the organization, the interests of the CNS, and the CNS's job responsibilities (Table 10–1 and Figure 10–1). Within each of the major subroles of clinician, teacher, consultant, and researcher, numerous opportunities exist for the CNS to demonstrate leadership and management skills. The primary focus for the new CNS will be at the far end of the leadership side of the continuum until more confidence is developed in the CNS role (Figure 10–2).

For the CNS in a staff position, leadership behaviors are utilized more frequently (Figure 10–3). As the CNS moves closer to or accepts

**TABLE 10–1. CNS Knowledge, Skills, and Processes**

| CLINICAL LEADERSHIP | LEADERSHIP/MANAGEMENT—OVERLAP FOR CNS/NURSE MANAGER | CLINICAL MANAGEMENT |
|---|---|---|
| • Clinical expertise<br>• Interpersonal competence<br>• Personal goals<br>• Role identity<br>• Recognizing generic recurring clinical problems<br>• "Massaging the system"<br>• Developing and implementing standards<br>• Recognizing and addressing ethical issues<br>• Support of staff nurse<br>• Consultation<br>• Patient advocacy<br>• Communication patterns<br>• Role model | • Organizational psychology (L/M)<br>• Understanding of organizational roles (L/M)<br>• Organizational communication—up, down, lateral (L/M)<br>• Time management (M)<br>• Group leader skills—committee (L)<br>• Group process skills (L)<br>• Program planning and development (M)<br>• Conflict resolution (L)<br>• Organization mission and goals (M)<br>• Collaboration (L)<br>• Problem-solving—analysis and insight (L)<br>• Change theory (L)<br><br>(L) = Leadership behaviors<br>(M) = Management behaviors<br>(L/M) = Behaviors used equally by leaders and managers | • Finance<br>• Personnel evaluation<br>• Marketing<br>• Program evaluation<br>• Personnel scheduling<br>• Hiring and firing<br>• Disciplinary actions |

233

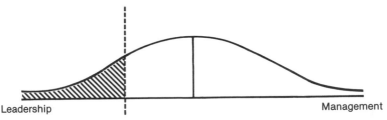

**Figure 10–2.** Range of behaviors on leadership/management continuum for beginning CNS.

a management position, the distribution between leadership and management behaviors becomes more equal (Figure 10–4).

Since most CNSs are not in line positions, effective leadership skills are vital if the CNS is to accomplish the goal of improving patient care both directly and indirectly. The CNS provides leadership in developing standards for new populations of patients (e.g., AIDS patients) or for populations requiring nursing care while undergoing a new therapy (e.g., patients receiving interleukin 2). Another demonstration of clinical leadership is recognition of a generic recurring event that requires modification of existing nursing care (e.g., evaluating an increased incidence of patient falls) or identification of deficiencies that are present in providing total patient care (e.g., strengthening family support systems).

One of the most difficult tasks for a new CNS is the acquisition and development of organizational knowledge, skills, and processes (Edlund & Hodges, 1983). These are the skills that help define who has formal and informal power in the organization, what the communication networks are that speed things through the system, and how the organization is influenced.

Knowing who to influence enables the CNS to alter behavior and opinions of nursing staff and administration to provide better patient care. Talking to the right person about a project or change in nursing care procedure can assist the CNS in accomplishing the task with the

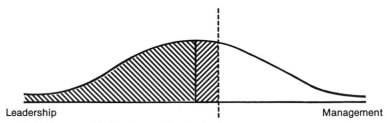

**Figure 10–3.** Range of behaviors on leadership/management continuum for CNS in a staff position.

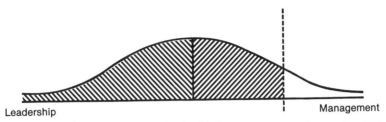

Leadership                                                                    Management

**Figure 10–4.** Range of behaviors on leadership/management continuum for CNS in a management position.

least resistance and possibly with a great deal of support. This skill is often refered to as "massaging the system" and involves developing a network of supporters throughout the organization who can help speed up the bureaucratic process (Fenton, 1985). Leadership skills strengthen the CNS's ability to argue, defend, explain, and justify the need for change within the organization.

These leadership skills are often interpreted as administrative skills. They are, however, more precisely survival skills. Without the knowledge of who is in control and how the daily operation is run, frustration becomes rampant and little is accomplished. Knowing how the organization is run helps the CNS to realize that there are various aspects of the system over which the CNS has little control (Farkas, 1982; Fenton, 1985). This permits assessment and control of the situation without wasting time on those aspects that are beyond the CNS's influence and actions. For example, when administration is under pressure to correct a critical nursing shortage, it is fairly certain that little attention will be given to those ideas that do not address this shortage. Failure of administration to respond to other issues demonstrates a shift in priority and does not necessarily imply lack of concern. The CNS who is involved in this "tug-of-war" of priorities is well-advised to remain objective and to be prepared when the priorities shift again.

Establishing oneself as a clinical expert and increasing one's knowledge of interpersonal, problem-solving, and organizational skills will serve to increase independent judgment and self-confidence. The CNS will be recognized as one who is credible and able to influence the behavior of others.

Knowledge of the clinical management end of the continuum (see Figure 10–1), which addresses financial and personnel issues, can be obtained by consulting those within the organization who have this expertise. As with the other behaviors, these processes can be valuable in assisting the CNS to accomplish goals and to survive within the organization. These clinical management concepts are not as alien to the CNS as might first be supposed. For example, the CNS is already using a basic marketing technique. Before presenting a staff inservice or educational offering, a needs assessment is often conducted. A needs assessment is a tool used routinely in marketing to determine the advisability of initiating a program. The CNS who can defend a patient program by presenting the financial benefits to the organization has a greater chance of succeeding than the CNS who argues only the issue of quality of care.

When one considers the breadth and depth of the capabilities of the CNS who can develop and combine leadership and management behaviors, it is no wonder that administrators want to place CNSs in management positions. There will be times in the CNS's practice when the CNS will move back and forth along the continuum to best meet the needs of the patient, the CNS, and the organization. The leadership/management continuum is expected to aid the CNS in making these transitions.

## Utility of the Continuum

The utility of the leadership/management continuum lies in its ability to: (1) assist CNSs and administrators to determine what mix of leadership and management knowledge, skills, and processes are needed to make a particular CNS position work well for the CNS and the organization and still maintain a clinical practice focus; (2) help CNSs determine if management factors are limiting their clinical roles; (3) enable CNSs to make career decisions; and (4) help CNSs, educators, and administrators develop plans and experiences to strengthen specific skills.

The utilization of the continuum affords both the CNS and administrator the opportunity to benefit from the leadership and management behaviors of the CNS. More importantly, the CNS can choose to enter a line position confident that the practice component of the CNS role can remain intact.

# ASSESSMENT OF LEADERSHIP/ MANAGEMENT BEHAVIORS

Before any decisions are made concerning the appropriateness of a particular position, the CNS must conduct both self- and organizational assessments in order to identify strengths and weaknesses that might prove advantageous or troublesome. Self-assessment is an important function for both the new and experienced CNS particularly because of the ambiguity of the CNS role and the differences in practice that exist from organization to organization. CNSs need to define the role for both the organization and themselves (Paulen, 1985).

The bases for a self-assessment are the behaviors listed in Table 10–1 along with the determination of how comfortable the CNS is in each component of the role. Areas that need to be considered are personal and professional goals and level of knowledge and skills in leadership and management behaviors. The ability to tolerate ambiguity and frustration and to be assertive in making one's needs known are two skills that prove helpful in the CNS's pursuit of clinical success. Self-assessment is the first step in becoming a successful leader (Holt, 1984). The next step is a careful assessment of the organizational structure and environment.

In conducting the organizational assessment, a critical factor to evaluate is the organization's and, specifically, the administrator's perceptions of and commitment to the CNS role. Other key factors that affect the CNS role are the organization's philosophy, goals, and objectives, and the CNS job description.

The organizations's philosophy and goals give a good picture of what the organization expects to accomplish now and in the future. They offer the CNS the opportunity to see the importance and integration of nursing activities within the organization and to evaluate the impact of a specialty area. The job description delineates the responsibilities of the CNS role, the authority of the CNS, the person to whom the CNS is directly responsible, and the amount of autonomy, flexibility, and accountability that is expected.

These self- and organizational assessments should be done when job hunting and on a periodic basis while in a CNS role. The purpose of such assessments is to determine the congruency of the CNS's personal and professional goals with those of the organization and to identify new learning needs related to acquisition of undeveloped leadership and management skills. Based on the assessment, a CNS may decide that there is a good match between personal and organizational goals and needs. The better the match, the easier it will be to use leadership behavior to everyone's advantage. The greater the disparity between CNS and organizational goals, the less likely it is that leadership behaviors alone will enable the CNS to be effective. In the latter case, the CNS may wish to explore with the administrator the possibility of a line position, or the CNS may make a decision that the goals are so disparate that it is not feasible to join or continue with the organization. There are times when both CNS and organizational goals may be congruent, but the nature of the goal demands that the CNS have some line authority such as that held by a program coordinator in cardiac rehabilitation or in oncology.

Thorough assessment facilitates this occurrence without jeopardizing the clinical practice component of the CNS role.

## ACQUISITION AND DEMONSTRATION OF LEADERSHIP AND MANAGEMENT KNOWLEDGE, SKILLS, AND PROCESSES

Many leadership and management behaviors are taught in graduate school and developed in the CNS practice. The CNS has ample opportunity to acquire and demonstrate effective leadership and management skills in day-to-day practice situations.

### Acquisition of Knowledge, Skills, and Processes

Graduate school offers the prospective CNS an introduction to leadership knowledge, skills, and processes that will be beneficial in the CNS's practice. Course content and practicum experience should provide the following: organizational psychology and structure; verbal and nonverbal communication patterns and techniques; change theory and an opportunity to apply change strategies to the clinical setting; opportunities to practice as a student CNS, after observing experienced CNSs, and to solve complex clinical problems successfully; and development, application, and evaluation of clinical standards for a patient population.

Graduate education should also provide management knowledge, skills, and processes that include group process skills and leadership, time management techniques, and a basic management language essential to successfully implementing the CNS role. Because of the emphasis on the clinical practice component of the CNS role, graduate education has been lax in offering the CNS adequate exposure to management behaviors.

Changes in health care organizations are prompting graduate schools to realize that more courses and experiences in management behaviors are essential for the CNS who practices in either a line or staff position (Poteet & Branyon, 1986). Such course work should give the beginning CNS self-confidence in discussing the CNS role and its benefit to the organization while learning how to incorporate the clinical practice component. Graduate school is an excellent opportunity for the CNS to merge leadership and management knowledge, skills, and processes with expectations of the CNS role. Continuing education and the workplace offer further opportunities for the CNS to acquire and then develop additional leadership and management behaviors.

## Demonstration of Knowledge, Skill, and Processes

With leadership and management knowledge, skills and processes acquired in graduate school, the CNS is prepared to further develop and demonstrate these behaviors in clinical practice. The CNS should actively seek opportunities to exercise clinical leadership in the workplace. This can be easily accomplished by caring for patients with complex problems and sorting out the accompanying clinical issues. Identifying recurrent generic problems and developing strategies to address these will demonstrate leadership behaviors to the staff. One example is that of a neurological CNS who noted an increased incidence of falls among elderly patients and instituted standards and a continuing education offering to help staff reduce the incidence.

CNSs can demonstrate management skills by assuming the role of chairperson on a committee that relates to the CNS's clinical specialty. This increases the CNS's organizational influence by giving an additional opportunity to demonstrate leadership and management skills as well as the opportunity to be in the forefront of any organizational changes that may affect the CNS's practice. Participation by the CNS in budget procedures may safeguard the staffing and equipment requirements of a clinical program. For example, an oncology CNS assessed and documented the need for a concentrated care unit for septic patients and others who required one-to-one but not ICU care, apprised the head nurse of the equipment needs, and elicited the head nurse's input on staffing needs. In this example, the CNS demonstrated both leadership and management behaviors, among which was the ability to recognize the authority of another and to work within that constraint while still accomplishing the CNS's goal

Another example of the need for a CNS to demonstrate leadership skills is shown in the following situation. With the head nurse on vacation, the charge nurse approached the CNS about a postoperative patient whose condition was very unstable. For two days the charge nurse had been trying to get the attending physician to transfer the patient to ICU without success. The physician believed that the patient was receiving appropriate care and did not need to be transferred. With the charge nurse present, the CNS reviewed the chart, assessed the patient, talked to the primary nurse, and then approached the physician. The CNS presented the patient's pattern of instability, including vital signs, laboratory data, and physical assessment data, and emphasized the advantages of placing the patient in the ICU. The physician agreed and the patient was transferred. This is an example of using clinical expertise and leadership to effect a change in patient care.

One of the major causes of financial concern for health care organizations is in the area of diagnostic related groups (DRGs) and the subsequent economic impact of early patient discharge from the system. The CNS can demonstrate organizational savvy and clinical leadership by instituting discharge planning procedures that meet the needs of the patient and staff while decreasing the length of hospital stay and saving the hospital potential lost revenue. By developing and instituting standards of care that include plans for the patient upon and after discharge, the CNS is able to incorporate the concepts of discharge planning into the system from the time of the patient's admission. One cardiovascular CNS was able to accomplish this by instituting a program in the coronary care unit (CCU) by which staff members, cardiac patients, and their families addressed the potential problems that the patient might encounter after discharge. Such a program continued as the patient progressed through the hospital system and served to better prepare the patient for discharge from the hospital as well as to give the staff a sense of what happened to the patient after being transferred or discharged from their unit.

There are abundant opportunities for the CNS to acquire and demonstrate leadership and management knowledge, skills, and processes in the workplace. The more these behaviors are utilized, the less difficulty the CNS will have in being identified as a clinical leader.

## THE CNS IN A MANAGEMENT POSITION

The CNS who assumes a management position must integrate both practice and management components and must be comfortable and confident in doing so. For the CNS who wishes to retain the CNS identity, the danger in a management position is the loss of the important clinical practice component. When the CNS stops functioning as a clinician, that part of the role is lost, and the CNS is no longer in a CNS role but is practicing instead as a manager. This is a critical issue for any CNS who enters into a management position and especially for the beginning CNS. A management position is not recommended for the new CNS who needs to develop role identity and confidence in the clinical practice component. However, in today's changing health care environment, the CNS may not have the option to fully develop the CNS role before being faced with a decision of whether or not to assume a management position. There are various criteria and strategies that should facilitate this decision process for both new and experienced CNSs.

## Criteria for a Workable CNS/Manager Position

For the CNS to function successfully in a management position while maintaining a clinical practice component, specific criteria must exist. The most important of all the criteria is that the organization is supportive of the CNS role. It is also necessary to establish the reason for the CNS being placed in a management position. A management position may serve to broaden the scope of the CNS's influence or it may be a means by which the organization can abolish the existing CNS position.

The organization's support for the CNS position is demonstrated by the manner in which the CNS is involved in patient care issues. The goals and objectives of the organization should include the CNS in the decision-making process concerning patient care issues and not just management ones. The job description should include direct patient care, consultation, education, and research as major responsibilities not merely as indirect functions. If this is not done, then the management position is designed to be solely an administrative one with only indirect patient care functions.

If the CNS is to have the necessary time to devote to clinical practice, the sphere of responsibility for the CNS in a management position must be limited in the number of patients and number and type of employees supervised. The guidelines that follow are based on the personal observations and experiences of the author and other CNSs who have been both successful and unsuccessful in maintaining a clinical practice as a CNS/manager.

For an inpatient unit on which the CNS has 24 hour accountability, the number of patients should not exceed 10. More than 10 inpatients would result in an increase in the degree of management responsibility for the CNS and a decrease in the amount of available clinical practice time. Obviously, both staffing and administrative tasks multiply with the addition of more patients. When management tasks require continual attention, the clinical practice component suffers.

It is possible for the CNS/manager to supervise a unit of more than 10 patients, if the CNS has a head nurse responsible for most of the unit's administrative functions. In this situation, the head nurse handles scheduling, performance evaluations, and unit management activities, while the CNS monitors clinical practice. Responsibilities between these two leaders must be carefully differentiated (Gresham, 1976). This arrangement allows the CNS to concentrate on clinical practice activities for a larger unit than would be possible if the CNS were the sole leader.

For an outpatient unit, the number of patient visits is not as crucial as the hours of operation and the staff to patient ratio. The hours of operation should be such that the CNS does not have to be concerned with around-the-clock staffing. Ideally, the outpatient unit operates on an 8- to 12-hour schedule. The staff to patient ratio should allow each patient to receive individualized care from the unit staff and from the CNS. An outpatient unit that has more than a 1:5 staff to patient ratio will prove troublesome for the CNS in a management position because of the problems that arise with coverage for sick or absent staff members.

The number of employees that the CNS supervises should be limited to 10 for both inpatient and outpatient units. Staffing problems for the CNS are then kept to a minimum, as are the accompanying personnel responsibilities, such as hiring, disciplinary counseling, and evaluating staff performance. As the experience and expertise of the staff increases, the CNS is able to supervise a larger number of patients or employees. Administrative tasks such as scheduling patients or staff and some aspects of budgeting and report generation can be delegated. This not only frees the CNS from many of the routine administrative tasks but also demonstrates a trust in the staff's abilities to perform these tasks. Fostering this behavior in the staff will encourge those with administrative ambitions to develop their management skills.

A definite advantage to any CNS who assumes a management position is the presence of another CNS who is in a similar management position in the organization and who has maintained a successful clinical practice. For the CNS new to this kind of position, it is essential to find a support person who can, in effect, act as the CNS's mentor and who can assist the CNS in implementing the position. The CNS who already has this same type of practice will prove most valuable in identifying the pitfalls and in suggesting effective tactics.

## Strategies to Integrate the CNS Role with the Management Position

If the CNS decides to assume a line position, a constant balance between the CNS subroles, particularly the clinician role and the management position, needs to be actively maintained. Several strategies are proposed to make the management position a successful one for the CNS and the organization and to protect the clinical practice component of the role (Table 10–2). This subrole is emphasized because it is the easiest to lose when one takes on management responsibilities.

It is to the CNS's advantage not only to continue professional development in the clinical specialty area but also to develop a firm base of management knowledge, skills, and processes as described in the leadership/management continuum. Although initially this may

**TABLE 10–2. Strategies for Successful Integration of Clinical Practice and Management**

1. Confirm that job description contains equal mix of clinical and management responsibilities.
2. Continue professional development in clinical practice specialty.
3. Develop strong knowledge base of leadership and management behaviors contained in leadership/management continuum through continuing education.
4. Conduct periodic evaluation of distribution of clinical and management responsibilities and tasks.
5. Develop rapport with an administrator who is supportive and could act as a mentor.
6. Establish reporting system that demonstrates both clinical and management accomplishments.
7. Develop management abilities of staff so they integrate various management tasks within their job responsibilities.
8. Structure work so that specific blocks of time are set aside for management responsibilities, for clinical practice, for education, and for research.

seem to further entrench the CNS in management behaviors, what really transpires is a CNS who is confident in both clinical leadership and management behaviors and who can create an equilibrium between the management and clinical practice aspects of the CNS role. With this confidence, the CNS is able to dictate the amount of time required for various management responsibilities and to defend those decisions.

Certain major management tasks require a time commitment only at specific months of the year. Although important, tasks such as budgeting, performance reviews, and financial reports require only a small, concentrated amount of the CNS's total annual work time to complete. With the use of good organizational and time management skills, information pertinent to completion of these activities can be collected over the course of a year and then finalized prior to their due dates, which are essentially the same each year. Any manager who attempts to start and finish a fiscal budget or a staff member's performance review the day before it is due will attest to the value of gathering the prerequisite information far in advance of the completion date. Once the major work on these are finished, they usually demand only short, periodic updates to keep them current. There are numerous continuing education offerings for nurses which can supply this basic knowledge and provide CNS/managers with the necessary tools.

The CNS needs to establish a reporting system that is beneficial to the CNS role but not time-consuming. The first step is to develop a rapport with the administrator to whom the CNS reports. A good relationship with this administrator is essential if the CNS is to establish the direction of the CNS role as well as the components to be included in the management position. When the CNS and the administrator share the same goal of quality patient care, both benefit from a relationship built on shared goals and mutual trust. Hopefully, the administrator is one who supports the actions of the CNS to other administrators, who upholds the importance of the CNS's clinical practice, and who could act as a mentor for the management role.

Having developed a rapport with the administrator, the next step is to decide on the reporting system itself. It is recommended that CNSs submit regular reports (i.e., quarterly, semiannually) to their immediate supervisors. Such reports can track CNS leadership/management activities and are useful for annual performance reviews and self-evaluations. These reports should be based on the goals and objectives that the CNS established for the year and should include both clinical and leadership/management behaviors. One or two sentences on the progress of each goal and objective is all that is required. Malone asserted that lack of documentation by the CNS is responsible for hospital administrators wondering what it is that the CNS does (1986). Regular reports keep administration advised of the management and clinical actions and successes of the CNS and provide an objective measure for evaluation. In addition, the CNS can structure the reports to contain those components that are important to the CNS role.

As with the CNS subroles, the amount of time spent on management behaviors has to be carefully determined. Time management skills, especially the ability to set priorities, are necessary for all CNSs but are imperative for the CNS in a management position. The management position must be structured so that time is set aside for management responsibilities, clinical practice, education, and research.

One way to look at the CNS/management position is to compare it to the joint appointment practitioner/teacher role that has gained acceptance in universities and medical centers. It is essentially two roles filled by one person. In the joint appointment practitioner/teacher role, the CNS must divide time commitments between the CNS subroles and formal teaching responsibilities. In the management position, the time is split between CNS practice and administrative components. If the two components are kept separate as they are in a joint appointment, then the clinical practice component remains intact while the CNS functions as an effective manager.

One way to separate the management and clinical components is to set aside segments of time for each specific component. The first few hours of each work day or a particular day of the week may be earmarked for management responsibilities, while the remainder of the time is spent on clinical matters. This is best conveyed to staff and colleagues by posting an activity calendar marked with the times or days designated for each component. In the beginning, the CNS must strictly adhere to this schedule so everyone becomes familiar with this pattern of clinical and management delineation.

It is critical that the CNS conduct periodic reviews of the management position by referring to the leadership/management continuum to determine the mix of responsibilities and tasks and to be alert for shifts in behaviors and activities that encroach on clinical practice. When increasing amounts of time are devoted to management, the CNS needs to recognize the risk of losing the clinical practice component. Regular monitoring of and reflection on the CNS/manager's practice and management roles are essential if the CNS wishes to both practice and manage effectively.

## Example of CNS in a Management Position

The following is offered as an example of successful integration of CNS practice with a management position. The author is the manager of a cardiac rehabilitation program with a five-member RN staff and a staff to patient ratio of 1:5 or at times 1:4.

The CNS/manager position evolved from a thriving inpatient cardiac rehabilitation service that originated with one part-time CNS responsible for education and counseling of cardiac patients. After a year of increasing patient caseload and physician requests for expanded services, another CNS was added.

As the cardiac rehabilitation program grew to include outpatient services, it became necessary for someone to assume the additional administrative responsibilities. At first this was done by the author on an informal basis so that control of the department would remain with those within the department. The author had been in practice for four years and was comfortable and confident with the leadership behaviors of the CNS role. After several months of performing the combined role and after careful self- and organizational assessment, the author submitted a CNS/manager job description to administration. The job description was designed to contain both clinical and administrative components. It had been previously determined that the administrator was supportive of the clinical practice component. The new combined CNS/manager position was accepted, and the author assumed this position on a formal basis.

The success of the position lies with the scheduling of management and clinical activities and with the composition and capabilities of the staff. The staff of the cardiac rehabilitation program just described consists of three Nurse Clinician (NC) IIIs and two CNSs in addition to the CNS/manager. Hospitalized patients are seen by the two CNSs on consultation. Outpatients are supervised by the CNS/manager and the three NC IIIs. Time is set aside on Tuesday and Thursday for management tasks. Every effort is made to have committee meetings scheduled on these days. All or part of Monday, Wednesday, and Friday are devoted to clinical practice issues. The CNS in the management position is able to act as a mentor for the other two CNSs and to provide clinical specialist practicum experience for graduate nursing students.

The staff are autonomous nurses who are responsible for their own coverage of sick and vacation time, and the CNS/manager is notified of their decisions or of any problems. The staff is also responsible for supply orders, requisitions for maintenance and equipment repairs, and supervision of the work area when the CNS is not available. This provides a sharing among all staff members of clinical and administrative tasks and gives the CNS/manager ample time to practice in the clinical setting. Leadership behavior is encouraged among all staff, and independent judgment based on strong problem-solving skills is fostered. The CNS/manager has become adept at management through continuing education, experience, and advice of other managers.

The advantages of the CNS assuming the management position have been the opportunities to: (1) maintain the clinical practice component of the CNS role as part of the management position; (2) maintain and increase the number of practicing CNSs in the organization; (3) increase the visibility and awareness of the CNS role among nursing and non-nursing administrators; (4) guarantee the quality and viability of the cardiac rehabilitation program; and (5) influence the decision-making process within the organization as it pertains to all cardiac services, especially those not directed by nursing personnel. The CNS has had little difficulty in maintaining the clinical practice component because of the assessments done prior to accepting the position and to the ongoing evaluation of the mix of clinical and administrative behaviors. The only problem initially encountered was gaining acceptance by other CNSs who were in staff positions. This was overcome through communication of the CNS's commitment to and success in maintaining the CNS role.

## EVALUATION

The evaluation of the CNS's leadership and management behaviors is accomplished through use of the leadership/management continuum. For the CNS in a staff position, evaluation will concentrate mainly on those behaviors on the leadership end of the continuum and on the CNS's ability to incorporate leadership behaviors into the practice of the CNS role. Indirectly the evaluation process is influenced by the CNS's leadership ability to communicate the success of goal attainment and other clinical accomplishment that might not be readily apparent. An excellent test of the CNS's leadership skills is to see whether the results of the CNS's actions have been noted and recognized by others in the organization.

For the CNS in a management position, the leadership and management behaviors that need to be evaluated will consist of those from all sections of the continuum and must also reflect clinical practice activities. Specific areas relating to effective accomplishment of leadership and management behaviors need to be included in the evaluation process. The areas to be considered are: (1) accomplishment of organizational goals and objectives; (2) accomplishment of personal goals and objectives; (3) involvement in organizational assessment, planning, implementation, and evaluation of projects involving specialty; (4) growth of programs initiated and/or coordinated by the CNS; (5) quality patient care as measured by quality assurance monitoring standards; and (6) cost-effectiveness of patient care activities in such areas as revenue producing ability, decreased length of stay for patients, decreased readmission rates, decreased staff turnover, and ability to stay within fiscal constraints. Use of the leadership/management continuum facilitates evaluation of the CNS's ability to utilize both leadership and management behaviors.

## SUMMARY

Regardless of placement, the CNS must possess and utilize leadership and management skills that influence the delivery of quality patient care and increase the value of the role to the organization. The CNS must continue to be viewed as a leader skilled in the use of leadership knowledge, skills, and processes. In addition, all CNSs must possess some knowledge of management processes to enhance their leadership behaviors. However, some CNSs, because of the nature of the job and the changes being experienced by health care organizations, must be equally skilled in leadership and management behaviors. For these CNSs, a balance between clinical and administrative responsibilities must be sought to protect the practice component of the CNS role in a line position. The future of the CNS within the health care environment depends upon the CNS's ability to identify those factors that strengthen or threaten the existence of the CNS role and clinical practice.

It is possible to protect and maintain the CNS's clinical practice in a competitive, cost-conscious environment. CNSs and administrators must work together to structure the CNS role in such a way that the

CNS's clinical leadership in patient care is not sacrificed and that organizational goals are met.

## References

Drucker, P. F.: Management: Tasks, Responsibilities, Practices. New York, Harper & Row, 1974.
Drucker, P. F.: Innovation and Entrepreneurship: Practices and Principles. New York, Harper & Row, 1985.
Edlund, B. J., & Hodges, L. C.: Preparing and using the clinical nurse specialist. Nurs Clin North Am 18(3):499–507, 1983.
Farkas, N.: The clinical nurse specialist in hospital organizations. In Marriner, A. (ed): Contemporary Nursing Management. St. Louis, C. V. Mosby, 1982, pp. 117–126.
Fenton, M. V.: Identifying competencies of clinical nurse specialists. J Nurs Admin 15(12):31–37, 1985.
Gresham, M. L.: Conflict or collaboration: A head nurse's view. In Chamings, P., and Markel, R. (eds): Symposium on the Clinical Nurse Specialist. Indianapolis, Sigma Theta Tau, 1976.
Harrell, J. S., & McCullough, S. D.: The role of the clinical specialist: Problems and solutions. J Nurs Admin 16(10):44–48, 1986.
Hershey, P., & Blanchard, K.: Management of Organizational Behavior: Utilizing Human Resources (ed 4). Englewood Cliffs, N.J., Prentice-Hall, Inc., 1982.
Hoeffer, B., & Murphy, S. A.: Specialization in nursing practice. In ANA (ed): Issues in Professional Nursing Practice. Kansas City, ANA, 1984 (ANA Publication NP-68B).
Holt, F. M.: A theoretical model for clinical specialist practice. Nurs Health Care 5(10):445–449, 1984.
Joel, L. A.: Master's prepared caregivers in line positions: A case study. In NLN (ed): Patterns in Specialization: Challenge to the Curriculum. New York, NLN, 1985 (NLN Publication # 15-2154).
Joel, L. A.: Preparing the clinical specialists for prospective payment. In NLN (ed): Patterns in Education: The Unfolding of Nursing. New York, NLN, 1985b (NLN Publication # 15-1974).
Lundborg, L. B.: What is leadership? J Nurs Admin 12(5):32–33, 1982.
Malone, B. L.: Evaluation of the clinical nurse specialist. Am J Nurs 86(12):1375–1377, 1986.
McFarland, G. K., Leonard, H. S., and Morris, M. M.: Nursing Leadership and Management: Contemporary Strategies. New York, John Wiley & Sons, 1984.
Naisbitt, J.: Megatrends: Ten New Directions Transforming Our Lives. New York, Warner Books, Inc., 1982.
Naisbitt, J., & Aburdene, P.: Re-inventing the Corporation. New York, Warner Books, Inc., 1985.
Paulen, A.: Practice issues for the oncology clinical nurse specialist. Oncol Nurs Forum 12(2):37–39, 1985.
Portnoy, R. A.: Leadership: What Every Leader Should Know About People. Englewood Cliffs, N.J., Prentice-Hall, 1986.
Poteet, G. W., & Branyon, M. E.: Clinical nurse specialist: Not every graduate nursing student qualifies. Nurs Educ 11(5):4, 1986.
Poulin, M. A.: Configurations of nursing practice. In ANA (ed): Issues in Professional Nursing Practice. Kansas City, ANA, 1985 (ANA Publication NP-68E).
Stodgill, R.: Handbook of Leadership: A Survey of Theory and Research. New York, Free Press, 1974.
Zaleznik, A.: Managers and leaders: Are they different? J Nurs Admin 11(7):25–31, 1981.

# PART III

# NURSING ADMINISTRATION AND THE CNS

# Justifying and Structuring the CNS Role Within a Nursing Organization

*Sally A. Sample*

## INTRODUCTION

Most clinical nurse specialists (CNSs) are employed within an organizational entity of the health care delivery system. The justification and placement of the CNS within an organization is based on a rational assessment of the corporate culture of the institution, the environment affecting the institution, a fundamental belief in the professional practice of nursing, and a vision of the future. The purpose of this chapter is to provide a process of deliberative inquiry as to the justification and placement of the CNS within the health care organization. It also has utility in reassessment of the prevailing CNS roles within an organization to meet the institution's goals.

## OVERVIEW OF ENVIRONMENT

The health care industry has been changing rapidly and will continue to change at a rate not seen in previous decades. The combination of technological advances with the resultant changes in medical practices and economic incentives have had a significant impact on professional organizations and health care service delivery. The current environment is turbulent, and the nurse executive is in the center of the vortex, striving to adapt the business of patient care within the organization of nursing services (Ripple, 1986). Nurse executives must seize the opportunity to assess, develop, and implement strategies for their organizations, which will determine standards of care within an integrated health care delivery system; must demonstrate nurses' efficiency and effectiveness in organizing and providing patient care services; must provide leadership that will motivate, educate, and negotiate for professional nursing practice; must strategically plan to meet their institution's goals; and, must market the value of nursing care.

This is an era for the CNS to be in demand. It is an era that values intellectual inquiry, creative insight, and a tolerance for ambiguity that retains a firm grasp on reality. It is an era of marketing specialized patient care services or product lines. It is an era in which clinical and administrative nursing leadership will determine the strategies for the survival, adaptation, and growth of professional nursing practice within organized nursing services.

Both nurse executives and CNSs require specialized skills to advance the practice of professional nursing. Such skills may be different but are complementary and necessary to the successful attainment of professional and institutional goals. However, there must be philosophical agreement on basic premises that will guide the development of the professional practice environment. These basic premises are: (1) nursing is a clinical practice discipline; (2) patient care is the heart of nursing; (3) research into the phenomena of nursing practice builds the foundation of the discipline; and (4) the management and organization of nursing services have as their aim the facilitation of the expert practice of nursing (Fagin, 1985).

## VISION AND VERSATILITY

To implement these premises is a significant challenge to both clinical and administrative leadership. It requires not only a set of skills but also a collaborative vision that determines the desired clinical productivity and patient care outcome.

Vision is a mental journey from the known to the unknown, creating the future from a montage of current facts, hopes, dreams, dangers, and opportunities. Vision helps nurse executives to position themselves and their organizations to create and take advantage of opportunities (Hickman & Silva, 1984). Vision is one way to rethink and reshape the dynamics of one's organization and to refocus the energies of nursing staff in the most productive and positive professional effort. At a recent nursing futures conference sponsored by the American Association of Colleges of Nursing and the American Organization of Nursing Executives, the participants engaged in visionary thinking toward nursing in the 21st century. A message that we can learn from futurists is that we can have the future that we want for our profession and our patients, provided that we take time from the present to engage in the necessary planning (*Journal of Professional Nursing*, 1986).

Vision and versatility are attributes essential for the nurse executive and the CNS. Each needs to anticipate change and develop the capacity to embrace and participate in this ever-changing world of health care and health policy.

Justification and placement of the CNS requires not only an assessment of the external and internal environment in which the institution or agency provides health services but also an assessment of commitment and support for the position within the nursing organization. The continuing evolution of clinical specialization in nursing has had a far greater impact on nursing practice than has any other movement to date. Yet our applause is weak, and our conviction is tested amid the economic environment of the health care industry.

## ASSESSMENT—EXTERNAL ENVIRONMENT

The nursing executive is faced with professional, clinical, and economic imperatives in the health care environment. It is critical for the nursing executive to assess the variables influencing the workplace in which nurses practice and for which the nurse executive has ultimate accountability. Such an assessment is ongoing and continuous. However, it is appropriate to do a more comprehensive assessment prior to placement of a CNS within the organization.

What are the data required of an environmental assessment and how is the information obtained? The nurse executive must prioritize time for reflection, data gathering, and analysis. Only upon reflection will the nurse executive be able to formulate the series of questions that will lead to the development of an environmental assessment. Excellent sources of data are state and national reports on significant health care issues. The state departments of public health generate information on demographics of populations and on reportable diseases and frequently make projections relative to health care needs within the states.

For example, what is the incidence of AIDS within populations that the institution serves? What is the anticipated population growth of elderly in the area, and what resources are available for their care? What target populations have unmet needs in the institution's referral base? Statistics on source of referrals, age of patients by service, and admission and length of stay profiles by case or by diagnostic related groupings (DRGs) within the institution confirm the reality and provide the foundation for forecasting future demands for nursing services.

Professional organizations at the national level have been instrumental in conducting major studies on nursing and health care. The American Nurses' Association (ANA) has produced two comprehensive reports on distribution and utilization of CNSs. These reports were developed by ANA's Council of Clinical Nurse Specialists and the Council on Psychiatric and Mental Health Nursing. Data described the work roles, practice dimensions, work with specific target groups, and factors associated with demographics and income (ANA, 1986). These data are useful in testing one's vision for the future role of the CNS.

Additionally, the ANA has published a series of monographs on Issues in Professional Nursing Practice which guide critical inquiry and future vision. The monograph on standards of nursing practice is directed to pursuit of quality as the intentional object of nursing action, to action for the good of the people served, and to professional renewal through the standards of nursing practice (ANA, 1985). Standards of practice have been developed for diverse practice environments, for generalist as well as specialty practice, such as cancer or rheumatology nursing (ANA, 1972, 1974, 1979, 1982, 1983, 1984, 1985, 1986). These standards have relevance in determining the desired patient care outcomes to be developed by the CNS in practice.

As the majority of CNSs are employed in hospital settings, the variables that attract and retain nurses within the work setting need reinforcement. The "magnet hospital" study provided data on the professional practice climate of hospitals that attract nurses to their agencies. High-quality leadership, primary nursing models, degrees of professional autonomy, and expectations of quality nursing perform-ance are key factors within the hospital environment (ANA, 1983).

The National Commission on Nursing report and the recently funded National Commission on Nursing Implementation Project are landmark initiatives on nursing. These projects critically examine the environment in which nurses currently practice and seek to define and develop future models of practice (NCNIP, 1983, 1986).

The data contained in each of these reports and standards provide input into the vision being developed to ensure a professional practice environment in which the CNS can excel.

## ASSESSMENT—INTERNAL ENVIRONMENT

The critical factors in the assessment of one's organization to determine the need for a CNS are similar to those factors in the nursing process: identification and determination of perceived need or vision, development of a plan or approach, implementation, and evaluation of outcome. The administrative process must be done with the same degree of expertise and attention which would be expected for a dynamic and complex patient care situation. Direct interaction with the nursing staff and with other significant patient care providers can provide essential information as to the need for a CNS within the organization.

Relevant supportive data from management reports would include demographics, educational preparation, written job descriptions, and performance evaluations for the CNS. Clinical data would include relevant statistics on the case-mix of patient populations, admission and length of stay profiles, accreditation surveys, risk management, and quality assurance reports.

The degree of commitment to and evidence of collaborative practice between and among health care providers gives an indication of the degree of trust and respect between professional groups within the institution. The degree to which education and expertise is valued may be correlated with participation at staff development or continuing education sessions by members of the nursing staff. Requests for clinical consultation by internal or external experts may also indicate the need for a CNS.

Assessment of the culture of the institution and analysis of the data relative to provider and patient mix brings the reality of the environment into focus for the nurse administrator. The case-mix may dictate the obvious need for an oncology CNS. The projected rise in teenage pregnancies may determine the need for a joint practice or shared CNS role with the Department of Obstetrics. The results of such an analytical effort are tested against the mission, goals, and objectives of the institution and the philosophy of nursing practice. An example of the assessment of both internal and external environments to determine CNS need was described by Hart, et al. (1987). The authors developed a four-step process: obtaining data from other teaching hospitals, surveying staff regarding CNS utilization, analyzing patient statistics in their agency, and ranking populations currently served or for whom a need was identified. Although the process was lengthy, the authors found it useful in gathering the information needed to equitably allocate their institution's CNS positions.

As the plan or vision begins to take substance and form, validation by respected colleagues within the institution or through one's professional network of nurse administrators confirms or challenges the plan. The critical indicator is that whatever organizational model is to be considered or whatever change anticipated, it must be congruent with the goals of the organizational structure in which it is to be implemented. It is at this juncture that the financial assessment and resource allocation process is developed, justified, and assured within the administrative budget. Negotiating progress toward the integration of the CNS into the institution requires perseverance with the influential providers of patient care, a delicate sense of timing, and unified support from within the nursing and medical staff organizations.

## THE DILEMMA AND THE DEBATE

The integration of the CNS into a nursing organization has evolved into different models over the past decade. The majority of specialists work in staff positions providing direct care, consultation, and teaching in continuing education programs. A smaller proportion function in line positions or in faculty roles. Recent studies identify that the consultation function is most frequently practiced and most highly valued (Campbell, et al., 1986). Nurse executives and CNSs within a metropolitan area were surveyed as to their perceptions of the specialist role. Both groups were in considerable agreement on three of the major CNS role components, i.e., clinical practice, education, and consultation. Administrators valued research more highly than did CNSs. These researchers also examined administrative components, which were the least valued (Tarsitano, et al., 1986).

Why the dilemma and the debate relative to the placement of the CNS within the organization? Why a controversy over a scarce and valued resource within the profession? Projections continue to forecast a need for specialists in a variety of settings. Yet, a degree of uncertainty and uneasiness as to the future role and viability of the CNS permeates the nursing profession. A partial explanation is the lack of reliable data regarding the cost-effectiveness of the CNS in the provision of patient care. Given the economic pressures to trim nursing budgets, the justification of the CNS must be directed toward the programmatic initiatives and objectives of the institution. Given the need to enhance productivity of the nursing staff, the activity of the CNS as a role model and expert practitioner could be justified on the basis of clinical leadership that motivated staff to improve their practice, eliminate knowledge or skill deficits, and increase job satisfaction. This would help to reduce turnover, the most costly element of any nursing organization.

A further explanation for the placement debate is the degree of role ambiguity generated by different utilization models, different expectations of job performance, and the varying degrees of impassioned rhetoric as to the merits of line versus staff placement within organizational settings. CNSs perpetuate these concerns as they are faced with perceived or real threat of job security. Nurse executives continue to discuss and debate the most cost-effective approaches to providing leadership in clinical practice settings. Despite uncertainty and ambiguity regarding the future of the CNS role, nurse educators continue to prepare clinical specialists for a situation that is rapidly changing.

## JUSTIFICATION AND PLACEMENT

There is no one "correct" placement for the CNS. Differences in organizations, specialties, and patient populations dictate different configurations. At the University of Michigan, the CNS position is organized to meet the needs of the institution, the client, and the individual practitioner. Clinical specialists function in both staff and line positions. Written performance plans determine job expectations and are evaluated and renegotiated annually. Role ambiguity is a constant, and individual CNSs must continually interpret the role in which they are functioning to professional colleagues, clients, and nursing staff.

The basic function and responsibility of the CNS at the University of Michigan Medical Center is described in the recently revised classification description:

> To provide expert and complex clinical nursing care to a specialized group of patients; to function as a consultant to health providers within the Hospitals and to the community; to develop and monitor implementation of new nursing techniques and standards of practice; to exercise clinical leadership through practice, staff development and research.[1]

Within this conceptual framework, the role of the CNS and the work that needs to be accomplished is negotiated. Different expectations are established to respond to changes in the environment, the political culture, and the institution's priorities. Programmatic initiatives, such as a transplantation center, eating disorders program, or primary care satellite clinics, frequently drive the need for clinical nursing leadership within the hospitals. CNSs are justified within the setting in a staff role to a director of nursing or a clinical manager. In the ambulatory setting, the specialist may be in a joint partnership with a member of the medical staff and have a reporting relationship to the director of ambulatory nursing services for nursing practice. The psychiatric liaison nurse works throughout the medical-surgical division, yet has a report-

---

[1]Reprinted with permission from the University of Michigan, Department of Nursing Services.

ing relationship to the director of psychiatric nursing. Her clients are nurses, patients, and families in the intensive care units.

Some CNSs choose to be in line positions. As long as the CNS negotiates a set of clinical expectations and continues to provide direct care to clients for a significant percentage of time, the individual can continue to use the CNS title. Professional and administrative authority are integrated by the CNS in the line position (Williams & Cancian, 1985). Combining clinical and management expertise provides the basis for assumption of power to justify, manage, and evaluate the resources necessary for clinical practice in the setting (Wallace & Corey, 1983).

In other situations, the CNS is selected for a managerial position and chooses the administrative role rather than the CNS role. In this case, the individual uses the line title, such as assistant director or head nurse, and is not considered a CNS. Clarity within the institution and faithfulness to the definition of the CNS require this change.

In either case, placement of master's-prepared clinicians in administrative positions is primarily a response to an organizational need for transforming leadership and change facilitation to achieve cost-effective nursing services. Selection of the CNS for a line position requires expanded leadership skills in the areas of personnel and financial management, strategic planning, and organizational development. The ability to inspire and empower nurses in their roles within the practice setting is a desirable leadership skill for the CNS who chooses to consider a line position.

An expansion of the consultation aspects of the CNS role resulted in a new position, the clinical nurse consultant, at University of Michigan Hospitals. This role became apparent when selected CNSs were delegated the responsibility to act as project directors for major system changes, such as primary nursing, quality assurance, and pain management. CNSs who moved into these positions had their titles changed to clinical consultant, as the focus of this role is the development of nurses' practice in the consultation subrole. Reporting directly to the director of nursing, the clinical nurse consultants facilitate the professional goals of the department, provide linkages and direction for major clinical efforts, and advise the nursing director on strategic clinical initiatives (Campbell, et al., 1986).

The individual with CNS experience who functions in the head nurse/manager role or the clinical consultant role is in a new and different position. This nurse brings to these positions the clinical expertise, the sense of inquiry, and the skills of teaching and mentoring acquired in the CNS role. However, the responsibility and accountability for a client-based practice is frequently not possible, so the individual cannot be considered a CNS.

The joint appointment position for the CNS is a model utilized for integrating practice and teaching as the context for advancing professional nursing practice. Established in the 1960s to provide links between nursing education and nursing services, the CNS/faculty role has had varying degrees of success. These roles require expertise in clinical practice combined with advanced education (Donovan, 1985). The dual reporting relationship to the dean of the school of nursing and the director of nursing services requires mutually agreed upon philosophy, goals, and outcomes to be achieved within time limitations. The balancing of work effort and the synthesis of the practice/teaching responsibilities is an awesome, but rewarding, task.

The economic imperatives within the hospital environment have stimulated new organizational models. A university medical center has organized their CNSs into a single consultation department to market nursing expertise both within the institution and in the community. Specific clinical services are contracted with the appropriate clinical director or agency; the contract forms the basis for service, productivity, and evaluation. This model provides access to the clinical units on a negotiated basis and a source of revenue from outside contracts (see Chapter 19; also Schwartz-Fulton, 1985).

## SUMMARY

The debate over placement of the CNS in a line or staff position is counterproductive to the justification of the role within any organized care delivery setting. Polarization of views as to the merits of one structure versus another leads to a win-lose outcome that creates confusion within the individual professional and promotes conflict rather than collaboration within the profession. Organizations need advanced clinical expertise in a variety of placements. The issue facing the profession is to promote, develop, and justify the utilization of the CNS in advancing the professional practice of nursing within whatever structural arrangement is most appropriate for the institution and the profession. To do less is to do a disservice to the cadre of professional nurse experts who function in diverse practice settings.

*References*

American Academy of Nursing: Magnet Hospitals: Attraction and Retention of Professional Nurses. Kansas City, American Nurses' Association, 1983.

American Nurses' Association: Clinical Nurse Specialists, Distribution and Utilization. Kansas City, American Nurses' Association, 1986.

American Nurses' Association: Psychiatric and Mental Health Clinical Nurse Specialists, Distribution and Utilization. Kansas City, American Nurses' Association, 1986.

American Nurses' Association: Standards of Nursing Practice. Kansas City, American Nurses' Association, 1972.

American Nurses' Association: Standards of Medical Surgical Nursing Practice. Kansas City, American Nurses' Association, 1974.

American Nurses' Association: Standards of Psychiatric and Mental Health Nursing Practice. Kansas City, American Nurses' Association, 1982.

American Nurses' Association: Standards of School Nursing Practice. Kansas City, American Nurses' Association, 1983.

American Nurses' Association: Standards of Practice for the Perinatal Nurse Specialist. Kansas City, American Nurses' Association, 1984.

American Nurses' Association: Standards of Nursing Practice in Correctional Facilities. Kansas City, American Nurses' Association, 1985.

American Nurses' Association: Standards of Child and Adolescent Psychiatric and Mental Health Nursing Practice. Kansas City, American Nurses' Association, 1985.

American Nurses' Association: Standards of Community Health Nursing Practice. Kansas City, American Nurses' Association, 1986.

American Nurses' Association and Oncology Nursing Society: Outcome Standards for Cancer Nursing Practice. Kansas City, American Nurses' Association, 1979.

American Nurses' Association and Arthritis Health Professions Association: Outcome Standards for Rheumatology Nursing Practice. Kansas City, American Nurses' Association, 1983.

Campbell, J., Behrend, B., Hunter, M., and James, J.: Clinical nurse consultants: Utilizing internal resources. Nurs Admin Q $10$(4):9–12, 1986.

Conference Proceedings on Nursing in the 21st Century. J Prof Nurs $2$(1):2–71, 1986.

Donovan, C.: Clinical nurse specialist practice in an acute care setting. In: Faculty Practice in Action. American Academy of Nursing, American Nursing Association, 1985, pp. 111–118.

Fagin, C.: Institutionalizing practice: Historical and future perspectives. In: Faculty Practice in Action. American Academy of Nursing, American Nurses' Association, 1985, pp. 1–17.

Hart, C.N., Lekander, B.J., Bartels, D., and Tebbitt, B.V.: Clinical nurse specialists: An institutional process for determining priorities. J Nurs Admin $17$:31–35, 1987.

Hickman, C., & Silva, M.: Creating Excellence. New York, New American Library, 1984.

National Commission of Nursing Summary Report and Recommendations. The Hospital Research and Education Trust. Chicago, 1983.

National Commission on Nursing Implementation Project. Invitational Conference Proceedings, Milwaukee, 1986.

Ripple, H.: The nurse executive: In the center of the vortex. J Prof Nurs $2$(1):275, 1986.

Schwartz-Fulton, J.: The clinical nurse specialist: Where the rubber meets the road. In: Faculty Practice in Action. American Academy of Nursing, American Nurses' Association, 1985, pp. 88–97.

Tarsitano, B., Brophy, E., Snyder, D., et al.: A demystification of the clinical nurse specialist role: Perceptions of clinical nurse specialists and nurse administrators. J Nurs Educ $25$(1):4–9, 1986.

Wallace, M., & Corey, L.: The clinical nurse specialist as manager: Myth versus reality. J Nurs Admin $8$:13–15, 1983.

Williams, L., & Cancian, D.: A clinical nurse specialist in a line management position. J Nurs Admin $15$:20–26, 1985.

# Administratively Enhancing CNS Contributions

Chapter 12

Susan B. Baird
Marilyn P. Prouty

## INTRODUCTION

Regardless of the practice setting or the assigned position within that setting, the clinical nurse specialist (CNS) is a valued commodity (Fralic, 1988). Depending upon the setting, the specialist may also be a very scarce resource. As with anything valued or scarce, very close attention must be paid to the use of the CNS. Through careful planning and insightful management, the full potential for contribution by this provider is more likely to be realized.

To focus actively on both the role of the CNS from an administrative point of view and the "fit" of this role in nursing organizations is appropriate at this point in the health care services revolution. The CNS has been actively incorporated into many practice settings for the past 10 to 15 years—time enough for the emergence of strong beliefs about the value of this role, its impact, and its future.

Given the pressures of health care economics within institutions and nursing services, there is substantial and pressing need to: match the value of the CNS role with the needs of an organization, articulate an organization's ability to extract everything possible from the role, and develop mechanisms that will yield quantifiable justification for CNS positions. It is immaterial whether an organization is just now preparing to incorporate the role of the CNS or whether the role is a longstanding one. Modifications can always be made to make the best possible use of this resource. Strategies can be placed or utilized to foster CNS role enhancement through the avenues of organizational structure, functional operations, and evaluation (Fralic, 1988).

# ENHANCEMENT THROUGH ORGANIZATIONAL STRUCTURE

Some things do not change, a reassuring thought to nursing administrators in these times of tremendous flux. *Structure still influences function.* As with anything to be built or to be built upon, careful thought must be given to the structure because it determines process. Structure sets the framework or staging for activity. This is just as true for the organization of services and people within an institution as it is for the physical plant of that institution. The structure makes a statement (DiVincenti, 1977, pp. 46–48).

The scrutinization of organizational structure yields information on the philosophy of that organization (DiVincenti, 1977, pp. 81–82). When reviewing the organization of a nursing service, for example, do role relationships appear sufficiently definitive for function, or are they rigidly conscripted? Does the flow between levels seem logical or slightly awkward? Is it a structure that promotes autocratic or democratic operations? The philosophy that is to guide the functioning of the nursing service should precede the design. For design to force philosophy is unfortunate and may prompt failure. The philosophy of the nursing administrator regarding the potential contributions of the CNS should guide the placement of that specialist within the structure. The previous chapter has defined parameters that guide the administrator in making that placement when initially considering the addition of a CNS. A variety of models obviously exist; the administrator can choose which model might best suit the needs and practices of the institution in order to enhance CNS contributions.

## Organizational Design

It is important to recognize that within the many organizational designs or structures that can accommodate the CNS, different placements can also exist within one design; i.e., all specialists may not function in the same way in a given institution and therefore may not necessarily share the same placement within an organizational chart. A limited survey of nursing department administrators, undertaken for the purpose of gathering information about variations in structural design, demonstrates this variability of placement within a structure (Table 12–1). Whether the CNS is placed in a line or staff position, whether the CNS is population- or unit-based, and who the CNS reports to within the administrative structure are all variables influencing function.

More telling than the actual structures and reporting functions were the comments of the administrators. Survey respondents repeatedly pointed to flexibility as being critical in order for the CNS to be

**TABLE 12–1. Placement of the Clinical Nurse Specialist**

| Summary of Nursing Administrators' Responses (N = 28) | | Number | Percentage |
|---|---|---|---|
| Respondents employing CNSs: | | 23 | 82 |
| Average daily census: | | 367 (range: 90–800) | |
| Average number of CNSs on staff: | | 7 (range: 0–25) | |
| Hospital type: | Community | 9 | 32 |
| | Teaching | 19 | 68 |
| Administrator CNS reports to: | Director of clinical area | 11 | 48 |
| | Director, other (e.g., of nursing education) | 4 | 17 |
| | Assistant Director of clinical area | 4 | 17 |
| | Vice President | 4 | 17 |
| Line vs. Staff responsibility: | Staff | 17 | 77 |
| | Line (supervise head nurses) | 3 | 14 |
| | Both (cover in Director's absence-1, supervise .4 FTE instructor-1) | 2 | 9 |
| Population-based vs. unit-based role: | Unit-based | 4 | 9 |
| | Population-based | 12 | 52 |
| | Both (unit-based but consult across divisional lines) | 7 | 30 |

optimally effective. Both the results of this limited survey and the nursing literature indicate that nursing departments are organized in a variety of ways and that administrators see both strengths and weaknesses within their own current or discarded structures (Fox, 1982; Kohnke, 1978). Representative comments include:

- Without line authority, effecting change is difficult or slower.

- In a line position, it may be difficult for the CNS to maintain a strong clinical base.

- The organizational model in current use may not provide enough structure for some CNSs. Although most are self-directed and do well, a few experience difficulty moving ahead.

- Because the CNS is a staff position here, authority and power to create change depends largely on personal or professional skills in the clinical setting and/or the degree of administrative support for their efforts.

- CNS comfort with the organization model varies depending on the quality of the relationship with their immediate supervisor.

Although a variety of organizational structures were identified by survey respondents, placing the CNS in a staff position reportable to the nursing director of a specific clinical area (Figure 12–1) was a

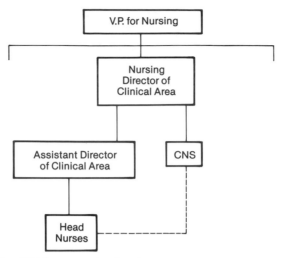

**Figure 12–1.** The CNS is commonly placed in a staff position reportable to the nursing director in a specific clinical area.

common staff placement. No clearly superior model emerged, however, and it seems less important which specific model is used than it is to have a sense of whether the model is allowing for the best possible functioning of the service.

Two models supported by the authors are highlighted here to demonstrate alternative placement approaches designed to enhance CNS contributions and accountability. Both place the CNS in a line position, an approach frequently easier to defend in such a cost-conscious era. Staff positions are frequently viewed, albeit erroneously, as superfluous resources.

### The Prouty Model

As shown in Figure 12–2, the Prouty model was envisioned as dividing departmental functions between two associate directors of nursing—one for administrative affairs and the other for clinical affairs. As first described by Prouty in 1983, administrative supervisors were responsible to the associate for administrative affairs, and the CNSs were responsible to the associate for clinical affairs. Both the administrative supervisors and the CNSs were in line positions. This meant that the nurses were responsible to the CNS for clinical matters and to the administrative supervisor for administrative matters. This structure symbolized Prouty's philosophy that the clinical component of nursing is as important and significant as the administrative component.

The Prouty model recognizes the CNS as an important leader in

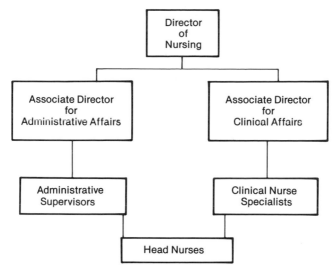

**Figure 12–2.** The Prouty model places the CNS in a line position recognizing the CNS as responsible for clinical practice in a specialty area.

the clinical arena of practice. As a line person responsible for clinical management in a specialty area, the head nurse manager has an identified clinical resource person available; and this is essential for realizing a holistic approach to the management of care on a patient unit. Critical to the effectiveness of this line placement, however, is the effective functioning of the administrative supervisor (or area director) with whom the clinical specialist is a peer. The formal identification of separate administrative and clinical functioning provides the CNS with real avenues for channeling the administrative components of care issues, without CNS attention being diverted unnecessarily from the clinical aspects of those issues. This design inherently provides the safeguard other administrators have sought through placement of the CNS in a staff position (O'Connor & Malone, 1983); the CNS need not get unnecessarily caught up in administrative functions because there is a ready peer for these concerns.

The Prouty model assists in preserving a clear focus on clinical expertise. Embodied in this model is the view that the CNS is the expert in clinical care and that loss of this expertise threatens the essence of the role. The CNS who loses clinical expertise loses two essential components of the role—practice and consultation (Baird, 1985). Traditionally, nurses with clinical expertise have been rewarded with administrative responsibilities. The pressure of these duties, however, may make it difficult for such nurses to retain their clinical skills.

Heavier reliance for clinical expertise than is realistic may be placed on the head nurse.

Alternatively, while some nursing leaders suggest that the role of the CNS can encompass both practice and administration, or middle management (Wallace & Corey, 1983; Williams & Cancian, 1985), others question whether the role can survive with this dilution (Barry, 1983). The Prouty model makes a strong statement about the division of labor within a practice setting and about the importance of the components of that labor. Administrative and clinical skills are recognized as equally important, and equal weight is given to both functions in this organizational structure.

The Prouty model recognizes the importance of the consultative role of the CNS but takes into account that the consultation process does not come easily or naturally to many nurses. Some CNSs, especially those new to the role, have to be "brought along" or helped to develop the consultant role component. Two direct consultative links are established by this organizational structure: a peer relationship with the administrative supervisor (or area director) and a clinical consultation link with the head nurse. Establishing credibility as a clinical expert is an essential step preceding the beginnings of consultative functioning; this structure forces that to happen. Once the CNS is viewed as a positive and supportive force, two changes begin to take place: the CNS takes further independent action to encourage consultation, and nurses themselves spread the word that assistance is available from the "new nurse."

To be most effective, the Prouty model requires a head nurse to view this reporting configuration as enhancing effectiveness and professional growth through the linking of resource people, rather than as two bosses. Effective communication is essential to the smooth flow of this model.

### Dual Leadership Model

In this model (Figure 12–3), used by one of the authors and some of the survey respondents, the head nurse and the CNS are peers. They are both in line positions at the same level. Both are prepared through education and experience for assuming a leadership role. This model is built on the assumption that few areas of decision-making on the patient care unit are either clearly administrative or clearly clinical. A similar assumption underlies the Prouty model, the difference being that in this model the clinical/administrative collaborative dimension occurs at the unit level. Who the CNS and head nurse report to depends upon the complexity of the organization. It may be an area assistant or

**Figure 12–3.** In the dual leadership model, the head nurse and CNS are peers. Depending upon the size and complexity of the organization, the position they report to may vary (indicated by the oblique parallel lines), but the reporting relationship and peer level are constants.

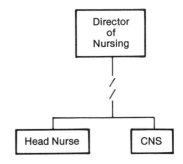

associate director. A shared responsibility provides an opportunity to identify those aspects best handled by each leader. For example, if a new type of treatment is to be initiated on the unit, and that treatment involves the delivery of new and complex care, the leaders can each identify and plan for those aspects within their purview. The head nurse will look at how this care can be delivered safely in such terms as staffing, equipment, and ancillary service requirements. The CNS will determine staff needs in terms of orientation, procedure definition and refinement, and clinical skill development.

This model is more likely to be practiced in settings where the CNS is unit-based. The strength of the model arises from pooled talents and energies as well as from shared responsibility. Both nurses provide the input they are best prepared to give, thus enhancing efficiency. There is a built-in inducement for using the complementary skills of the two leaders. When responsibility and accountability are shared, it is more likely that these leaders will create a work environment of mutual support rather than one that puts the CNS and head nurse in competition with each other.

Success with this model depends, in part, upon having two skilled leaders. Traditionally, head nurse positions have been filled by selecting a highly skilled clinician from the unit's staff, a person who has seemingly demonstrated potential for leadership. The role of the head nurse has changed and now demands a different mix of skills. The head nurse, increasingly and more appropriately being called a nurse manager or unit director, is held accountable for a high level of skill and knowledge in a variety of areas: the economics of the patient unit, the management of people, personnel functions, performance evaluation, unit organizational problem-solving, adherence to regulatory body standards, and the shaping of unit and nursing department policy. To accomplish these functions puts tremendous time demands on the head nurse leaving little time to concentrate on the clinical needs of the unit's staff. The CNS in the dual leadership model serves as a rich complement to the nurse manager. The roles are not competitive; smooth functioning and growth of the unit and its staff depend upon integrated actions. The potential for expanded use of this role seems likely given the increased demands on the head nurse in terms of management responsibilities coupled with the increased complexity of care inherent in today's acutely-ill hospitalized patient.

Success with this depends upon two prepared professionals who are comfortable in their positions and committed to working together. This model is sensitive to role jealousies and inequities in performance; competitiveness can easily undermine its effectiveness.

## Structural Decisions

Two decisional factors seem at the crux of enhancing the contributions of the CNS through organizational structure: line versus staff placement and population-based versus unit-based assignment. Which configurations enhance role performance? Few administrators would say there is only one clear answer to these two related questions, but administrators responding to the survey described earlier seemed to link enhanced flexibility with organizational structures where the CNS was *staff* rather than *line* and where the CNS was *population-based*.

### Line Versus Staff Placement

Some respondents considered that the nurse placed in a staff position was perceived as less threatening to staff level nurses, and that this appeared to increase the utilization of the CNS by the staff nurse. Further, it was expressed by survey respondents that placing the CNS in a staff position seemingly protected the CNS from being seduced into management and administrative problems. Thus, they were more accessible for clinical issues and clinical assistance (Metcalf, Werner, and Richmond, 1984). The question has arisen, however, whether accountability and responsibility can be adequately ascertained in a staff position (Edlund, 1983). Many nursing administrator respondents emphasized the demand and value of consultant skills and identified these as the rationale behind population-based assignments. Reporting lines varied and appeared to be a function of institutional size.

Some of the survey respondents placed the CNS in a consultative staff position based on the belief that this gave the CNS more freedom to function, a broader sphere of influence, and more opportunities to influence practice. This placement may be more appropriate for a nursing department that is learned about the role of the CNS and very sophisticated about the effective use of the consultative process in nursing. To have a placement that formally allows for, and even depends upon, appropriate use of the consultative process requires a certain maturation in practice. The more complex and varied the patient population within an organization, the more crucial the need for consultative services between units and settings.

The models previously described place the CNS in a line position, and many of the advantages of this placement have already been discussed. There appears to be a beginning tendency to tighten organizational structures and clarify reporting linkages for enhanced accountability. It is generally easier to defend line positions; staff positions may be viewed as more expendable. Reporting relationships, which can influence both formal and informal communication patterns, are clearer where few staff positions exist.

Whether or not staff placement actually gives the CNS more autonomy than line placement is debatable. Freedom to function within a prescribed role is more a function of the philosophy of a nursing service than placement (Poulin, 1984). For example, a nursing service philosophy that purports autonomy of practice as part of the professional nurse role and recognizes that leadership has its own special autonomy will accommodate and nurture autonomy in practice regardless of placement. The authors support administrative approaches that encourage participative management, management by objectives, decentralized decision-making, accountability, and autonomy of practice. These assist the individual nurse to emerge as a more confident and prepared practitioner. A changing focus from autocratic to participative leadership is based on the assumptions that skilled leadership people can be developed at different levels within the organization and that this capacity for leadership must be in both administrative and clinical leaders. The authors believe these tenets of organizational behavior are best accomplished by placing the CNS in a line position. Having both clinical and management leadership in line positions makes a loud statement within nursing and within the larger organizational structure about the expected impact of these professionals.

### Unit-Versus Population-Based Assignment

Whether the CNS can make a greater contribution from a unit-based or population-based appointment depends upon the size of the population to be served and the expectations of that service. A medical-surgical CNS, for example, will have little impact when population-based in a large facility. There is simply no way the CNS can concentrate activities sufficiently to serve the many units or many disease entities falling within the confines of medical-surgical care. A population-based, medical-surgical CNS could perhaps have more impact focusing on specific subpopulations such as those with diabetes or gastrointestinal disorders. Alternatively, a unit-based, medical-surgical CNS will probably have a greater impact on practice. Even if the unit serves a variety of diseases, the CNS quickly becomes familiar with the skills of the nurses on that unit and the types of problems that frequently arise. The style of the staff in terms of problem-solving, the strengths and weaknesses of the staff, and the approaches that have facilitated transfers of knowledge in the past are well known.

In general, assignment should accommodate easy and direct access to the patient population by the CNS. The more specialized and complex the specialty, the more imperative that access becomes. The CNS belongs with the patient population to be served. If patients are concentrated on one unit, a unit-based assignment will enhance productivity. If the specialty is scattered, population-based is probably the best assignment for the CNS, keeping in mind that role diffusion is a distinct possibility.

A contributing variable to the success of the CNS in either placement is experience. The unit-based approach gives the CNS defined boundaries for operation and a more limited sphere of responsibility. The unit provides structure, which may enhance a sense of security. As the CNS gains experience and credibility within the role and within the institution, the less structured parameters of population-based assignments may be quite workable and even desired by the CNS ready for expanded horizons.

To enhance the contribution of the CNS regardless of placement, the structure should make sense to the organization in terms of its philosophy, be workable in terms of change and decision-making, and demonstrate effectiveness. Introducing the role broadly and thoughtfully rather than in prescribed terms of *line* or *staff* and *population-* or *unit-based* will enhance flexibility in functioning. Such placement decisions need not be permanent. They make sense only as long as they work to the advantage of the practitioner and the department. Modifications can easily be made as care demands shift. For example, a new medical-surgical CNS might initially be placed on one medical-surgical unit where the patient mix is both general and gastrointestinal surgery. After a year's experience, the CNS may well feel ready to assume responsibility for the ambulatory care components of these services and to add an additional medical-surgical subpopulation such as arthritis. This broader practice base may reflect a change from a unit- to a population-based assignment.

# ENHANCEMENT THROUGH STRUCTURING FUNCTIONAL OPERATIONS

Once placement decisions are made and a model has emerged to define role operations, attention should shift to additional aspects of departmental functioning which have the potential to influence CNS output. Carefully preparing the organization for a new CNS, developing communication networks, and identifying potential problem areas can go far in ensuring that CNS contributions will be enhanced.

## Preparing the Organization

Although the CNS is a veritable institution in some nursing service departments, others still function without them. Economic reasons may be the underlying reason for this decision, but a negative previous experience may also be guiding present actions. Other departments may not add to their existing cadre of CNSs because the value of the CNS role has not been made apparent. Certainly there are cases in which a nursing service has been unsuccessful in utilizing the CNS well. The difficulty may have been with the individual, the nursing service, the role, or all three.

Being cautious about the dangers of generalization, it still seems legitimate to make the statement that CNSs are, without doubt, a difficult force with which to reckon. They work hard, well, and skillfully but still have motivation and energy left over to present yet another new idea or an analysis of one's ailing department, complete with solutions. They may not always balance their freely shared advice with any insight into what is actually happening in the department or what has changed for the better. Occasionally, there is a perceivable tendency for their presence to be viewed as elitist or purist, or both. Fortunately, this view is tempered with another: CNSs are highly motivated, committed, and educated specialists who recognize the potential of their specific role with the nursing department and who also demonstrate commitment to their profession in the broader sense by serving on committees, publishing, and planning relevant workshops.

Providing an environment that will be the most conducive to the work of the CNS is not an easily achievable task but is one that requires conscious attention and refinement over time. Elements of developing this environment include: gaining nursing department commitment; building physician support; orienting the staff to the CNS role and skills; orienting the CNS to the staff's strengths, weaknesses, and goals; and promoting CNS visibility. Certainly this task is easier today than when CNSs were a relatively new professional force, and when few providers, even within nursing, were really aware of their education and practice skills. Most providers today have at least heard of the CNS role; many will have worked with them in other agencies and be aware of their potential contribution.

Whether introducing the first CNS into an organization or adding to an existing complement, attention to several basic steps will facilitate the introduction or expansion of the role (Table 12–2).

It is easiest to prepare an organization for the addition of another CNS position if there is already a successful model in place. Being able to present concrete examples of how practice was influenced, how change was made easier, or how staff use this person as a resource in problem-solving go far in making the institution receptive to the possibility of adding another such resource. Another useful approach would employ an outside CNS as a consultant to describe how the addition of a CNS in a specific specialty could make a measurable difference.

Building on a bad experience is obviously more of a challenge. A careful analysis of what went wrong in the past and what could have been done differently is a useful beginning. If it was a poor fit between the CNS and the service, this needs to be acknowledged. If administration let the previous CNS down by not adequately preparing the organization or by not being sensitive to early signs that trouble was brewing, then openly acknowledging this and analyzing how things could be different is an essential step in understanding and working through the past.

Gaining nursing department commitment depends upon understanding the role, its competing demands, and its vagaries. The CNS

**TABLE 12–2. Basic Steps to Facilitate Introducing or Explaining the Role of the CNS Within an Organization**

- Involve key people—head nurses, assistant and associate directors of nursing, and physicians, for example—in early discussion of the role and critique of the position description.

- Prepare the position description, redrafting until the elements of the role are clearly encompassed in outcome expectations.

- Guide the nursing staff through the process of understanding the role and the assistance they can provide in incorporating the role into the organization.

- Enhance networks with colleagues in other institutions who have utilized the CNS to provide avenues for future consultation if difficulty in implementing the role occurs.

- Move slowly but deliberately toward planning for this addition in the next budget year rather than trying to sell this budget addition without preliminary groundwork.

needs considerable freedom; the nature and substance of the role demands flexibility in its performance. There are variables in the practice setting which specialists must be free to respond to as they occur. For example, CNSs understand that their guidance and assistance are needed on evening and night shifts as well as on day shifts, and that working hours may change. Others in the department may need help to understand why the CNS seems to have this unusual freedom in scheduling.

Another area that frequently gives rise to questioning from disciplines within the institution is concern that the CNS is frequently off the unit or involved in activities that do not seem directly related to issues within the department or specialty. "Where are they?" and "What are they doing while we're in the middle of this mess?" are common questions when the CNS role is not understood. The nursing administrator needs to help others to see that the CNS possesses a sense of responsibility to the growth of nursing as a profession in addition to a sense of responsibility for their specific charge within the organization. This responsibility occasionally takes time away from the unit or population base.

Although there needs to be a sense of priority and balance among activities, the CNS also needs freedom to perform a variety of functions. Promoting understanding among leader and staff of the competing demands for the attentions of the CNS may help them to understand, for example, why the CNS is not always on the unit. It is the joint responsibility of the nursing administrator and the CNS to negotiate this balance as part of the annual work plan with activities undertaken on the basis of that agreement. The CNS has communication responsibilities as well—the unit should be aware of the CNS's schedule and how to reach the CNS.

When a CNS is new to an institution, whether the first CNS or an addition to a cadre of many, the administrator works quickly and deliberately to help establish that CNS as an important part of the nursing leadership team. Early visibility is important. By taking the CNS along to certain regular meetings, especially those at which key physicians and administrators may be met, the nursing administrator ensures that this person is seen, known, and recognized as a vital addition. Introducing the new CNS at a department head level meeting and briefly explaining the role and the preparation that it involves may also be useful. Sending notices throughout the institution to introduce the CNS is also useful. A variety of methods can be used, but the important action is that high visibility is pushed within the first two weeks to two months. From there, the CNS will carry the momentum.

These brief examples demonstrate that preparing the organization can make a difference in role implementation and in achieving the best mix between CNS performance (output) and CNS satisfaction (growth). Giving this aspect of preparation inadequate time or sidestepping it completely under pressure to "get the position filled" may result in later difficulties.

## Developing Communication Networks

To ensure that the contributions of the CNS are maximized, communication linkages need to be developed on several levels: between the nursing administrator and the CNS, within the nursing department, with physicians and other disciplines, and among CNSs within and outside the facility. The CNS is more likely to be fully productive when the organization's officials understand and support the role to the extent that they willingly provide the freedom necessary for role functioning, without being overly concerned with what the CNS is producing in any one hour or on any one day.

To impose a rigid structure for CNS practice is to dilute the potential effectiveness of the role. Provision of such freedom is difficult, particularly if the nursing administrator still has some remnants of an autocratic attitude or if that is the general administrative climate within the institution.

There are obvious risks that the administrator must be willing to take. A regular forum for communication must be established between the CNS and the administrator, and the need for this regular communication must be respected despite busy schedules or "crises" on either side. An inexperienced CNS or one new to a setting will need more frequent contact. Regularly scheduled conference times keep the administrator apprised of potential problem areas on the service and serve as a barometer of how the CNS is functioning. Communication links must also be established with the medical staff, especially with key members of that staff who may be less familiar with the role and the potential contributions of the CNS. Gaining physician support for the CNS is essential and is best done through establishing open communication between the CNS and the physicians involved. Support comes more easily when physicians are helped to realize that CNS contributions will benefit the care delivered to their patient population. If tangible evidence of this occurs rapidly, support will most likely be forthcoming. The credibility of the individual CNS will be recognized even if true understanding of the concept of the role comes less readily.

There is certainly potential for conflict. The knowledge of the CNS in clinical matters, for example, in many instances is close to that of the physician. The CNS may not always agree with the patient orders left by a physician and may be quite verbal in making suggestions, especially in areas of symptom management. CNSs are frequently very skilled in their sensitivity to the patient and to the nurse caring for that patient and will speak out openly on behalf of either. They are generally persistent and do not shy away from shallow reasoning, misdirected anger, or procrastination from physicians or those in other disciplines. For the nursing administrator, this can mean visits from vexed physicians who question the right of the CNS to persistently question medical management approaches, from administrators who do not want the "boat rocked," or from the head of dietary or housekeeping, for example, who wonder why the work of their department employees is being challenged.

Nursing administration may thus be placed in a difficult position, needing to support other disciplines but also needing to assist the CNS in making necessary changes that will yield better care. Occasionally, an administrator may need to help the CNS assess or modify a chosen approach. More often, however, the CNS is identifying and facing problems or situations in the organization which should have surfaced or been recognized long ago. If multiple problems surface too quickly, and there is apparent need for simultaneous change in many directions, anxiety and anger can result. These are times when the CNS needs to receive support and appreciation for exposing problems but may also need assistance in setting priorities and pacing the solutions.

## Identifying and Addressing Problems

As the CNS (or group of CNSs) begins to assess the practice situation and identify areas for change, the potential for conflict increases. Although specific problems will vary, the sources of problems may have some commonalities: interdisciplinary conflict, overextension, decreased accessibility/availability, role jealousy, conflict over direct care expectations, leadership conflicts and power struggles, and boredom or stagnation. These problems are obviously serious but hardly insurmountable. Some may seem only bothersome in their intensity, but left unaddressed, they can seriously undermine the CNS's effectiveness. Other problems can be overwhelming in their impact on the functioning of the CNS. The nursing administrator must be alert for major problems: signs of obstructionism either by or against the CNS, CNS incompetency, or evidence that there is truly a bad fit between the CNS and the role expectation or organizational philosophy.

### Interdisciplinary Conflicts

It is not uncommon for physicians to question the authority of the CNS who questions medical practice. Sometimes that approach seems easier than adequately addressing the care concerns raised by the CNS. In preparation for addressing care issues with physicians, the CNS may need assistance in developing a plan that considers approach, timing, and setting. Nursing administrators can frequently assist the CNS in joint care planning that is collegial instead of competitive in nature. At other times, the physician may need assistance in understanding the time or approach needed to make change. For example, when oncologists requested that nurses take over chemotherapy administration for inpatients, they had difficulty understanding why it could not happen at once. Responding to the oncologists' request, the CNS devised a time plan that outlined the practice expectations and the educational and practice sessions necessary for safely changing practice. By seeking input from the physicians about the plan and even asking for their assistance in presenting a portion of the content, the CNS gained their commitment.

When tensions arise between disciplines, the administrator can often be useful in determining whether the situation itself warrants these tensions or whether there are other underlying problems. The administrator should not be regarded as an ever-ready mediator but as one who can serve the CNS as an objective listener and interpreter of actions. The administrator may be able to guide the CNS into a course of action for directly confronting situations.

### Work Load

Many problems encountered in the CNS role can be traced to a common source of conflict, i.e., trying to do too much at once. The CNS who demonstrates competency and skill in making change quickly becomes very sought-after. Often without realizing it is happening, the CNS finds the day filled with committee meetings, informal consultation requests, speaking engagements, and myriad details to be attended to. Staff may begin to complain that the CNS is not on the unit as often as before and that it is harder to make contact or get time to discuss care problems. Staff on an especially hectic unit, initially understanding of the many demands on the CNS, may begin to express concern that the CNS does not seem to be sharing in direct care or never seems to be on the unit when "things are at their craziest." Staff who had formerly asked the CNS for assistance with a new procedure or piece of equipment may now ask another staff nurse who seems to be more readily available. Alternatively, the head nurse may receive more of these requests, and tensions between the head nurse and CNS may build. The head nurse begins to see the CNS as someone who has far more freedom and who can leave the unit when the going gets tough. The head nurse may long for such seeming luxuries as "library time."

On the other hand, the CNS may be feeling terribly stressed. Less seems to get crossed off the "to do" list each day. When few projects are actually completed, the satisfaction that comes from seeing change in place or tasks completed is greatly diminished. Jumping from crisis to crisis leaves the CNS frustrated. The CNS may long for earlier days when practice could be concentrated in fewer areas, when depth rather than breadth of practice prevailed. In addition, the CNS may begin to realize that the majority of time is spent on what has to get done, and that there is no time to investigate new areas or problems or to develop or pursue individual research or teaching interests. The CNS may begin to feel frustrated in the role, seeing few opportunities for activities that could represent professional development. Likewise, the CNS whose role is tightly bounded and who is offered little opportunity for professional development may also experience frustration and/or stagnation.

Administrative support has been identified as a key element in the successful implementation of the specialist role (Baird, 1985; Poulin, 1984). A plan for the continued professional growth of the CNS should be negotiated between the administrator and the CNS and should be a formal part of the actual work plan. Doing so demonstrates the administrator's recognition of the value placed on professional growth and reassures the CNS that these activities will be recognized and safeguarded. On the other hand, formalizing this part of the work plan provides an opportunity to negotiate the focus, direction, and time commitment for professional development.

### Conflict Management

The CNS can become quite skilled at recognizing early signs of role stress or conflict. Recognizing that there is a problem or potential problem in the making is important. Major disasters can be avoided by addressing small tensions. A realistic work plan, developed annually and reviewed periodically, is one approach to placing some reasonable guidelines on performance. Setting priorities within the work plan is also vitally important—all problems cannot be dealt with to the same degree at the same time, yet the CNS can juggle many projects at once if given some forecast of how far and how fast that project can move. Setting intermediate points of progress is useful so that satisfaction can be realized along the way, even when a project is a long-term one. For example, the CNS may have several ideas about how to improve the clinical practice of the staff of a particular unit. Issues that can be identified, such as addressing a problem with the delivery of safe care or overcoming difficulties encountered with implementation of a care regimen, would take precedence over developing a patient education booklet for a patient population or assisting staff with writing an article for publication. Although the CNS may not see a completed patient education booklet as soon as may be desired, reviewing what is already available or determining what it is patients need or want to know can be used as intermediate progress points yielding satisfaction.

The CNS and nursing administrator must strive to maintain an open relationship so that the reasonableness of the workload can be appraised at any point in time. The desire of the CNS to undertake new projects when existing ones are seemingly mired in organizational red tape must be tempered with the needs of the organization. When conflict arises with others in the organization, the administrator can objectively appraise the situation and guide the CNS in preparing an approach for openly addressing the issue. Sometimes, there is more organizational history or politics in the situation than the CNS may be aware of, and the administrator can assist the CNS to place current conflict within this context and plan appropriate responses.

Occasionally, it becomes clear to the administrator (and often to the CNS as well) that there is a bad fit between the organization or its expectations and the skills of the CNS. The CNS may not be able to appreciate or work within the philosophy of the organization, may be the source of obstructionism, or may not be competent in the role. It would be a highly unusual situation if this becomes apparent to the administrator but is a shock to the CNS. The administrator and CNS can work together to determine how serious the situation is and whether it can be remedied.

The CNS who has some insight into the power of the role and the extent to which the CNS can influence how the role works has a far better chance at working out serious difficulties than the CNS who feels victimized or feels that everyone else is at fault. A plan to help restore competency and credibility needs to be jointly established and implemented. The administrator has as much to lose as the CNS if resolution cannot occur. The administrator may not only lose this particular CNS and the investment made in the orientation of that CNS but also stands to lose support for the position itself. For this reason, an administrator will usually work hard with the CNS to monitor and resolve problems.

## ENHANCEMENT THROUGH EVALUATION

The administrator has obvious expectations for each CNS's performance; others in the institution or service will have their own expectations. The CNS will have yet another set of expectations. How congruent these expectations are and whether they are being met is important to all. Developing and implementing a framework for evaluating performance and using that evaluation to enhance performance is a vital component of the role (Fenton, 1985).

One of the more interesting paradoxes in this modern era of clinical nursing specialization is that while there is a common cry from administrators and CNSs for quantitative evaluation approaches, almost none exist. One administrator in our survey, noting the use of an evaluation based on the position description, said, "We think we need something else but we're not sure what it should be." This appears to be a common sentiment.

Two avenues of evaluation are needed: performance evaluation and impact evaluation. It is probably safe to say that every institution has some form of performance evaluation but few, if any, undertake impact evaluation. Additionally, little evaluation research has been undertaken. Anecdotal rather than quantitative evidence is often the only data available to demonstrate the positive impact of the CNS on the nursing staff (e.g., orientation, satisfaction, and turn-over), on patient care (e.g., quality and safety of care, and patient education), and on interdisciplinary care (e.g., communication and joint planning). There is general agreement among administrators, educators, and CNSs that the development and testing of quantitative evaluation approaches is probably one of the most pressing needs in clinical nursing specialization.

## Models for Performance Evaluation

No one model emerges as being outstanding for performance evaluations. The few approaches that exist are fairly simplistic. Many CNSs keep logs that can form the basis for a self-evaluation. Ongoing information accrual is obviously much more reliable than trying to recollect activities just prior to an annual evaluation. Noting consultations, staff problem-solving activities, and interdisciplinary communications can be useful in identifying both levels of activity and emerging trends. This information can be linked with outcome objectives. For example, if an objective is to increase consultation between the unit-based oncology CNS (OCNS) and staff nurses caring for cancer patients on other units, tracking the number and nature of such consultations provides the needed objective data.

The majority of respondents in the administrators' survey previously mentioned use a criteria-based evaluation. These frequently evolve from the position description. Several administrators noted that their evaluation process is being revised; their comments indicate that the development of evaluation processes specific to the CNS may be emerging. Comments offered provide additional insights:

- The system for CNS evaluation is a peer review model. This is accomplished by yearly formal evaluation using the competency based tool. The CNSs compile portfolios of work accomplished. This work is presented to their peer review committee.
- The evaluation is weighted in allocated time and outcomes based on education, consultation, research, and service (the patient caseload).
- The evaluation uses a management performance appraisal system that includes personal and department goals.
- The most frequent and important job duties are selected and the CNS is evaluated on these duties.
- We currently use the formal organizational evaluation process mandated by personnel but are testing a peer review process.

In general, an annual work plan should serve as the basis of evaluation. Work plans written in a format of measurable outcome objectives are most useful. The objectives should be specific enough to guide actions and to measure their achievement but not be so prescriptive as to hamper creativity and flexibility. Although work plans usually forecast a year, periodic review should allow for modification. Work plans should encompass avenues of professional growth as well as professional performance.

## Impact Evaluation

The First National Invitational Conference of Oncology Clinical Nurse Specialists (Donoghue & Spross, 1985) was one setting where impact evaluation was a clear focus of interest. In both the addresses and discussion sessions, interest in this subject was apparent and was noted as crucial to survival. Hamric identified that necessity by showing positive changes in nursing and/or patient behaviors attributable to the CNS (Hamric, 1985). Yasko noted that through facilitating the coordination of patient care, the CNS will assist in decreasing the use of agency resources, the cost of supplies and equipment, and the length of hospitalization. She stated that lowering the cost of care will ensure the viability of the role (Yasko, 1985). The key question here is not whether that can happen but how anyone will know that it has. Baird noted that part of CNS survival depends on making the role absolutely indispensable. The most effective and indisputable approach to do that, she adds, is being able to document the effects of the OCNS on patient care (Baird, 1985). Impact evaluation is the key.

What is being done in this area? Administrators participating in our survey were asked how they measured the impact of the CNS role within their nursing department. Several respondents indicated they had not measured it or that they had no specific mechanisms but rather relied on informal feedback. Descriptive methods were noted by some respondents who stated that they looked at such things as the quantity and quality of educational programs presented, numbers of consultations, and involvement of the CNS in meetings and projects. Others noted such diverse indicators as:

- how well Joint Commission on Accreditation of Healthcare Organization (JCAHO) standards were met
- turnover in nursing
- relationships with physicians
- job satisfaction of the staff
- quality of written policies and procedures
- quality of care
- patient satisfaction.

Information was not included on specifically how some of these factors were measured or on how outcome was attributed to the CNS and not to a myriad of other possible influences. Obviously attributing the cause is far more difficult and yet more important.

A number of indicators were identified which might be used to measure CNS impact: staff turnover, job satisfaction, nursing practice (quality of care), and evidence of interdisciplinary practice (role acceptance). Each has potential in terms of value, but each also has its particular measurement difficulty. Hopefully this difficulty will be seen by researchers as a challenge and not as a deterrent.

An outcome of the oncology CNS conference mentioned above was a series of recommendations relating to practice, education, and administrative support. Three recommendations relate to evaluation and appear appropriate for all CNS populations:

1. Evaluation must proceed out of the goals and objectives mutually established by the CNS and administrator in the work plan.

2. Cost effectiveness as well as patient outcomes must be included. (Each CNS must work on identifying and quantifying their effectiveness in practice. Quantifying needs to include cost, patient outcomes, [nurse retention, effect on implementation of the nursing process], effect on length of patient stay, etc. Quantifications must include structure, process and outcome.)

3. Evaluation instruments should be developed with consideration given to the CNS's effect on agency mission, quality of care, and patient care costs. (*Oncol Nurs Forum*, 1985).

Administrators need evaluation data for a number of purposes. Its most obvious use is with CNS performance counseling. In addition, evaluation data is useful in substantiating changes of focus or functions of existing positions, individuals, or programs. Data can also be used to substantiate the need for new positions. Finally, evaluation data can be used relative to practice—forecasting trends in practice, identifying deficits in practice, or documenting practice initiatives.

## PLANNING FOR FUTURE ENHANCEMENT

This chapter has outlined avenues for enhancing CNS contributions through organizational structure, functional operations, and evaluation. Although there are obvious difficulties and challenges in being committed to these avenues, there are also obvious rewards. The value of the CNS is underscored repeatedly throughout the chapters of this book. Administrators who take deliberate steps to enhance the contributions of the CNS benefit from their investment in terms of departmental functioning and productivity.

Unquestionably, this role is to be safeguarded. Although relatively well established and understood, it would be a mistake to view the role as permanently defined. To continue to be valuable, the CNS role and its implementation have to be reflective of current practice trends and responsive to current needs. Organizational structure and functional operations are useful mechanisms for the enhancement of the role. Evaluation can then determine whether these initiatives are working. It seems crucial to find new ways to review the CNS position and then use the findings from that inspection to strengthen it in all aspects— from the conceptualization of the role to preparation, implementation, and evaluation.

*References*

Barry, K.: A step backwards? (letter). J Nurs Admin *13*(11):7, 1983.
Baird, S.B.: Administrative support issues and the oncology clinical nurse specialist. Oncol Nurs Forum *12*(2):51–54, 1985.
DiVincenti, M.: Administering Nursing Services. Boston, Little Brown and Company, 1977.
Donoghue, M., & Spross, J.: The oncology clinical nurse specialist, role analysis and future projections. Oncol Nurs Forum *12*(2):35–36, 1985.
Edlund, B.J., & Hodges, L.C.: Preparing and using the clinical nurse specialist. Nurs Clin North Am *18*(3):499–507, 1983.
Fenton, M.V.: Identifying competencies of clinical nurse specialists. J Nurs Admin *15*(12):31–37, 1985.
Fox, D.H.: Matrix organizational model broadens clinical nurse specialist practice. Hosp Prog *61*(11):50–69, 1982.

Fralic, M.F.: Nursing's precious resource: The clinical nurse specialist. J Nurs Admin *18*(2):5–6, 1988.

Hamric, A.B.: Clinical nurse specialist role evaluation. Oncol Nurs Forum *12*(2):62–66, 1985.

Kohnke, M.: The development of the clinical nurse specialist. *In* Kohnke, M. (ed.): The Case For Consultation in Nursing. New York, John Wiley and Sons, 1978.

Metcalf, J., Werner, M., and Richmond, T.S.: The clinical nurse specialist in a clinical career ladder. Nurs Admin Q *9*(1):9–19, 1984.

O'Connor, P., & Malone, B.: A consultation model for nurse specialist practice. Nurs Econ *1*(5):107–111, 1983.

Poulin, M.A.: Future directions for nursing administration. J Nurs Admin *14*(3):37–41, 1984.

Prouty, M.P.: Contributions and organizational role of the CNS: An administrator's viewpoint. *In* Hamric, A.B., & Spross, J. (eds.): The Clinical Nurse Specialist in Theory and Practice. New York, Grune & Stratton, 1983.

Recommendations for administrative support of the oncology clinical nurse specialist. Oncol Nurs Forum *12*(2):72, 1985.

Wallace, M.A., & Corey, L.J.: The clinical specialist as manager: Myths versus realities. J Nurs Admin *13*(6):13–15, 1983.

Williams, L.B., & Cancian, D.W.: A clinical nurse specialist in a line management position. J Nurs Admin *15*(1):20–26, 1985.

Yasko, J.M.: The predicted effects of recent health care trends on the role of the oncology clinical nursing specialist. Oncol Nurs Forum *12*(2):58–61, 1985.

# Supportive Supervision of the CNS

*Chapter*

**13**

*Sarah Jo Brown*

## INTRODUCTION

One portrayal of the CNS's work environment is that it is composed of two subcultures: an administrative culture and a caregiving culture. While these subcultures are both parts of the larger nursing culture, forces exist in health care which hamper mutual understandings between administrators and caregivers. Changing health care regulations, financial pressures, the necessity of competing with alternative provider organizations, and the high number of nursing position vacancies consume much of the time and attention of nursing administrators. Addressing these issues can reduce the amount of time available to nursing administrators for direct nursing care issues and staff concerns. Similarly, direct care providers are confronted with heavier workloads, more complex nursing care situations, the trend toward shorter hospital stays, expanding bodies of clinical literature, and many new technologies. All of these demands absorb clinicians' time and energy so that they are less likely to be able to keep abreast of changing priorities and regulations in the health care industry or to have professional involvements outside the immediate caregiving setting. There is a risk that the members of the two subcultures may have little contact with one another, and that when they do meet regarding common concerns, they will have difficulty appreciating each other's perspectives and priorities.

### "Shuttle Diplomacy"

CNSs often find themselves interpreting economic realities and administrative decisions to nursing staff and clinical realities to administrative staff. The CNS can, indeed, be the person in the middle, a person expected and required to speak the language of both subcultures, understand the issues and dilemmas of each, and participate in the problem-solving of both arenas.

When organizations are stressed and changing quickly, relationships between CNSs and the nursing administrators to whom they report become vital communication links in nursing departments. Each person in the relationship has information and perspective derived from a different arena of involvement, which the other needs to consider in order to make sound decisions. Within the context of the relationship, the CNS and the administrator can explore strategies for joining the seemingly disparate realities of economic pressures and changing patterns of health care with the actualities of patients who need competent and caring nursing services.

In addition to providing a link, the CNS-administrator relationship can and should provide the CNS with meaningful interpersonal and substantive support. This support is in part collegial support of the person in the role but is also organizational support for the purposes and activities of the role. In reality, the two forms of support are inseparable, but it is sometimes helpful to distinguish between them.

Organizational support for the purposes and activities of the role was well described in a 1984 national survey of oncology nursing CNSs (Spross & Donoghue, 1985) and an associated article by Baird (1985). Specific forms of administrative support which are relevant to the CNS role were identified: role clarification and integration of the position into the leadership and clinical systems of the organization; economic justification of the role; commitment of resources (space, clerical support, funds for continuing education, travel expenses, time for research and professional development); anticipatory and problem-solving guidance; and provision for peer support. Some of these forms of support for the role will also be examined in this chapter; however, the emphasis will be on forms of interpersonal action which constitute administrative support.

The discussion will commence with the proposition of a framework for CNS supervision. The general characteristics of that supervision will be set forth, and the rationale for its use will be offered. Specific adaptations will be described and illustrated. Issues that must be incorporated into the deliberations of CNSs and the nursing administrators to whom they report will be discussed. Finally, organizational conditions that affect the providing and receiving of administrative support will be examined.

# A FRAMEWORK FOR CNS SUPERVISION

## A CNS Profile

In the first edition of this book, a framework for supportive supervision of CNSs was proposed (Brown, 1983). An important assumption of that framework was that many, if not most, CNSs are committed professionals who are motivated toward achievement (McClellan, et al., 1953). That is to say they aspire to bring about a high level of care in the nursing setting in which they work, are able to set difficult but potentially achievable goals for themselves, and will work diligently toward those goals. By nature of their clinical background and education, many CNSs possess personal and problem-solving skills that enable them to work well with others. They are motivated to obtain personal success within the framework of the nursing organization (Hinrichs, 1966).

## Supportive Supervision

A person with the work orientation and talent profile just described is the ideal CNS; while not all CNSs match this profile, many do, and those who do should be provided with supportive supervision. This variety of supervision assumes that employees are responsible, motivated, and creative when they are trusted and appreciated and when they are enabled to participate in organizational goal setting, decision-making, and problem-solving (Likert, 1961). Supportive supervision creates an environment in which employees are given freedom to determine many aspects of their role. This freedom is, of course, modulated by organizational goals and needs.

The freedom provided in this form of supervision is not an end in itself, rather a way of allowing flexible and innovative responses to organizational situations. Freedom does not mean that CNSs can do whatever is of personal interest without regard for organizational relevance or can proceed without consulting or informing their supervisors. Certainly, CNSs and their supervisors should discuss the appropriateness of proposed changes in clinical practice, implementation plans and timetables for new clinical programs, and decisions to get involved in major multidisciplinary projects. Prospective communication of plans ensures consideration of relevant organizational factors and coordination with other programs.

Supportive supervision does mean that CNSs' activities are not completely directed by the person to whom they report. The CNS and administrator should seek agreement regarding the goals on which the CNS should focus. In pursuing this agreement, all facts, as well as the opinions of both persons, should be considered, and conflict should be resolved through a combination of confrontation and commitment to mutual understanding. Imposition of the organizational authority of the administrator should be used only when earnest dialogue does not produce compromise or emergence of a new alternative. Once agreement regarding the CNS's job priorities has been reached, the CNS should be given a great deal of autonomy in enacting the role and pursuing the agreed-upon goals.

Some administrators to whom CNSs report are reluctant to use supportive supervision because they believe it does not hold one accountable or it is too laissez faire to ensure effective performance. These concerns are legitimate in certain situations, but the individual CNS's characteristics must be taken into account before dismissing this style of supervision. CNSs are a diverse group: some are new to the role, others have been in the role for many years; some are headstrong or intent on "doing their own thing," but many others are sensitive to the needs of the department and to the work pressures of others; some are self-serving, but a majority strive to enhance patients' experiences and other nurses' job satisfaction. Given this diversity in motivation, ability, and performance, it is illogical to assume that they all will benefit from the same form of supervision. Some need structure and specification of expectations, while others perform admirably with a great deal of autonomy. Some need a great deal of direction, while others need a sounding board, suggestions, or a modicum of administrative facilitation. Supervision must be fitted to individual maturity, commitment, and performance levels; one style will not fit all CNSs.

Some administrators believe that they must deal with all employees on the same basis. The logic behind this position is that if autonomy is given to one CNS, it will have to be given to all, and this could lead to disorder. While the administrator should be honest, impartial, and open-minded in dealing with all CNSs, the forms of supervision provided need not be identical for all individuals. Those who have consistently demonstrated the ability to perform competently and effectively have earned the right to supervision that is more collaborative, i.e., less advisory and directive in form. Those who have not demonstrated a sensitivity to characteristics of the organization when planning and prioritizing or an ability to affect smooth implementation of changes must be helped to see that the credibility of the department and that of the CNS role depends upon an acceptance of continued, advisory supervision by the administrator.

This adaptation of supervision to the professional and role developmental level of the CNS could be described as differential supervision, since the specific form of supervision is tailored to the individual's aptitudes, experience, and past performance. Differential supervision does not constitute partiality or inconsistency but rather acknowledges differences in professional maturity and degrees of contribution. It could be argued that differential supervision is crucial to both equity and incentive because it appropriates autonomy according to readiness for it and recognizes successful past performance. To avoid misunderstandings, the supervisor who affirms a philosophy of differential supervision should inform employees of this early in their relationship, so that the means of acquiring greater autonomy are clear to all.

## An Alternative Characterization of the Relationship

As was evident in the preceding discussion, the concept of supportive supervision implicitly assumes a hierarchical relationship between two persons. In the first edition of this book, the author called for minimal emphasis on the hierarchical aspects of the CNS-administrator relationship and for the establishment of a collegial relationship between them (Brown, 1983). Since that time, the author has thoughtfully considered Styles' (1982) description of collegiality and has deliberated whether collegial support is a more accurate description of the mutual advocacy that should characterize the CNS-administrator relationship.

Styles defined collegiality as a *sharing* of responsibility and authority and as an attitude of collaboration with another individual. The sharing of responsibility and authority is based on recognition of the fact that "elements of primary and secondary responsibility may operate in every situation, rotating among us as time and circumstance require" (Styles, 1982, p. 144). The collaborative attitude is based on the necessity of bringing together administrative and professional (clinical) expertise. This characterization of collegiality de-emphasizes the hierarchical status difference that may exist between two individuals by focusing on mutuality of purpose and shared responsibility.

The assumption that there is mutuality of purpose is often valid for the CNS-administrator relationship. However, the assumption that responsibility is shared is somewhat incompatible with the hierarchical chain of responsibility and authority which is fundamental to organizational structures, job descriptions, and operations of most hospitals and nursing departments. To represent the relationship between CNS and administrator as collegial denies that the CNS is organizationally accountable to, or reports to, the administrator. Therefore, the author will continue to use the term supportive supervision, as it allows for a great deal of sharing of responsibility and authority (collegiality) yet retains the notion that specified responsibilities and authority in most organizations are ultimately vested in one individual (Robbins, 1980).

## Practical Suggestions

It is easy to underestimate the need for clarification of expectations, feedback, and guidance required by the novice or new-to-the-setting

CNS. A weekly, one-hour appointment between the CNS and the supervising administrator has been found to be valuable by many CNS-administrator dyads (Fife & Lemler, 1983); such frequent and regular meetings enable problem exploration, airing of frustrations, and sharing of "little" accomplishments. At first, planning for change will need to be at a very specific level with the administrator probing issues such as alternative strategies, possible sources of resistance in the organization, and systems implications. Further, the administrator might request such clarification aids as a brief, written statement of the problem and objectives, a time-anchored flow chart of the implementation plan, or class objectives and outline. Such adjuncts to dialogue ensure that the issue under consideration has been thoroughly considered and is mutually understood.

Once a CNS has demonstrated the ability to set appropriate goals, plan exhaustively, and execute implementation of a new program or project with interpersonal and organizational adeptness, the administrator will not need to review and discuss subsequent proposals in such detail. Instead, the dialogue will be more collegial, with the two individuals focusing more on strengthening the proposal, considering all contingencies, and deliberating as to how to maximize the program's chance for success. It may be very important to the CNS's self-esteem that increased competency in role performance be recognized and honored by a change in the administrator's supervision.

## Mutual Planning of Goals and Activities

An important component of the supportive supervision framework is planning the work goals of the CNS. In fact, planning goals together may well be the heart of the relationship between the clinical specialist and the administrator. Through goal-setting dialogue, the organization (represented by the administrator) and the individual CNS find the mutuality of purpose that binds them together. In these deliberations, the CNS and the administrator agree that "of all the problems that we face and of all the goals you could pursue, these are the most important ones." Such dialogue ensures that the CNS is pursuing goals that are sanctioned by the department and releases the CNS from any guilt that may result from problems not being addressed or requests for involvement which must be declined.

The process of objective setting has been well-described elsewhere (Ganong & Ganong, 1980; Brown, 1983); however, several additional suggestions will be offered. The goals developed by the CNS and supervisor should pertain to enhancement of individual performance as well as to programmatic objectives; both issues are relevant to the

CNS's performance. A second suggestion is that six-month goal setting may be more useful and relevant than annual goal setting. The annual timeframe used to work well, but the current fast-changing health care scene introduces so many unforeseen forces that it is becoming difficult to project goals a year ahead. Lastly, the CNS's work goals should be shared with others whose roles interface with the CNS so that they will know what to expect, and what not to expect, of the CNS; this clarification of priorities can be very helpful in preventing misunderstandings and conflicts.

An important framework for the goal-setting dialogue of the CNS and the administrator is the setting of general, departmental goals and priorities. These departmental goals should be translated into individual job objectives; thus, departmental goals should determine some *portion* of the individual's objectives and activities. This relay of focus is particularly important in work settings that are bombarded by many requests and demands from sources outside the department. By setting general priorities and goals, nurse executives create a sense of order and priority amidst multiple pressures and increase the likelihood that members of the department will not become overwhelmed or work at cross-purposes.

Some goals of the department will pertain to changes in administrative structure or procedures, but others should address issues aimed at improving staff performance or nursing care delivery. The latter type of goal usually applies to all or many clinical areas and is one in which CNSs will provide leadership, either individually or as a group. A secondary benefit from these goals, which cut across clinical areas, is that the activities directed at their attainment often bring the CNSs together in common effort; and this can contribute to an esprit de corps amongst them.

## THE ADMINISTRATOR AS A SUPPORTIVE SUPERVISOR

Providing meaningful support and helpful supervision for the CNS is a demanding undertaking. It requires that administrators have a commitment to being available to CNSs as they experience frustrations. It requires the capacity to truly enter into another person's planning and problem-solving thinking, the willingness to serve as an advocate for another person's aims, and the fortitude to promote unappreciated values and causes.

In addition to these personal attributes, administrators who aim to support CNSs will be more effective in doing so if they possess organizational influence and savvy. The administrator who is a credible member of the administrative team and who has skill in negotiating cooperative agreements with other disciplines and departments has a sphere of influence which is different from that of the CNS. In addition, the administrator who is familiar with both the executive and operational workings of the organization usually has influence over a greater range of organizational resources than does the CNS. Thus, the administrator can often facilitate certain aspects of a clinical program or project for the CNS.

Clearly, the administrator to whom the CNS reports must have managerial expertise as well as an appreciation for nursing care and nursing care delivery issues. Most often these qualities are found in persons with prior direct care and unit-level leadership experience, a master's degree in nursing administration, and a leadership style that is open to collaboration with direct care providers. While such a profile is not absolute, it is a very reliable guideline in selecting a person to whom a CNS will report.

## DEVELOPMENT OF ESSENTIAL CNS SKILLS

Both novice and experienced CNSs will need ongoing feedback regarding their clinical and leadership performances to encourage them as they attempt to affect nursing care in a fast-changing and financially pressured environment. Novice CNSs and CNSs new to the setting should be assisted to evaluate their clinical skills relative to the demands of the setting and be given opportunities to remedy any weaknesses. This is important because clinical credibility is essential to this role, which carries the title of "specialist"; deficiencies will be quickly noticed by other practitioners and could restrict the CNS's clinical influence. Even CNSs with advanced clinical skills should be required to identify mechanisms for periodic peer review. Every practitioner, regardless of expertise or years of practice, should be willing, even eager, to submit their clinical practice to the review of peers to ensure continued refinement of, and new perspective on, clinical knowledge and skills.

From the beginning, the administrator should also assist the new CNS to reflect on and evaluate leadership behaviors. Self-interest, interpersonal insensitivity, and excessive aggressiveness are behaviors that have been mentioned by staff and nursing administrators as causing organizational conflict and limiting the effectiveness of individual CNSs. If these or other disruptive behaviors are noticed, they should be discussed at the time they occur so they do not impede role success. Naturally, behaviors that contribute to good communication and work relationships should be recognized and discussed also, as this contributes to insight and self-confidence.

# ADDRESSING PERFORMANCE PROBLEMS

Deficiencies in performance should not be allowed to continue without candid discussion. For example, if the administrator learns from a head nurse that the nursing staff view the CNS of the ICU as a "bungler" in performing physiological monitoring, this should be discussed with the CNS so a plan can be made to increase proficiency or address what may be unrealistic expectations of the staff. Failure to discuss it is unfair to the CNS as it denies opportunity to plan self-improvement and potentially subjects the CNS to ridicule or anger from the staff. When persons who have titles that imply advanced expertise and who are known to earn substantial salaries do not perform well, the matter is more discussed and more resented than when a staff nurse or assistant head nurse performs poorly. Failure to address obvious incompetence in leaders implicitly communicates that high level performance is not expected and weakens the department's commitment to quality nursing care.

Deficient or problematic performance can arise from many sources, and it should not be assumed that the sole source is the abilities or attitude of the CNS. The following questions are some the administrator should consider when confronted by problematic CNS performance:

- Are the expectations of CNS performance clear, agreed upon and understood in the same way by all parties in the conflict? Is the problem what the CNS does or how it is done?

- Does the problem stem from: lack of information, clinical inexperience, organizational inexperience, interpersonal insensitivity, inadequate resources, too much responsibility, ambiguity of organizational structure, lack of organizational priorities or goals, inadequate guidance and supervision, or professional territorial conflicts?

- Would it help to document the time the CNS spends in various activities so as to gain a clearer idea of how the CNS is implementing the role?

- Would it help to have a respected peer spend a week with the CNS as a source of ideas and feedback?

- Does the organization have the resources (including time) to remedy the problem?

## CAREER PLANNING SUPPORT FOR THE CNS

Concern for the CNS's career is an important form of support which should be addressed explicitly, rather than assumed. Many of the CNS's career goals can be advanced within the context of the organization. Kleinknecht and Hefferin (1982) maintained that career planning can benefit both the organization and the individual and identified the elements of a career development process.

To bring the CNS's career goals and the organization's resources and needs into alignment, the CNS and administrator may need to discuss issues such as:

- What career aspirations the CNS holds and which ones could be met within the context of the organization.
- How the CNS will be assisted to acquire clinical skills associated with emergent forms of health care management.
- What multidisciplinary or professional involvements will provide the CNS with the opportunity to impact health care issues relevant to the CNS's specialty.
- How the CNS can refine skills, particularly subrole skills such as classroom teaching or consulting.
- How the CNS will be assisted in conducting clinical research, e.g., arranging or contracting for consultation with a skilled nurse researcher.
- Whether the CNS will need help in writing for publication and, if so, who in the organization or nursing community could guide such writing endeavors.

All of these questions pertain to activities that are of career interest to most CNSs and also could result in capacities and outputs of benefit to the organization as well.

## ORGANIZATIONAL STRUCTURE AND CNS SUPPORT

Decisions regarding organizational structure have implications for how CNSs receive support from nursing administrators. Various structures involve different delegations of responsibility, authority, and accountability which, in turn, affect the CNS–administrator relationship. Essentially, CNSs can report to different nursing administrators or they can all report to one nursing administrator.

The former alternative is frequently found in decentralized departments that incorporate decision-making power close to the practice level of the organization. In this organizational structure, a common arrangement is for the CNSs to report to clinical area or clinical service directors. This arrangement is advantageous because both leaders have responsibilities that contribute to the delivery of the same patient care services; thus, they share objectives and familiarity with the operational problems of the service or area. In the course of performing their respective functions, they are likely to confer frequently; such contact often results in mutual understanding and recognition of the constraints and problems of the other person's job and, ultimately, in a solid working relationship. There are many advantages of the CNS reporting to an area or service director, but they all hinge on the nursing administrator being committed to including the CNS in the planning and decision-making for the service.

Potential drawbacks to this accountability arrangement arise from the multiple administrative responsibilities of the area or service director. The administrator's relationship with the CNS is often one of many important relationships (e.g., several head nurses, other area directors, physicians of the involved services) that must be attended to. The administrator may inadvertently neglect the relationship with the CNS because there is an assumption of mutual understanding between them. Over time this assumption can result in the underutilization of a supportive relationship that is potentially valuable to both persons.

Under regulatory conditions, which are requiring greater fiscal accountability, considerable administrative attention is focused on costs, documentation of services, and budget monitoring. There can be a tendency for administrators to settle for sustaining the extant quality of nursing care rather than striving for its improvement. As a result, they may not be truly receptive to ideas for improving nursing care unless they are obviously cost-saving or revenue-generating. The CNS may become frustrated if clinical concerns consistently fail to receive attention amid the myriad issues facing nursing administrators.

Another potential problem is that a particular director may not be accustomed to having a person who is educated at the master's level report to her or him; this could represent a threat to the administrator or it could result in inappropriate supervision. It should not be assumed that, because CNSs are educated at graduate level, they will not require guidance and encouragement to perform well.

When all CNSs report to one person, such as an associate director or a director of nursing consultation, nursing executives are able to select a person with the right blend of experience, education, and style to work with the CNSs. This has advantages in that the administrator who accepts such a responsibility would presumably have a commitment to the CNS role. Further, the administrator would have significant time to devote to CNS concerns because responsibility for CNS supervision would be a major part of the job. Such an arrangement also enables the administrator to use insights and successful ideas gained from working with one CNS in guiding another who encounters a similar situation. Lastly, it facilitates the building of a cohesive CNS group with peer support and shared goals.

The obvious disadvantage to all CNSs reporting to one person is that the CNS may not be viewed as an integral member of the group that makes patient care decisions in the CNS's area or service. This arrangement sets the CNS outside the decision-making processes of the service and makes the CNS somewhat dependent upon the decision-making style of the administrative person for the area. The possibility exists that the CNS will be excluded from dialogue and decisions regarding those clinical services even though the CNS is a contributor to them. The interpersonally and organizationally competent CNS may be able to gain access to these decision-making groups, but the less savvy CNS may be excluded. This exclusion could severely limit the CNS's ability to affect nursing care in the area.

Two other organizational placements deserve mention from the perspective of administrative support—the CNS reporting to a director of nursing and the CNS reporting to the medical director of a clinical service. Small hospitals have reported success with the CNS reporting to the director of nursing (Mummah, 1981). The director of nursing may be the most appropriate person to supervise the CNS, particularly if the director possesses a broad professional perspective, educational credentials, commitment to the CNS role, and organizational influence. However, in large departments, directors of nursing may be so involved in hospital administrative matters that they are unable to devote much time to supervising CNSs. If the CNS's access to the director of nursing is limited to infrequent, scheduled meetings, or if the director of nursing does not know much about how operational activities are conducted, the CNS may feel unsupported even though reporting to a top-level administrator. The drawbacks of this reporting arrangement will probably be most acutely felt by novice or new-to-the-setting CNSs as they will not receive the type or amount of supervision they need.

Some CNSs are being hired by medical staff services or private medical practices to provide nursing care and/or to coordinate complex patient care programs (Burford & Wey, 1980; Littell, 1981; Chamorro, 1981; Weiland, 1983). This arrangement has the advantage to patients of ensuring that the doctors and nurses coordinating their care are in close communication. From the perspective of administrative support, these roles have been problematic because the incumbents often stand apart from the nursing department. Frequently, persons in these roles experience a distinct lack of cooperation from some nursing managers and administrators or from staff nurses who resent their intrusion on what have been traditional staff nurse responsibilities. Depending on the medical director and the administrative support system of the medical service, CNSs in these positions can either feel isolated and left to tackle organizational issues on their own, or highly supported by members of their service. These arrangements seem to be most successful when the CNS is an experienced and mature individual, capable of negotiating responsibility agreements among caregivers.

The potential benefits of this kind of organizational placement of the CNS to patient care demand that it be given thoughtful consideration. Many of its problems can be overcome if a plan for interfacing this kind of position with the general nursing staff and with nursing managers and administrators is formulated at the time the role is implemented. A joint appointment to the medical service and to the nursing department with clearly delineated responsibility and accountability may facilitate the CNS's relationships with members of the nursing department and promote coordinated and comprehensive patient care.

Chapter 11 addressed justification and placement of the CNS role within a nursing department. It should be recognized that these administrative activities are forms of administrative support for the CNS role and its incumbents. In fact, they may represent the most fundamental form of support in a resource-competitive environment. Structuring the CNS role in ways that closely link it with patient outcomes and recognized nursing functions may decrease the role's flexibility; however, it may be an essential strategy for ensuring continuation of the role in the most basic sense.

## SUMMARY

In the context of the CNS-administrator relationship, the caregiving culture and the administrative culture can interface successfully. Nursing services and products that are economically viable and clinically relevant can be formulated, and effective ways of delivering nursing care in a resource-limited environment can be realized. Together, CNS and administrator can foster the creation of work environments that enable the practice of nursing to maximize patient outcomes.

*References*

Brown, S.J.: Administrative support. *In* Hamric, A.B. & Spross, J. (eds): The Clinical

Nurse Specialist in Theory and Practice. New York, Grune and Stratton, 1983, pp 149–170.

Baird, S.B.: Administrative support issues and the oncology clinical nurse specialist. Oncol Nurs Forum 12(2):51–61, 1985.

Burford, C., & Wey, J.M.: A clinical nurse specialist–social worker team on a cardiovascular surgery service. Heart Lung 9(5):841–845, 1980.

Calkin, J.D.: A model for advanced nursing practice. J Nurs Admin 14(1):24–30, 1984.

Chamorro, T.: The role of a nurse clinician in joint practice with gynecological oncologists. Cancer 48(2):622–631, 1981.

Fife, B., & Lemler, S.: The psychiatric nurse specialist: A valuable asset in the general hospital. J Nurs Admin 13(4):14–17, 1983.

Ganong, J., & Ganong, W.: Nursing Management (2nd ed). Germantown, Md, Aspen Systems, 1980.

Harrell, J.S., & McCulloch, S.D.: The role of the clinical nurse specialist: Problems and solutions. J Nurs Admin 16:10):44–48, 1986.

Hinrichs, J.: High Talent Personnel: Managing a Critical Resource. New York, McGraw-Hill, 1967.

Kleinknecht, M.K., & Hefferin, E.A.: Assisting nurses toward professional growth: A career development model. J Nurs Admin 12(7):30–36, 1982.

Likert, R.: New Patterns of Management. New York, McGraw-Hill, 1961.

Littell, S.C.: The clinical nurse specialist in a private medical practice. Nurs Admin Q 6(1):77–85, 1981.

McClellan, D.C., Atkinson, J., Clark, R., et al.: The Achievement Motive. New York, Appleton-Century-Crofts, 1953.

Mummah, H.: Role of the gerontological clinical nurse specialist at Whittier Hospital. J Gerontol Nurs 7:(10):600–602, 1981.

Robbins, S.P.: The Administrative Process (2nd ed). Englewood Cliffs, N.J., Prentice-Hall, 1980.

Spross, J.A., & Donoghue, M. (eds): OCNS conference conclusions, recommendations for administrative support of the oncology clinical nurse specialist. Oncol Nurs Forum 12(2):71–73, 1985.

Styles, M.M.: On Nursing: Toward a New Endowment. St. Louis, C.V. Mosby Company, 1982.

Wallace, M.A., & Corey, L.J.: The clinical specialist as manager: Myth versus realities. J Nurs Admin 13(6):13–15, 1983.

Weiland, A.P.: Physicians and nurse joint practice: A description of nurse practitioners on a cardiac surgery service. Heart Lung, 12(6):576–580, 1983.

Williams, L.B., & Cancian, D.W.: A clinical nurse specialist in a line management position. J Nurs Admin 15(1):20–26, 1985.

Zander, K.: Second generation primary nursing: A new agenda. J Nurs Admin 15(3):18–24, 1985.

# Chapter 14

# Peer Support and Peer Review

*Anne Edgerton Winch*

## INTRODUCTION

The support of the CNS by other CNSs is an important issue that cannot be overemphasized. Peer support, in combination with support from administrators and nursing staff, is instrumental to both professional and personal development. Initially, discussion of the CNS in the literature emphasized role definition and educational preparation. The need to explore pressures and frustrations faced by all CNSs has emerged as the role has evolved. This chapter will discuss first the importance of peer support to the CNS and will suggest strategies for the development of peer support. Discussion of peer support provides a foundation for consideration of the concept of peer review and its importance to the CNS. Strategies for actualization of a CNS peer review process will be presented.

## IMPORTANCE OF PEER SUPPORT TO THE CNS

While the CNS experiences the same basic need for support as any nurse, issues related to practice of the CNS color the matter of peer support differently. Brown (1983), in discussing the CNS's unique need for administrative support, identified issues that are equally powerful in contributing to the CNS's unique need for peer support. The CNS role continues to lack uniformity from one setting to another and within the same setting. The lack of uniformity among CNS roles creates some ambiguity, which typically does not exist with more established roles, such as the head nurse role. In addition, confusion regarding the CNS role can result from the dynamic and flexible nature of the role and the variability in the strategies chosen by individual CNSs in implementing the role. CNSs are at risk for professional isolation. Support

**299**

from CNS peers is essential if the CNS is to confront what are often intense emotions resulting from role ambiguity and confusion and to be successful and satisfied personally and professionally in the role.

The role responsibilities of the CNS often include activities that other nurses have viewed as their responsibility. This intraprofessional territoriality may cause conflict. For example, the CNS may be perceived as interfering when primary nurses become possessive of patients and are resistant to intervention by or consultation with the CNS. Head nurses who have worked on a particular unit for a number of years may promote themselves as the only clinical expert available to the staff and attempt to undermine the role of the CNS. CNS support in helping peers deal with intraprofessional conflict can be invaluable.

In the role of patient advocate, the CNS interfaces with many disciplines in clarifying and coordinating patient care and is likely to be confronted by differences of opinion and role territoriality that may cause interprofessional conflict. Johnson and her peers (1982), who are all psychiatric CNSs practicing in Washington State, identified this issue of role overlap and territoriality between the CNS and those in other mental health disciplines as one that uniquely affects the need for professional support among CNSs. Support from peers is vitally important in enabling the CNS to problem-solve with regard to territoriality, both intra- and interprofessionally. Peer support fosters a sense of belonging. Professional growth is thus enhanced and reinforced by interaction with peers.

Johnson, et al. (1982) also identified multilevel demands for support inherent in the role as contributing to the CNS's unique need for peer support. These multilevel demands for support exist in the practice of all CNSs and are addressed in the literature. Holt (1975) described the CNS as a kind of "super nurse" (p. 83). Fenton (1985), in exploring the competencies of advanced nursing practice by CNSs, described in detail the multilevel demands for support made upon the CNSs she interviewed and observed. "Building and maintaining a therapeutic team in order to provide optimum therapy" was a very significant competency required of the successful CNS (pp. 32–33). Within this competency, the provision of emotional support for nursing staff and dealing with change and resistance to change were described as daily activities by CNSs. For CNSs to be responsive to these demands for support by individuals and by the system, CNSs must identify sources of support for themselves. Peers are one fundamental source of this support.

Another issue, addressed by Brown (1983), is that presently most CNSs are women, who are often well-educated, articulate, and confident and who express well-developed ideas about patient care and the role of nursing in the delivery of care. In some settings, this profile of the female nurse may lead to resistance to the CNS role or to the CNS's ideas, particularly among male physicians and hospital administrators.

Gender issues may also influence the giving and receiving of support by CNSs. In coping with numerous demands and potentially unrealistic expectations of others and of self, the CNS is at risk for "Type E" behavior, a concept recently described in high-achieving women by Braiker (1986), a clinical psychologist and management consultant. Type E women derive this label from their effort to be "Everything to Everybody." They have difficulty accepting the fact that needs for nurturing and support can and do coexist with parallel needs to be autonomous, self-reliant, and independent. It is easy to see how this might describe the characteristics of some CNSs!

Both informal discussion and the literature (Metzger, 1985) imply that nurses, CNSs included, fail to support one another professionally and personally. Concern for peer support among nurses is evidenced by recent attention in the nursing literature to the concept of mentoring (Campbell-Heider, 1986); Hagerty, 1986) and discussion of its importance in promoting individual and professional growth. Although mentoring has been described from a variety of perspectives, these different frameworks suggest that "mentoring is the cultivation of young talent and the promotion of career development through the lending of organizational, role, or interpersonal support and teaching" (Hagerty, 1986, p. 17). Historically, CNSs have had no one to serve as mentors for them because in most systems the CNS represents the top of the clinical hierarchy. CNS peer support represents the beginning of a mentoring relationship between individuals who occupy similar positions in the work hierarchy. Professional growth is encouraged, especially for the beginning or novice CNS, and is reinforced for all CNSs by the peer group. Additionally, in implementing their role, CNSs serve as mentors to other nurses. Support of one another enhances the ability of the CNS to enter into a mentoring relationship with other nurses.

A final issue influencing the CNS's need for support which was identified by Brown (1983) is the dependence of the CNS in many systems on nursing administration for power and influence in organizational matters. Again, support from CNS peers provides an avenue for problem-solving. Perhaps more important is the power base that a group identity may provide for CNSs, enhancing their ability to have input into the system, to communicate with nursing administration, and thus to influence the standards of care within the institution.

In exploring predictors of employment success, Fenton (1985) recognized the successful CNS as one who is able to develop a support system and generate job satisfaction without expecting the job or the system to supply it. The importance of peer support for the functioning and role development of the CNS is also substantiated by the survey findings reported in Chapter 3.

There are many benefits of peer support for the CNS. It is clear that peer support can significantly influence role implementation and development for all CNSs, regardless of the time spent in the role. Some of the other benefits of peer support are less obvious but are equally important and thus warrant attention.

Peer support provides CNSs with a means to validate their perceptions. These perceptions may be related to specific nursing care issues, to needs within a particular practice setting and/or the nursing profession in general, and to actions and reactions of self and others to the needs and issues at hand. Primarily an interpersonal process, *support* is a seeking or desiring by one individual of assistance, guidance, recognition, or encouragement from another (Brown, 1983). Although not mutually exclusive, professional support and personal support differ from one another in their primary purposes. Professional support has as its focus the accomplishment of professional growth through stimulation of ideas, provision of practical help and opportunities for sharing of professional experiences, and enhancement of the profession, while the goal of personal support is self or personal enhancement (Johnson, et al., 1982).

It is logical to argue that personal growth will lead to professional growth and vice versa. Much support and growth do emerge from informal contact among CNS peers meeting for coffee, lunch, or outside of the work setting for socialization, or through telephone calls to one another to share good news or "crisis" situations. However, the distinction between the central purposes of these two types of support is crucial to the successful provision of professional support. The provision of support requires an interaction between at least two persons and is often provided by a group of individuals or peers. Educational preparation, qualifications, and/or position are qualities that determine who is a peer. As support is often provided in a group setting, further discussion of peer support will be considered in a group context.

Clarification of the purpose of a group at the outset is most important. Kirschenbaum and Glaser (1978) identified confusion regarding the purpose of the group as a major pitfall of the professional support group and cautioned against the group becoming an encounter group. In a professional support group, a small number of professionals with common interests meet periodically to learn together and support one another, thus fostering professional development (Kirschenbaum & Glaser, 1978). Purposes of the professional support group include provision of practical help to group members, stimulation of ideas, sharing of professional experiences, and serving as a forum for exchange of relevant information with one another.

With clarification of the purposes of the professional support group, acknowledgment of the overlap between personal and professional needs can occur without threat to the group's existence. Professional support groups can and should be safe places where much camaraderie exists and CNSs are encouraged to share and validate their feelings and perceptions.

A final benefit of peer support for the CNS is the provision of a power base. This benefit is of particular importance to the CNS in a staff position. The power ascribed to the CNS in a line position is derived from the administrative responsibilities of hiring, firing, and supervising employees. While the CNS in a staff position derives power from clinical expertise, this clinical power remains something of an unknown. A recent nursing resource study by an outside consultant group at a university hospital employing multiple CNSs in staff positions disclosed that the CNSs were perceived as a group, and as a group with considerable power (Deloitte, Haskins, and Sells, personal communication, March 1986). Some CNSs in the group were concerned about this perception, which they regarded as negative. Other CNSs viewed it as positive and indicative of arrival at a developmental milestone, with power derived from their clinical expertise. The group continues discussion of the meaning of this perception and action that it may require.

## STRATEGIES FOR DEVELOPMENT OF PEER SUPPORT

The initial step in developing peer support for CNSs is acknowledgment and acceptance of the need for support. It is important to clarify that support needs do not conflict with the need and desire for independence and autonomy in practice as a CNS. In acknowledging their need for peer support, CNSs must be prepared to invest considerable time and energy into developing that support.

Establishing regular contact with CNSs is a step that occurs early in the process of developing peer support. The frequency of contact may vary, from weekly to monthly to bi-monthly depending largely on the geographical proximity of the members of the peer group. Membership in the peer group will be discussed later and is less important than the commitment of the members to meet or contact one another at the agreed intervals and to be available to one another on an informal basis. While some CNS groups, such as the institution-based CNS group at the University of Virginia, feel strongly about the importance of weekly group meetings, the literature contains little information regarding the frequency of contact. The experience of the author, supported by that of CNS colleagues, suggests that contact should not be any less often than every other month. When CNSs want to be perceived as a group having influence, meetings should be at least once a month and ideally twice a month. When group impact is less important, meetings every other month are acceptable. This does not negate the importance of contact with other CNS peers at intervals longer than every other month—for example, an annual gathering of CNSs with the same specialty practice. However, this less frequent contact should be viewed as supplemental, not as a primary source of peer support.

Kirschenbaum and Glaser (1978) viewed the leadership role in a professional support group as being shared by all members. They used the term "convener" in referring to the person(s) who takes initial action in bringing the group together. This author's experience recommends the use of an agenda in keeping the professional support group focused; the agenda can be the responsibility of the convener or can be established by consensus of the membership for the following meeting. Minutes of professional support group meetings should be kept for reference by the group and for the benefit of absent members.

An additional aspect of professional support groups considered unique by Kirschenbaum and Glaser (1978) was familiarity with and use of four learning modes. An awareness of these four learning modes is helpful in guiding the group's activities and the support provided. Because a developmental relationship exists between peer support and peer review, strategies for the development of peer review will be discussed within the context of these four learning modes later in the chapter.

First is the teaching-learning mode in which group members teach and learn from one another. Sharing of experiences and resources, presentations, lectures, and discussions are examples of ways a group functions in this mode. The second learning mode of professional support groups is the problem-solving mode. Challenges experienced by the CNS in the practice setting are presented to the group for discussion. The third learning mode is practice and allows members to practice a skill or endeavor and receive feedback in a supportive environment. The fourth and final learning mode is the action-project mode. This mode involves group members actively in projects designated to bring about changes in their professional environment. Of note is the potential of an action-project to either unite or divide a group; such a project influences the development of trust, which is a prerequisite to peer review.

## Sources of Peer Support

Peer support for the CNS is derived from two different but equally important CNS peers: CNSs with the same specialty practice and CNSs with varying specialty practice. Issues related to practice in a particular specialty area are best addressed by peers sharing the same specialty area. Issues common to CNSs because of similar role elements regardless of specialty area, as well as more global issues of importance to the profession, can be addressed by peers with varying specialty practice. If peers whose specialty areas differ fail to look at the challenges they share in their practices, provision of support is hindered. Education and enhancement of practice takes place in interaction with both kinds of CNS peers. CNSs are often surprised at the benefits of exposure to peers practicing in differing specialties.

Within the same institution, peer support among CNSs is facilitated if all CNSs report to the same individual (Malone, 1986). Similarities rather than differences may be emphasized when all members share the same boss. The formation of a group identity may occur over a shorter time period when this condition exists.

Use of a "buddy system," pairing a new CNS with a more experienced CNS, is another useful strategy for developing peer support within an institution or agency in which multiple CNSs practice. This strategy potentially creates a bond between the two individuals and between the new member and the group. At regular intervals, for example, at three, six, and nine months, developmental issues can be addressed by the "buddy" and by the group. Initiation of the new CNS into the role and the system is thus facilitated.

When more than one CNS is employed in an institution or agency, as is often the case in university hospital settings, CNSs have a readily available source of peer support. When a CNS is the only one in the institution or agency, the CNS must look beyond the institutional setting for peer support. Primary support for this individual will come from those identified by the individual as peers within the immediate work environment. Clarification of who is a peer is important for all CNSs but particularly for the CNS who is geographically isolated from other CNSs. Equality of education, qualifications, and/or position are attributes of a *peer*, with educational equality perhaps most important. Who one defines as a peer may be influenced by a value judgment; i.e., a peer of the CNS is one whose clinical judgment and expertise are respected. Or, a peer may be defined for the CNS as a result of the reporting structure within the organization. Each CNS may thus define and select peers individually.

While support from CNS peers may become secondary or supplemental for the geographically isolated CNS, it remains essential to growth and development in the CNS role. Obtaining and maintaining this support, however, may require more energy. Potential sources of CNS peers include other institutions, agencies, and organizations in the community, the state, and the nation. The professional support group developed by Johnson and her colleagues (1982) was composed of psychiatric–mental health CNSs in a metropolitan area who had a need for support among peers sharing the same specialty. They described an arrangement that their group developed in response to the needs of a psychiatric CNS in a remote geographical area; this CNS met with the group once and subsequently enjoyed the privileges and benefits of membership "in absentia" by raising issues and receiving group responses via written correspondence. The effectiveness of this arrangement was not addressed. However, this is a strategy that other CNSs may find beneficial.

Peer support may also be found at the state level, through state nurses' associations and councils, or groups of CNSs established as interest or practice groups. At the national level, the ANA Council of CNSs provides opportunities for contact and support among CNSs with the same and differing specialty practice. Other groups organize annual meetings; for example, a group of maternal-child CNSs in St. Louis, who obtained grant funding for further exploration of their specialty practice, have organized an annual meeting for the last three years for maternal-child CNSs. Specialty organizations provide an additional source of peer support for the CNS. Participation in specialty organizations is an effective way of ensuring contact with CNSs with the same specialty practice. For example, a CNS whose specialty is otolaryngology enjoys support from CNS peers with specialties different from her own employed at the same institution. This CNS was excited, however, to meet several other otolaryngology CNSs at a national meeting of the Society of Otorhinolaryngology and Head-Neck Nurses, Inc. (OHN) and to experience the benefits of peer support from CNSs who share a common specialty practice. Conferences, seminars, and continuing education offerings provide opportunities for networking and support among CNSs at the local, state, regional, and national levels which may continue long after the planned program.

The journal *Clinical Nurse Specialist,* whose focus is general issues related to the CNS role and role implementation and development, was first published in the Spring of 1987. The journal should provide additional opportunities for CNS peer support, particularly for the CNS who is more isolated in the practice setting. Networking among CNSs may be facilitated and a forum for dialogue provided via journal articles and letters to the editor.

## Variables Influencing Peer Group Effectiveness

The size of the peer support group is a variable about which little is known. Johnson, et al. (1982) suggested that the formation and development of the professional support group generally parallels that of any small group. A small group is defined as 2 to 20 persons who interact with each other, each one influencing and being influenced by one another (Shaw, 1976). It is hard to conceive that a group much larger than this could fulfill primary support needs for the CNS. Groups whose membership numbers more than 20 can and do meet needs for support. However, primary support is usually provided by smaller groups that exist within the large group. In considering size, it is important to acknowledge that groups are fluid and dynamic and move through stages of development from introductory or orientation stage, to working stage, and on to termination stage (Luft, 1984). The importance of size as a variable is determined by other variables such as the purpose(s) of the group and interpersonal characteristics of group members. It is important to note here that changes in the membership of the group and, consequently, the size of the peer group may significantly affect the development and maintenance of support in any peer group. CNS groups may need to spend time processing these changes when members are added or leave the group.

There is a potential danger in the "safety" of the peer support group. As members of a support group, CNSs should expect to receive as well as to give support. Failure to define the purpose(s) of the peer support group and develop guidelines for group functioning can lead to misuse of the peer support group, a factor that undermines its effectiveness and leads to its demise. For example, a CNS may find inappropriate support in the peer group and "dump" problems and concerns on peers. CNS peers may encourage further "dumping" by their behavior, listening and empathizing with the experiences of their peer but not engaging in any problem-solving with this individual or as a group. The response of the group may encourage this CNS to continue a pattern of "dumping" on the group; the group requires no change in behavior by this CNS and is not really providing support. This type of relationship prohibits growth of the CNS and is unfair to all parties.

A CNS experiencing difficulty in role performance may also seek protection in the peer support group. Failure of CNS peers to confront this individual while offering help may have potentially significant legal ramifications. Ultimately, a CNS must be held accountable for individual professional development. However, despite the popularity of the concept of accountability both within and outside of the nursing profession over the past two decades, the concept remains for the most part an unrealized achievement. In holding peers accountable for their nursing practice, group members must wrestle with difficult questions such as accountability on whose part? Accountability for what acts? Accountability to whom? Perhaps most important are difficult questions regarding the relationship of peer support to supportive supervision. What is the role of a peer within a professional support group in confronting issues of accountability? Is it a peer's responsibility to report the professional behavior of the CNS peer in question to the supervisor? Are there situations in which failure to confront a peer about questionable professional behavior has legal ramifications for the one who fails to report?

It is the responsibility of the peer support group to deal with these questions and make decisions with regard to the issues they raise. The author does not believe that the decisions themselves are most important. Most vital is that the group has clarified for itself and its members how it chooses to function. Making these decisions strengthens the group's position with respect to being able to accomplish peer review successfully later.

In the truly professional support group, CNS behaviors that need to change should be confronted. Members of a professional support group should be committed to providing constructive criticism to one another as well as positive feedback. Still, how far a group will go in addressing the behavior of a member who is using the group inappropriately remains a decision to be made by individual groups. Peer support groups may not be willing to take responsibility for corrective action. Groups that choose to act may find a useful model in the concept of clinical supervision currently used in psychiatric–mental health nursing (Critchley, 1985). The relationship of the supervisor to the one being supervised in this model moves through four developmental stages. The relationship begins as teacher-pupil and progresses to teacher-apprentice, with the focus on the client. The focus then becomes personality issues and increased self-awareness for the trainee and finally a relationship characterized by mutual consultation. Creative adaptation or use of this model may be helpful to CNSs regardless of specialty. Problems related to clinical practice or to implementation of CNS subroles can be identified. Use of the model may help to provide structure in dealing with the problem and with developing independent role behaviors for the CNS once in question.

An example of a situation in which problem-solving occurred through the use of clinical supervision may be helpful in illustrating application of the concept. A CNS in an institution in which primary nursing was practiced became quite distraught over a period of months as the nursing leadership and staff on one of the units with whom she worked accused her of being meddlesome and interfering and made her feel more and more unwelcome on the unit. While the CNS confided in her peer group at weekly meetings, she blamed the unit's nursing staff for the problem; the situation continued to worsen until it became a crisis for the CNS. A more experienced CNS in the group intervened, offering to provide role consultation to the distraught CNS. Together, they reviewed activities and behavior of the CNS in question, discussed new approaches that they role played, and evaluated the strategies after implementation. Self-awareness was enhanced when the CNS realized that her style and approach had frequently been in direct competition with the primary nurses. This CNS was then able to examine with the unit staff their needs and priorities and to renegotiate role expectations. Professional and personal growth resulted from this role consultation between the two CNSs.

## IMPORTANCE OF PEER REVIEW TO THE CNS

For the CNS, the issue of evaluation poses unique and additional challenges primarily as the result of the independence and autonomy of the role and the variability in role expression among CNSs. Peer support provides the CNS with the opportunity for constructive feedback related to role performance and encourages professional growth. The relationship between peer support and peer review is developmental. Peer review that is helpful to those involved in the process and that will stand the test of time must be built on peer support.

To *review* is "to give and write a critical report and evaluation of" (Webster's New World Dictionary, 1970). In response to public demand for an organized medical review system to ensure standards of health care, the concept of peer review was introduced in the medical literature in the 1960s. Influenced by this trend in medicine, the nursing profession recognized its own accountability for practice and responsibility to the public by establishing peer review as a priority at the 1972 convention of the American Nurses' Association (ANA). The ANA promoted peer review as a means of maintaining standards of care. The development of the concept of peer review is highlighted in Table 14–1 and is discussed by Leibold (1983). Leibold defined peer review for the CNS as "the critical evaluation of one's clinical practice by colleagues who are equal in education, qualifications and/or position and therefore are able to make qualitative judgments concerning clinical performance" (p. 219).

**TABLE 14–1. Historical Development of the Concept of Peer Review in Nursing**

| | |
|---|---|
| 1972 | Peer review established as a priority at American Nurses' Association (ANA) Convention. |
| 1973 | *Guidelines for Peer Review* drafted by ANA Congress for Nursing Practice. |
| | Appointment of task force by ANA to revise and update local and national peer review programs. |
| | Development of generic and specialty standards of nursing practice begun. |
| 1976 | Peer review gained further support with publication of ANA's *Code for Nurses.* |
| 1977–1979 | Support for peer review system based on evaluation of individual nurse's actions found in the literature. |
| 1980 | Professional mandate for peer review in nursing firmly established in *Nursing: A Social Policy Statement.* |

Peer review has special significance for the CNS. On the basis of their level of expertise, CNSs assume greater responsibility for direct care practice and for the advancement of the nursing profession. In accepting this responsibility, specialists are charged by the profession (ANA, 1980) to seek periodic review of clinical data from an equally prepared expert in the same specialized area of practice. By utilizing peer review to evaluate and improve performance, the CNS models the value of peer review for other nurses, who may also adopt it as a mechanism for evaluation and improvement of performance. An ongoing process for evaluation and improvement of nursing care is thus established.

Through peer review, individual accountability is facilitated. This aspect of peer review assumes greater importance at a time of heightened awareness of legal liability issues and increased accountability to the consumer. Bennett (1985) warned nurses in leadership positions with responsibility for hiring and supervising of the importance of peer review. He cited three cases in which hospitals and/or individual nursing personnel have been held liable for improperly employing an individual whom they knew, or had reason to believe, was incapable of performing the task for which the individual had been employed. As leaders in nursing, CNSs are not immune to issues of legal liability whether or not they are in positions with line authority. As a process that facilitates individual accountability, peer review offers protection to the individual nurse as well as to the consumer.

The advent of DRGs has encouraged and promoted the study of nursing care in an attempt to decrease patient's length of stay and thus costs. Peer review, by serving as a tool for evaluation and documentation of nursing practice, focuses on the quality of nursing practice. However, quality, quantity, and cost of care are reciprocals; changes in one of these dimensions of care affect the other two dimensions. Inherent in concern for quality of care is attention to quantity of care, so that patients receive only the care needed at the lowest cost compatible with quality. One focus of peer review activities is determination of the appropriateness and timeliness of individual practice decisions. Thus, peer review has implications for cost-effectiveness, efficiency, and productivity as practice decisions are reviewed. Participation in peer review by the CNS demonstrates awareness and concern for cost-effectiveness in providing nursing care and promotes a mechanism for ensuring that standards of care are met. Participation in the process of peer review provides a means for justifying the merits of the CNS role to the health care delivery system and the consumer. Effective peer review will help to foster the survival and growth of the CNS role.

## STRATEGIES FOR DEVELOPMENT OF PEER REVIEW

In examining strategies for development of peer review by CNSs, the experience of selected CNSs throughout the country, who are currently involved in developing and/or implementing peer review, will be included. Discussion of strategies for the development of peer support provides a foundation for discussion of strategies for the development of peer review, as peer review evolves from peer support.

Ramphal (1974) identified two types of peer review: individual peer review and agency review. Individual peer review involves evaluation of the quality of nursing care given by an individual nurse, while agency review assesses general patterns of care provided to patients within an agency. Historically, the concept of peer review has been utilized in the design of quality assurance programs within agencies, most commonly in the nursing audit and the patient care audit. These measures evaluate the quality of nursing care and reflect the standards of practice developed by a group of nurses, usually on a given nursing unit. Evaluation is accomplished by either a retrospective review of the patient record after discharge or a combination of direct observation, patient and nurse interviews, and chart review of selected patient records during hospitalization.

These forms of evaluation are important quality assurance mechanisms. However, they neither evaluate individual accountability for nursing practice nor are they particularly helpful in examining the practice of the CNS. The CNS has multiple contacts and associations within and beyond the system which are not necessarily documented in a given patient record or patient outcome. Individual peer review must then involve the use of alternate ways of gathering information for evaluation. In conducting either type of peer review, Anderson and Davis (1987) noted that disagreements abound as to whether measurements of structure, process, or outcomes should be examined.

In defining *review* and *peer review*, both Webster (1970) and Leibold (1983) included the word *critical*, which for many has a negative connotation. Given this negativity, peer review has the potential to be viewed as punitive or disciplinary and thus in opposition to support. This negative perception of peer review as a threat to the individual nurse is discussed in the literature (Hauser, 1975; Gold, et al., 1973; Lamberton, Keen, and Admoanis, 1977; McClure, 1978) as one of the major pitfalls of peer review. A peer review instrument should thus be devised and implemented with respect for the confidentiality of participants, while providing useful information about practice. The fact that peer review evaluates job-specific performance criteria and not personal characteristics or worth may require emphasis throughout the process.

Fundamental to implementation and success of peer review is the establishment of trust. Identification of the need to establish trust is easier than surmounting the problems the lack of trust pose for successful peer review. Interaction with a peer group for the purpose of support is one strategy that allows for trust to develop.

Professional passivity is an issue that is closely related to the establishment of trust and that must be addressed in order for peer review to be successful. Peer review of an individual's practice too often operates in accordance with laissez-faire principles. Individuals, although professionals, are too often reluctant and unwilling to pass judgment on one another. Gold, et al. (1973) noted that this is especially true for those who are creating and functioning in new roles, i.e., the CNS role. McClure (1978) cautioned that identifying the problem of passivity is much simpler than overcoming it. She noted that passivity also seems to be a function of female sex role identity, which makes it understandable that a field so dominated by women should suffer from such a handicap. Surely this handicap is not an insurmountable one.

Socialization of students and young graduates into a more active approach to the role of "nurse" is a strategy that addresses the issue of professional passivity and indirectly addresses the issue of trust. "To be accountable means to be willing to seize responsibility, not to wait until it is thrust upon us" (McClure, 1978, p. 49). Lamberton, Keen, and Admoanis (1977) described peer review with students in a family nurse clinician program based on the belief that if nurses are to function independently in the role, they must not only develop a sense of responsibility for the outcomes of their practice but also learn ways to demonstrate accountability. In learning the principles of peer review, students moved through four phases: personalization, implementation, formalization, and actualization. While evaluation of the peer review component of the curriculum was not addressed, students did verbalize that the process helped them to improve their practice and was a useful learning experience for both reviewers and reviewees. It would be interesting to know how many of the graduates of this program continue to participate in peer review when it is no longer a course expectation. Such socialization efforts may be most successful when they are valued by more educational programs and begin early in the educational process.

Given the issue of trust and the potential for threat, it is crucial to establish goals for peer review and to prioritize those goals when developing a system of peer review. The process of goal-setting clarifies misconceptions and allows for expression of hopes and fears by those who will be participants. Goals for peer review will guide the selection or development of a peer review tool and implementation of the process.

Along with establishing and prioritizing goals, decisions must be made initially about how peer review will be used. The following questions should guide group decision-making. Is participation in the peer review process voluntary or required? Will peer review become a part of evaluation of the CNS by the one to whom the CNS reports? If peer review is incorporated into the formal evaluation of the CNS, how is it to be used? What weight will peer review carry in the evaluation process? How can the process be made most reliable? The experience of groups who have wrestled with these issues will be discussed in the following paragraphs.

In describing peer review by and for the CNS, both Leibold (1983) and Blanton, et al. (1985) indicated that the decision to share peer review data with the supervisor was left to each CNS. Blanton and her colleagues stated that "the reason we chose to separate the peer reviews from the supervisor's evaluation was to keep the peer review honest and open without making each CNS feel her job was in jeopardy" (p. 1284). However, they noted that, to date, each specialist has chosen to have her supervisor present in a peer conference in which each reviewer's written evaluation was shared.

Because a developmental relationship exists between peer support and peer review, it is helpful to view further strategies for the development of peer review within the context of the four learning modes described by Kirschenbaum and Glaser (1978) and introduced earlier in the discussion of professional support groups. Approaches that fall within the teaching-learning mode of group functioning, e.g., sharing experiences and resources, presentations, lectures, and discussions, can also provide a beginning for the development of peer review. Members of one CNS group, whose long-term goal is to implement peer review for all dimensions of practice, currently give presentations to the group. Some members have presented patient care studies in which individual and/or groups of similar patients are presented and reviewed by the group with attention to application of the nursing process, use of nursing diagnoses, and adherence to standards of care. Other CNSs have shared paper or poster presentations for critique and feedback before delivery at a workshop or conference. To date, presentations have been done on a voluntary basis. All CNSs have found this method to be supportive and to be an initial step toward peer review.

Oncology Nurse Associates, a professional corporation formed by a group of practicing oncology CNSs in New York State, described a similar form of peer review. In accomplishing one of their goals, that of generating quality, comprehensive lectures on any aspect of oncology nursing, this group refined its material by a peer review process. Members of the group reviewed a planned presentation before it was given to ensure that the speaker was clear about objectives and that the material presented accomplished those goals ("Oncology clinical nurse specialists," 1986). Presentation review is also a part of the peer review process described by Blanton and her colleagues (1985).

While both the second and third learning modes, problem-solving and practice, allow for provision of support, they also have the potential to provide a basis for peer review. For example, CNSs often consult CNS peers in the same or differing areas regarding patient care issues. Reviewing clinical practice by accompanying the CNS in the care of patients and reviewing patient charts and/or case presentation allows for problem-solving while providing for individual accountability, improvement of practice, and assurance that standards of care are met. Review of practice should focus on implementation of the CNS role in the specialty; if the reviewer has the same specialty area, specialty content can also be addressed.

An additional example of the problem-solving mode operating in a way that may lead to development of peer review is illustrated by members of the author's CNS group who developed and use a structural instrument based on their job description, which they call Quantum (Crigler, et al., 1985). The instrument was originally developed proactively in response to a perceived need to document how CNSs spent their time and to describe their practice. These CNSs code their time daily during a two-week period of each quarter with respect to the four categories of their job description—clinical practice, consultation, education, and scholarly activities. Currently, Quantum continues as a group project; development and use of Quantum has provided information on how CNSs implement the role and changes in emphasis over time. By helping to describe CNS practice and defining practice emphases, the Quantum instrument is viewed as an initial step toward development of the criteria for peer review. Because of the variability in role expression, such structural instruments provide a means of identifying practice emphases. CNSs can build on this structure, developing peer review in a way that evaluates the process of how the time is spent. Groups who are interested in peer review should consider starting with a structural instrument such as Quantum. Working together on a project that examines structure is an activity that is group-building and less threatening than beginning with process evaluation. Projects have the potential to unite groups, allowing for the development of trust which is vitally important to successful peer review. Sharing of projects such as Quantum also provides networking opportunities for CNS groups.

The fourth learning mode, the action-project mode, positively influences the development of peer review in a way that can best be illustrated by an example. Psychiatric–mental health CNSs practicing independently in the state of Maryland have developed a peer review process that has enabled them to obtain third-party reimbursement for their services (S. Jimerson, personal communication, September 4, 1986, October 16, 1986). The development of this process was a survival response to the need for recognition and reimbursement by third-party payers. These practitioners developed criteria for peer review based on the ANA standards of care for psychiatric and mental health nursing practice. While their peer review mechanism has yet to be tested, these CNSs, who are primarily independent practitioners, have provided a measure of protection for themselves and their specialty practice and are now recognized as reimbursable providers by third-party payers in the state.

With goals for peer review established and prioritized and decisions made regarding the use of data gathered in the peer review process, criteria for use in peer review must be developed. Use of criteria in the peer review process which are succinct, definitive, and articulate expectations for performance clearly is recommended by experiences described in the literature. Review of the literature also suggests the use of three different kinds of criteria: criteria specific to a particular clinical area or patient population; criteria based on the nursing process and proficiency with its use; and criteria based on the CNS's job description or enactment of CNS subroles. Examples of each type follow.

Gold and his colleagues (1973) suggested that "peer review . . . be primarily specific to a clinical area or discipline, with the nurse specialists in that area having the option to involve nurses from other clinical areas as appropriate" (p. 636). Leibold and her colleagues (1983) acknowledged the importance and validity of this idea but did not believe it was practical in their agency. They chose to include in their peer review a faculty member with master's preparation in the review-ee's specialty, who could validate any clinically related questions that CNS peer reviewers with differing specialty practice might have. It is a strategy that may be helpful to other CNSs in developing peer review but that presents challenges in implementation for the individual CNS or group of CNSs who do not have readily available nursing faculty or a pool of nurses with master's preparation in a specialty area of practice.

The nursing process served as the basis of the narrative tool initially used in the CNS peer review process described by Leibold and her colleagues (1983). The results of the narrative tool were later analyzed, and specific behaviors were identified which defined the essential aspects of CNS practice within their institution. Analysis resulted in identification of seven categories of CNS practice: assessing, problem-solving, communicating, providing care, supporting, teaching, and evaluating. These seven categories formed the basis of an objective tool. Specific actions were then identified within each category to be used as parameters for evaluating the CNSs' clinical practice.

Blanton and her colleagues (1985) recommended against the use of specific criteria in peer review because of differences in the way each CNS interprets and fulfills the expectations of the role. This group used a combination of all three criteria in their peer review process. They began with their job description as the basis for peer review with documentation of CNS performance in the roles of practitioner, re-searcher, consultant, and change agent. Evaluation of performance in each of the subroles was accomplished through direct observation of the CNS by a CNS peer. A second evaluation form based on components of the nursing process followed soon after in the development of peer review by this CNS group. Integration of knowledge and communication skills were also included to evaluate application of the nursing process. Evaluation of lectures, demonstrations, and group discussions led by the CNS were evaluated by a third form designed to look at style of delivery, content, use of group dynamics, and communication skills. This group did not view the lack of uniformity in criteria as hampering evaluation.

Differences in expression of the role seem to be characteristic of the CNS. Role expression is influenced by the emphasis placed on the various role components in response to system needs and the CNS's personal and professional developmental needs. Although experience with peer review specific to the CNS is limited, it would appear that criteria for review should be derived from the nursing process and components of the CNS role as defined in the literature and by the peer group. The goals for peer review and the prioritization of those goals will provide structure for the development and use of the criteria for review. Peer review with a goal of specialty practice review will require the use of criteria directly related to that specialty practice. When the goal of peer review is review of an individual's performance in the CNS role, the use of less specific criteria will be required. The characteristics of the peers conducting the review, i.e., all CNSs with the same specialty area or CNSs with a variety of specialty areas, will also affect the utilization of criteria in the peer review process. Regardless of which of the three types of criteria or combination of criteria are chosen for peer review, the challenge of writing behavioral criteria that are objective and measurable remains.

## Variables Influencing Peer Review Effectiveness

As CNSs struggle with how to actualize the concept of peer review and learn from the experience of other CNSs, there are several issues related to implementation of these strategies which warrant discussion. The most critical problem in actualizing the concept of peer review is the failure of peer support development to a stage advanced enough to sustain peer review. When an attempt is made to "graft" a peer review process on a less-than-cohesive group, the graft is not likely to be successful. This is an important issue that cannot be overemphasized.

While well-developed and firmly established peer support is the variable that dictates the success of peer review, there are other factors that also significantly influence actualization of a peer review process. The first of these is the time commitment involved in conducting peer review. Blanton and her colleagues (1985), a CNS group with six members, used their system to evaluate each CNS yearly. The five peers were all involved in the review process; each CNS had a different role in the review process for each peer, with tasks varying from year to year. The time spent by each CNS in peer review averaged 40 to 48 hours a year, approximately 2 per cent of each CNS's time. This figure includes time spent writing reports and in the feedback session. While Leibold (1983) did not give a specific amount or percentage, she did note that the only negative comment made by reviewers in reacting to use of their narrative tool for peer review was that writing the summary was "time-consuming" (p. 226). The large time commitment involved in the evaluation of CNS practice is a potential threat to peer review given the current scrutiny of productivity and obsession with cost-effectiveness in today's institutions.

CNSs should involve themselves with peers within their own institution or agency, if they are fortunate enough to have peers in their practice setting, as well as peers in other institutions and agencies in the community, state, region, and nation. The issue of time is particularly significant to the CNS engaged in peer review with peers outside of the employing institution or beyond the local community. Review among those peers may involve additional time and money as a result of geographical separation.

If peer review is to survive and grow, it must be developed in a way that is neither cumbersome nor time-consuming, and must demonstrate the value of the time spent. Creativity is a requirement in overcoming these hurdles. CNS groups committed to actualizing peer review might contract for time to develop a peer review process. Through utilization of peer review as a process measure—evaluating criteria specific to a particular patient population or clinical area, criteria based on the nursing process and its use, and/or criteria based on the CNS's job description or enactment of subroles—CNSs may be able to concomitantly demonstrate change in patient outcome. Such changes may be reflected in length of patient stay, occurrence of complications, or frequency of readmission to health care settings.

Another possible approach would be to pursue resources for funding of a project to develop, implement, and evaluate the effectiveness of peer review in a specific setting. Emphasizing the potentially measurable benefits to the consumer of nursing care subjected to such a review would conceivably facilitate funding. The use of peer review by psychiatric–mental health CNSs in Maryland in securing third-party reimbursement for their service might lend itself to further development if subjected to such study. Further study of peer review will move CNSs, and nursing as a profession, closer to actualization of the concept.

The time frame for implementation is another factor influencing development of peer review strategies. Leibold (1983) believed that a CNS new in the role should not be involved in peer review until after six months to a year. Blanton and her colleagues (1985) did not recommend involvement of a new CNS in the peer review process until after a year in the role. These recommendations are supported by current knowledge of the role development of the new CNS.

In discussing strategies for development of peer review, it is clear that peer review has the potential to influence role implementation and development. Individual strengths and weaknesses in implementing the CNS role can be identified. Peer review has the capability to increase awareness of the influence of the CNS on a number of levels, beginning with the individual CNS and extending to society at large. Self-evaluation may assume a different status in the evaluation process. Customarily, self-evaluation has been an important component of the evaluation process, whether formal or informal. While Blanton and her colleagues (1985) used self-evaluation as a formal part of the peer review process, Leibold (1983) discovered unexpectedly that each reviewee had done an unwritten self-evaluation following each observation by a reviewer. Leibold's observation suggests that self-evaluation is valued more by CNSs participating in peer review and is thus undertaken with added thought and care. The quality of care delivered to patients should improve as a result of direct peer input. Opportunities are provided for CNSs to develop expertise in giving and receiving constructive criticism and for positive change to be effected through open communication.

Blanton and her colleagues (1985) addressed these latter benefits, noting the helpful criticism and suggestions for improvement that are offered by reviewers and the increased cohesiveness of the group. "We realize that when we help one another improve the quality of care we give, the group as a whole benefits" (Blanton, et al., 1985, p. 1287). They commented specifically on the value of the process of peer review and the recognition of this value by nurses "the **process** of peer review, and performing it with honesty and true concern for each other, are more important than the forms that are used or the words used to describe the forms" (p. 1287). Although the peer review model described by Leibold (1983) is not currently in use as described, the experience of developing a peer review mechanism is significant, regardless of the success or failure of the mechanism itself. Participation in the process of peer review provides an opportunity for CNSs to work and grow together through evaluation and documentation of their contributions to patient care, to nurses, and to nursing. While peer review may not always accomplish its stated goals, the process of peer review is perhaps more important today, given nursing's developmental stage and our current struggle to actualize the peer review concept. By engaging in peer review, CNSs contribute to the development of nursing knowledge, refine use of the nursing process for ourselves and our colleagues, and help to define and refine nursing diagnoses and interventions.

## SUMMARY

Support of the CNS by other CNSs is an important issue that cannot be overlooked or overemphasized. Peer support not only acknowledges a basic human need but, for the CNS, also significantly influences role implementation and development. The success of effective peer review is founded on peer support. As a specialist or expert nurse, the CNS has a responsibility to be actively involved in peer review. In an era of cost containment and at a time when the CNS role continues to evolve, participation in peer review provides an opportunity for CNSs to justify the merits of the CNS role to the health care delivery system and to the consumer thus fostering the survival and growth of the role. The CNS can thus be instrumental in establishing an ongoing process for education and the improvement of nursing care.

Peer review is presently a concept that few would argue with but that few have actualized. CNSs need to continue to work together to meet the challenges of developing and implementing effective peer support and peer review.

### Acknowledgment

Special thanks to the Clinical Nurse Specialist Group at the University of Virginia Hospitals.

### References

American Nurses' Association: Code for Nurses with Interpretive Statements. Kansas City, ANA, 1976.

American Nurses' Association: Guidlines for Review of Nursing Care at the Local Level. Kansas City, ANA, 1976.

American Nurses' Association: Nursing: A Social Policy Statement. Kansas City, ANA, 1980.

American Nurses' Association: Nursing Quality Assurance Management/Learning System. Kansas City, ANA, 1982.

American Nurses' Association: Peer Review in Nursing Practice. Kansas City, ANA, 1983.

American Nurses' Association: Perspectives on the Code for Nurses. Kansas City, ANA, 1978.

American Nurses' Association: Quality Assurance Workbook. Kansas City, ANA, 1976.

Anderson, P.A., & Davis, S.E.: Nursing peer review: A developmental process. Nurs Management 10(1):46–48, 1987.

Bennett, H.M.: Effective credentialing and peer review of nursing personnel. Crit Care Nurs 5(1):104, 1985.

Blanton, N.E., Bogner, J., Collins, H., et al.: Putting peer review into practice. Am Nurs 85(11):1284, 1287, 1985.

Braiker, H.B.: The Type E* Woman: How to overcome the stress of being *Everything to Everybody. New York, Dodd, Mead & Co., 1986.

Brown, S.J.: Administrative support. In Hamric, A.B., and Spross, J. (eds): The Clinical Nurse Specialist in Theory and Practice. New York, Grune and Stratton, 1983, pp. 149–170.

Campbell-Heider, N.: Do nurses need mentors? Image 18(3):110–113, 1986.

Crigler, L., Hurt, L., Burge, S., et al.: Quantifying the clinical nurse specialist role: A pilot study. Virginia Nurse 52(3):37–39, 41–42, 1985.

Critchley, D.L.: Clinical supervision. In Critchley, D.L., and Maurin, J.T. (eds): The Clinical Specialist in Psychiatric Mental Health Nursing: Theory, Research and Practice. New York, John Wiley & Sons, 1985, pp. 495–510.

Fenton, M.V.: Identifying competencies of clinical nurse specialists. J Nurs Admin 15(12):31–37, 1985.

Gold, H., Jackson, M., Sachs, B., and Van Meter, M.J.: Peer review—a working experiment. Nurs Outlook 21:634–636, 1973.

Hagerty, B.: A second look at mentors. Nurs Outlook 34:16–19, 24, 1986.

Hauser, M.A.: Initiation into peer review. Am J Nurs 75:2204–2207, 1975.

Holt, F.M.: Clinical nurse specialist—supernurse?? Symposium on the clinical nurse specialist. Sigma Theta Tau Monograph Series 75:83–89, 1975.

Johnson, R.M., Richardson, J.I., Von Endt, L.L., and Lindgren, K.S.: The professional support group: A model for psychiatric clinical nurse specialists. J Psychos Nurs Ment Health Serv 20(2):9–13, 1982.

Kirschenbaum, H., & Glaser, B.: Developing Support Groups. La Jolla, University Associates, 1978.

Lamberton, M., Keen, M., and Admoanis, A.: Peer review in a family nurse clinician program. Nurs Outlook 25:47–53, 1977.

Leibold, S.: Peer review. In Hamric, A.B., and Spross, J. (eds): The Clinical Nurse Specialist in Theory and Practice. New York, Grune and Stratton, 1983, pp. 219–233.

Luft, J.: Group Processes: An Introduction to Group Dynamics (ed 3). Palo Alto, Mayfield Publishing Co., 1984.

McClure, M.L.: The long road to accountability. Nurs Outlook 26(1):47–50, 1978.

Malone, B.: Working with people: Evaluation of the clinical nurse specialist. Am J Nurs 86(12):1375–1377, 1986.

Metzger, N.: Support: Do you give it? Do you get it? Nursing '85 15(5):98–101, 1985.

Mullins, A., Colavecchio, R., and Tescher, B.: Peer review: A model for professional accountability. J Nurs Admin 9:25–30, 1979.

Oncology clinical nurse specialists form independent corporation. Oncol Nurs Bull July 1986, p. 11.

Page, S., and Loeper, J.: Peer review of the nurse educator: The process and development of a format. J Nurs Educ 17:21–29, 1978.

Passos, J.Y.: Accountability: Myth or mandate? J Nurs Admin 3:21–29, 1973.

Ramphal, M.: Peer review. Am J Nurs 74(1):63–67, 1974.

Shaw, M.E.: Group Dynamics. New York, McGraw-Hill, 1976.

Spicer, J., and Lewis, E.: Intensive care staff nurses develop peer review criteria. Nurs Admin Q 1:57–61, 1977.

Webster's New World Dictionary of the American Language, second college edition. Guralnik, D.B. (ed). New York, The World Publishing Co., 1970.

Zimmer, M.: Evaluation using patient health/wellness outcome criterion variables and standards. In American Nurses' Association (ed): Issues in Evaluation Research. Kansas City, ANA, 1976, pp. 57–73.

# PART IV

## ISSUES
## AND
## TRENDS

# Educational Preparation of the CNS

*Mariah Snyder*

## INTRODUCTION

The educational preparation of students currently in clinical specialist programs and of those soon to enter these programs is critical to the further development of the CNS role in this rapidly changing health care system. Reviewing the evolution of graduate education will provide guidance in planning for the future. After discussion of the diverse clinical specialist programs in existence, several models that could be used in the educational preparation of the CNS will be presented. It is incumbent on the nursing community to devise and implement plans now to ensure that the graduates of clinical specialists' programs will have an impact on health care in the 21st century.

## GRADUATE EDUCATION IN NURSING

"We've come a long way, baby," a phrase often used in the women's movement, can aptly be applied to graduate education in nursing, particularly when one considers that in 1952 only 1,449 nurses had graduate degrees (Kelly, 1985). The following factors contributed to this low number of nurses with graduate degrees: (1) professional careers for women were not commonplace; (2) few baccalaureate programs in nursing were in existence; (3) funding for graduate education was lacking; and (4) the body of nursing knowledge was only beginning to be defined. The number of nurses holding a master's degree increased to 11,500 in 1962 and to 25,000 in 1972. Over 95,000 nurses currently have a master's or doctoral degree (ANA, 1987).

Through the years, numerous studies have examined nursing and nursing education in the United States. A major conclusion of many of these studies was that nursing education should be provided in colleges and universities, thus removing the control of nursing from hospital boards. A recommendation of the Goldmark Report (Goldmark, 1923) supported the establishment within universities of postgraduate programs in administration, education, public health nursing, and private duty nursing. While this latter category may seem inappropriate in today's health care settings, at that time private duty nurses were the chief caregivers for acutely ill patients. The Brown Report (Brown, 1948) reiterated many of the statements of the Goldmark Report including the need for nurses to be educated in institutions of higher learning. Lysaught (1974) noted that future studies were indicated to determine how the nurse clinician could be used more effectively in improving health care. It has taken nursing and the health care community considerable time to implement these recommendations. This may be partially due to hospitals' reluctance to give up control of nursing education. Also, because nursing was a new academic discipline, universities were hesitant to provide wholehearted support to graduate nursing programs.

One factor that has had an immense impact on increasing the number of nurses with graduate degrees has been the Nurse Training Act (NTA), which was part of the Health Services Act. The NTA was initiated in 1964; since then it has been renewed by Congress at periodic intervals—often because of intense lobbying efforts by nurses. In addition to providing tuition and stipends for individual nurses, the NTA has supported construction of nursing education buildings and the development of specialty and practitioner programs. Federal funding for nursing education has been significantly reduced in recent years. This has resulted in a shift to part-time students and the development of fewer new specialty programs to meet emerging needs.

## Master's Education

Today there are 129 accredited master's programs, with the majority offering opportunities for clinical specialization (NLN, 1984). Recognition by nursing service administrators of the impact that clinical specialists have on the improvement of patient care, the availability of federal funds for the development of clinical specialty programs, and federal traineeships to support nurses pursuing graduate education accelerated the inauguration of graduate programs with clinical specialization focus areas.

The number of specialty areas has expanded drastically from the original psychiatric-mental health, medical-surgical, and pediatric programs. Williamson (1983) examined offerings of graduate programs and found more than 130 specialty titles. This large number may be the result of schools applying unique titles to traditional specialty areas (i.e., child health maintenance as opposed to pediatrics). Many subspecialty areas have evolved such as burns/emergency/trauma, oncology, gerontology, women's health, perinatal, critical care, and neuroscience.

## Doctoral Education

There has been a rapid increase in the number of nurses holding doctorates; currently nearly 4,000 nurses have doctoral degrees with the majority of these degrees obtained in disciplines other than nursing (ANA, 1987). Nurses have thus brought the knowledge and methodologies of the other disciplines in which they were educated to the discipline of nursing. While this phenomenon has contributed to the richness of the discipline of nursing, it has also created problems. Some nurses who have received their education in disciplines outside of nursing have found it difficult to focus on nursing and nursing problems, and they continue to view nursing as secondary to the discipline in which they were educated. Differences in language and methodology have created communication problems.

Two doctoral programs in nursing existed in the United States in 1946 (Kelly, 1985). Since then 32 programs have been initiated, and a significant number are in the planning stages. Currently, programs are found in 23 states and in the District of Columbia; thus, many nurses find these programs quite accessible. Doctoral programs prepare nurses to be theoreticians, scholars, administrators, health policy teachers, planners, and clinicians. Nurses with doctoral preparation are, foremost, scholars and researchers. The knowledge that emanates from the research is aimed at improving nursing care of patients.

Three types of doctoral degrees are offered in nursing: Doctorate in Philosophy (Ph.D.), Doctor of Nursing Science (D.N.S.), and Doctorate in Education (Ed.D.). Recently, nurse educators have begun to debate the differences between the expected outcome for graduates of Ph.D. and D.N.S. programs. Students in Ph.D. programs are prepared to be nurse researchers. The curriculum focuses on assisting the student to obtain the knowledge and skills needed to carry out research in a specified area of nursing. The curriculum of D.N.S. programs, on the other hand, aims to prepare graduates for the scholarly practice of nursing as a clinical specialist or nurse therapist (Kelly, 1985).

Doctoral education in nursing is still in a developmental stage. Decisions about the number and focus of programs and distinctions between graduates with particular types of degrees need to be made. An overriding concern must be to maintain quality programs.

Although the number of nurses with advanced degrees has increased markedly in the past two decades, this number falls far short of the need projected by 1990. A study by the Institute of Medicine (IOM, 1983) stated that 256,000 nurses with master's degrees and 14,000 with doctoral degrees would be needed by 1990.

## New Educational Programs

Several institutions have initiated a professional doctorate in nursing (N.D.) as the basic preparation for entry into nursing practice, similar to medicine, law, and other professions. Students entering the program possess, at the minimum, a bachelor of science or arts degree in another discipline. Thus, the curriculum of the N.D. program is devoted solely to nursing, and the program is usually three years in length. The N.D. degree is not a graduate degree; graduates of the programs are prepared to be beginning practitioners.

Generic preparation also exists at the master's level. Several schools, such as Yale University, admit students who have a non-nursing baccalaureate degree and are not nurses. The length of the program is extended from the usual two years to three years. After their first year, students in the Yale program select one of the specialty areas offered (Diers, 1976).

The generic preparation in the N.D. and master's programs permits students to pursue nursing without obtaining a second baccalaureate degree. Because of the increasing complexity of the health care system and the heightened acuity in hospitals, nursing educators are questioning whether it is possible to provide both a liberal education and nursing education in four years. Changes in the basic preparation of nurses, such as with the N.D. or generic master's programs, will have an impact on the education for clinical specialization.

# EDUCATIONAL PREPARATION OF CLINICAL SPECIALISTS

Society and the health care system are characterized by constant change. Education of clinical specialists must anticipate change so that graduates are prepared not only to function effectively but also to be able to provide leadership in the delivery of health care.

## Competencies

One problem that has plagued clinical specialization since its inception has been the lack of commonalities in graduate programs regarding the content of programs and the expected outcomes. Table 15–1 lists the outcomes of graduate nursing education promulgated by the National League for Nursing. These outcomes provide overall direction for nursing curricula. However, to date, a basic core to be included in programs has not been developed.

McLane (1978), in a study of deans of schools of nursing with graduate programs, directors of nursing services, and graduate students, determined seven core areas to be included in master's nursing programs: interpersonal relations, research, accountability for nursing practice, change agent, educator, philosophy of nursing, and means that support graduates to be "humanizers." These competencies are not specific to the preparation of CNSs, but they are clearly ones that are needed for this role. The competencies suggest core coursework in nursing theory, research, change theory, teaching-learning, and leadership.

Recent attempts have been made to differentiate expectations for nurses with basic entry preparation and those with advanced education. Benner's differentiation between novice and expert provides direction for considering skills/competencies that should exist for the expert practitioner (1982). Benner stated, "the expert nurse's performance is holistic rather than fractionated, procedural, and based upon incremental steps" (p. 406). She contended that both experience and formal education are necessary for developing the competencies of an expert.

Fenton's ethnographic study (1985) of clinical specialists sought to specify more precisely Benner's domains of nursing practice as they

**TABLE 15–1. Characteristics of Graduates from Master's Programs in Nursing**

A master's degree in nursing provides students with an opportunity to:
- Acquire advanced knowledge from sciences and humanities to support advanced nursing practice.
- Expand knowledge of nursing theory as a basis for advanced nursing practice.
- Develop expertise in a specialized area of clinical nursing practice.
- Acquire the knowledge and skills related to a specific functional role in nursing.
- Acquire initial competence in conducting nursing research.
- Plan and initiate change in the health care system and in the practice and delivery of health care.
- Further develop and implement leadership strategies for the betterment of health care.
- Actively engage in collaborative relationships with others for the purpose of improving health care.
- Acquire a foundation for doctoral study.

(Reprinted with permission from National League for Nursing, Division of Baccalaureate and Higher Degree Programs: Characteristics of Graduate Education in Nursing Leading to the Master's Degree (Publ. No. 15–1759). New York, NLN. Copyright 1979 by NLN.)

apply to the CNS. In addition to Benner's domains of helping role, administering and monitoring therapeutic interventions, managing rapidly changing situations, diagnosing and monitoring function, teaching/coaching function, monitoring/ensuring quality of health care practices, and organizational and work-role competencies, clinical specialists in Fenton's study added the domain of consultation. The CNSs in her study were experts in delivering nursing care to patients, analyzing the system, implementing change, consulting with nurses and other health care workers, and motivating and providing support to nurses on the unit.

Because of advancements in technology, particularly in tertiary care settings, and the extension of technology to home care settings, a need exists for clinical specialists to have competencies related to caring for patients who depend on high technology for survival. According to McCormick (1983), course content in computer science, biochemistry, physics, immunology, and genetics—in addition to the traditional science courses—will be necessary for nurses to function effectively. Use of high technology in the delivery of health care requires renewed emphasis on the use of humanizing elements such as touch by health professionals, particularly nurses (Powell, 1984). High technology creates associated ethical issues. Expertise in dealing with ethical issues and assisting others in making decisions is assuming greater importance in the CNS role.

Since the inception of the CNS, controversy has existed over whether the CNS should be in a line or staff position. The increasing economic crunch faced by many hospitals has caused more agencies to hire the CNS for a line position. While the clinical specialist role was envisioned to be one of leadership, it was in terms of patient care and not in the direct managing of a unit. Administrative functions detract from involvement in patient care and in working with the staff for quality care. However, having administrative electives available in an academic program will provide CNS students with the opportunity to learn how to function in a possible line position.

Many CNSs provide care to specific patient populations. Some nursing specialty organizations have defined competencies and knowledge for specialists in their particular area. In 1985, the Oncology Nurses Society documented specific knowledge and skills required by clinical specialists in oncology. These detailed recommendations should be considered by faculties that have oncology specialty programs. Educators need to give attention to the recommendations formulated by specialty organizations to help ensure that graduates will have the necessary skills and knowledge for providing care in specialty areas.

## Programs of Study

Vast differences exist in the course of studies found in the 129 National League for Nursing (NLN) accredited graduate nursing programs. Differences exist in length of program, types of courses offered, and type of degree offered. Comparison of length of programs is difficult because some programs are on the quarter system while others use the semester system. Programs vary from 9 to 28 months of study (Sills, 1983). Approximately one-third of the master's programs take two full academic years to complete (Feild, 1983).

The content included in a course of study for a clinical specialist should be related to the competencies addressed in Chapter 1 and in Part II of this book. While the content of a program for clinical specialization can be defined at a specific point in time, the program must be dynamic to meet the changing needs of society (Reed & Hoffman, 1986). Content on nursing theories, research, moral and ethical positions, change theory, health delivery systems, nursing issues, and the clinical area of specialization is essential in all CNS curricula.

A framework for practice assists CNSs to function in an effective manner. Knowledge of nursing theorists provides CNSs with a background from which to choose a nursing theory that can serve as the basis for practice or suggests a background from which a framework can be constructed. Meleis (1985) noted that few nursing theories have been utilized and tested in the practice realm. If nursing theories are to serve as the basis for practice, CNSs must play an integral role in introducing these theories to the practice area and translating their sometimes esoteric terms into concrete premises that can be tested. According to Murphy and Hoeffer (1983), practice-generated theory guides practice once the theory is validated; likewise, theoretically based practice serves as the basis for further theory refinement.

Research courses are also an essential component of CNS education. Table 15-2 provides the ANA's expectations for the research capabilities of master's-prepared nurses. With the increase in doctorally prepared nurses, there is less expectation for the master's-prepared nurse to be an independent researcher. However, the CNS's role in evaluating projects and in critiquing research findings for use in the clinical area does not lessen the emphasis on research content necessary in the curriculum. The CNS must recognize the limits of research knowledge possessed and seek consultation whenever necessary.

A number of programs have recently added courses on moral and ethical decision-making. Our health care system has produced many situations in which ethical issues are prominent, i.e., keeping a person

**TABLE 15–2. Research Capabilities of Graduates from Master's Programs in Nursing**

- Analyzes and reformulates nursing practice problems so that scientific knowledge and scientific methods can be used to find solutions.
- Enhances the quality and clinical relevance of nursing research by providing expertise in clinical problems and by providing knowledge about the way in which these clinical services are delivered.
- Facilitates investigations of problems in clinical settings through such activities as contributing to a climate supportive of investigative activities, collaborating with others in investigations, and enhancing nursing's access to clients and data.
- Conducts investigations for the purpose of monitoring the quality of the practice of nursing in a clinical setting.
- Assists others to apply scientific knowledge in nursing practice.

(From American Nurses' Association Commission on Nursing Research: Guidelines for the Investigative Function of Nurses. Kansas City, American Nurses Association, 1981. Reprinted with permission of the ANA.)

alive on a respirator, caring for persons with AIDS, and using scarce resources. Having a framework for making ethical decisions, such as the one proposed by Crisham (1985), assists CNSs as they work closely with staff, families, and patients in determining the course of action to be taken. Many hospitals and health care agencies are establishing ethics committees. Clinical specialists with knowledge about ethics can provide valuable leadership to these institutional committees.

Content related to the area of specialization, including courses taken in other disciplines, is a critical component of CNS programs. However, specific nursing courses in which this content is translated into the context of nursing are needed. For example, the student in a neurophysiology course (that is part of a neuroscience clinical specialty program) acquires knowledge about the causes of increased intracranial pressure. Application of this knowledge to the nursing care of severely head-injured patients is made in nursing courses in which nursing activities that can decrease intracranial pressure are explored. It cannot be assumed that students are able to make the applications without specific assistance from the faculty.

CNS education necessitates content on overall role theory, usual role expectations for the CNS, functional dimensions of the CNS role, role ambiguities and conflicts, and strategies for successfully implementing the role (NLN, 1978). Ideally, this content would precede or be concurrent with clinical experiences for role development. Such placement would enable the student to test the content in clinical situations while guidance is available.

Changes in the health care delivery system resulting from the institution of diagnostic related groupings (DRGs) have, in some regions, made it more difficult for clinical specialists to obtain positions. Agencies are also reluctant to hire persons with advanced degrees when they can staff the agency less expensively with nurses having lesser preparation. Inclusion of content on marketing strategies will prepare graduates to "sell" their expertise to hospitals, home care agencies, and/ or business organizations. Nurses, including CNSs, have traditionally not had to market themselves because jobs have been plentiful. However, nurses now need to seek new and innovative ways in which to practice and market their expertise (Coleman, Dayani, and Simms, 1984).

A number of authors have identified areas in CNS programs which they believe require strengthening. Lewis (1980) suggested seven areas: leadership and management skills, group process skills, organization theory, ability to negotiate, ability to debate, ability to develop support systems for self, and faith in one's own abilities. In addition to these areas, Edlund and Hodges (1983) added course content on how to effect change; Sills (1983) suggested teaching-learning theory and methods for teaching. Implementing change to improve patient care, particularly through utilizing research findings, is a key component of the CNS role.

The list of competencies elaborated as necessary for the CNS is mammoth. Programs of at least two years in length are necessary for acquiring the knowledge and skills needed to master these competencies. Programs of shorter length result in graduates not being adequately prepared for the role and in frustration experienced by both the CNS and the employer.

## Clinical Experience

One criterion for admission into a number of graduate specialty programs is that the applicant must have one, two, or three years of clinical practice in the specialty area. McKevitt (1986) found that significantly more programs in 1984 than in 1979, 25.5 per cent as compared with 16 per cent, required clinical experience for admission to specialty programs. Faculty in these programs believe that additional skills beyond the basic preparation are required so that the student will have direction in pursuing advanced knowledge.

Clinical practice is a very important element in the educational preparation of the CNS. The experience is best placed after didactic courses to enable the student to transfer and apply the advanced knowledge acquired in classes. The abilities to work with a selected patient population and to have role modeling by a clinical specialist are key elements in clinical experiences. The amount of time spent in clinical areas varies from program to program. It is imperative, however, that programs provide at least three quarters or two semesters of clinical experience. Students need this amount of time to be able to gain an understanding of the new role they will assume.

Innovations in nursing education (generic preparation in a N.D. or master's program) may alter the requirement of prior clinical experience. Those who pursue nursing in one of these ways are different from the typical graduate of a baccalaureate program. Often these students bring maturity in addition to the knowledge and skills from other disciplines, giving them a broader perspective of health care and nursing. The initiation of residency programs, similar to medical residency programs, for doctorally or master's-prepared nurses who have educational preparation but who lack clinical experience is one model for assisting these graduates to become specialists. Other innovative approaches need to be considered in order to facilitate specialization of the nontraditional graduate.

Specialization in nursing has largely taken place in academic settings, whereas medical specialization has utilized preceptors in the clinical area. This may be the result of the differences in the amount of basic preparation between the two disciplines. Adequate role modeling, ideally provided by faculty members, is an important aspect of the clinical experience of the CNS student. According to Lewis (1980), graduate faculty members need to spend time and energy and be in the clinical areas with students; clinical conferences with the student are not sufficient for accomplishing clinical goals. Faculty members are thus able to evaluate the performance of the student and serve as the gatekeeper to practice, permitting only those who are qualified to become clinical specialists (ANA, 1980).

The profession is experiencing a renewed focus on faculty practice. Cason and Beck (1982) hypothesized that the lack of homogeneity that faculty members in their study expressed regarding the CNS role was due to the increased attention being given to faculty practice. Further evidence of this increased interest is the annual conferences on faculty practice sponsored by the American Academy of Nursing. If this trend persists, more faculty will be involved in the clinical experiences of CNS students. The unification model presented in Chapter 16 is an example of one mechanism for role modeling and supervision by qualified faculty members.

In addition to supervision by faculty members, every attempt should be made to have clinical experiences in agencies that utilize CNSs. Immersion in the role and seeing the CNS perform various role functions provide critical learning experiences.

### Certification

An outcome of a CNS course of study should be that the graduate is eligible for certification in the specialty area. Certification is defined by Fickeissen (1985) as "a process that validates nurses' knowledge and expertise in a defined functional or clinical area of nursing" (p. 265). Sixteen nursing groups offer certification in 35 areas of nursing. The requirements for certification vary for each area; many do not have advanced formal education as a requirement but merely require that the nurse have "x" years of clinical experience in the specialty area and possess the knowledge needed to pass the certification examination. The number of nurses becoming certified has increased significantly in recent years. Over 82,000 nurses have been certified by the American Nurses' Association and specialty organizations (ANA, 1987).

The American Nurses' Association believes that practicing specialists need to meet two criteria: advanced formal preparation at the master's or doctoral level and certification in the particular specialty area (ANA, 1980). Educational programs need to provide students with information about the purposes for certification and the means for obtaining it. Certification of nurses by the profession guarantees the public that these nurses possess advanced knowledge and skills. Certification also allows for the comparison of nurses from various CNS programs (Feild, 1983).

## Areas of Specialization

Traditionally, areas of clinical specialization have been congruent with medical specialty areas. Hospitals are organized in this manner, and medical specialty divisions is a logical way for using clinical specialists within the hospital. In addition, nursing had given little attention to the organization of its knowledge base when the first specialty programs were established. While in some instances the medical categories are usable and proper for nursing specialization, the time has come to evaluate current areas of specialization and determine if they are adequate for delivering quality nursing care.

Nursing diagnoses provide one possible means for categorizing specialty education. Nursing diagnoses are, however, in a developmental stage. Use of nursing diagnoses helps to place the emphasis on nursing and the role nursing plays in working with health problems. Nursing diagnoses also help to decrease overlap of services between specialty areas. For example, stress is common in many patient populations. If the nursing diagnostic category of stress was an area of specialization, the specialist would be available throughout an institution and would be truly knowledgeable in this area. There would be specialists in pain, skin integrity, and so forth.

Nursing interventions are another possible way to reorganize nursing specialization. Nurses adept in specific strategies would be called in much the way medical specialists are today. Interventions such as teaching, stress management techniques, or nutrition are possible areas for organizing clinical specialization in the future. *Independent Nursing Interventions* by Snyder (1985) or *Nursing Interventions for Nursing Diagnosis* by Bulechek and McCloskey (1985) delineate numerous interventions in which nurses could specialize.

Functional status and using the categories proposed in *Nursing: A Social Policy Statement* (ANA, 1980) are other possible ways for organizing specialty areas. Nurses could specialize in mobility problems, communication problems, and the like. This framework is consistent with nursing's emphasis on optimum patient functioning. Carrieri, Lindsey, and West (1986) have specified physiological phenomena that could also serve as the basis for organizing specialties in nursing. These phenomena are closely aligned with functional status.

## PERSPECTIVES ON THE FUTURE

The functions currently being performed by CNSs are very diverse. It is anticipated that this diversity will continue. In addition, new specialty areas, such as space health, will be needed. Demands for CNSs to be consultants in home health agencies and in other community areas are increasing. Changes in mechanisms for reimbursement may see an increase in specialists establishing independent practices.

Feild (1983) provided recommendations regarding CNS education. A number of these addressed the need for more uniformity in programs so that employers would have a better idea of the competencies of the beginning CNS. Lack of commonality across programs continues to exist—in fact, it is probably increasing. The National League for Nursing criteria for accreditation of master's programs provide only general directions for curriculum content. The American Association of Colleges of Nursing in *Essentials of College and University Education for Professional Nursing* (1986) delineated specific knowledge and expertise expected of graduates of basic education programs. A similar document would be useful in specifying expectations for graduates of CNS programs.

Cutbacks in federal sponsorship of specialty education programs and the reduction in traineeships have had a profound effect on graduate nursing education. The majority of graduate students go to school on a part-time basis. Developing educational programs that provide quality learning experiences for part-time students will further the effectiveness of graduates. Lobbying efforts to increase funding for graduate nursing education need to be continued.

Changes in the health care system, such as an increase in acuity in tertiary care centers, an increase in the amount of nursing care required in homes, an increase in the elderly population, and evolving health care problems such as AIDS, may demand a different type of knowledge and skills than is presently being taught in graduate specialty programs. Interactions between nursing education and service will help in creating programs for CNSs who will be adept in these areas. (See Chapter 16 for an in-depth discussion of the collaborative relationship between nursing education and nursing service.) Long-range projections must become part of nursing education so that trends can be detected and programs developed.

As the discipline of nursing evolves, the nature of specialties will change. Specialties that more truly reflect the nature of nursing rather than mirror the medical model will become more common. This will facilitate the development of a knowledge base in nursing.

Nurses with basic preparation at the N.D. or generic master's levels may have very different educational needs than nurses prepared at the baccalaureate level. Knowledge about the graduates of these programs will assist educators in modifying courses of study for students who pursue specialization. Graduates of these programs may elect to bypass the master's program and pursue specialization at the doctoral level.

Several articles have addressed the possible merger of nurse practitioners and clinical specialists (Aherns & Norris, 1983; McCarty, 1986). Initially, practitioners functioned in clinics and community settings, while CNSs worked in hospitals. Because of changes in the health care system, nurses prepared in practitioner programs are now assuming CNS roles in hospitals and specialists are assuming positions in the community (Lynaugh, Gerrity, and Hagopian, 1985). Do enough similarities between the roles now exist for these two advanced practice programs?

Program evaluation in individual programs is routinely done; however, evaluation of CNS programs at the national level would be invaluable. Data would provide a basis for revision of programs and shaping of new initiatives.

Program evaluation and discussion of some of the preceeding issues may lead to different models for preparing the CNS; the author provides perspectives on three possible models. They are meant to serve as an impetus for discussion and planning and should not be considered as the best or only system. The three are not mutually exclusive but rather address the following issues that the author believes need to be paramount in discussions: paying attention to cost-effectiveness while still having an educationally sound preparation; decreasing confusion about graduate education in nursing; and providing the student with adequate preparation so that the CNS and the employer are not frustrated. The three models proposed for educational prepa-ration of the CNS are a combined CNS/practitioner model, a preceptor model, and a doctoral preparation model.

## Unification of CNS/Nurse Practitioner

The CNS and nurse practitioner roles were developed to serve very different populations. Practitioners were found in clinics, offices, and community settings, while CNSs were situated in hospitals. Grad-uates of some practitioner programs received degrees; others received certificates. With changes in the health care scene, the demand for practitioners to function in their established mode has lessened. This has resulted in more practitioners seeking positions in hospitals. As the acuity level of patients in home care settings and nursing homes has increased, CNSs are beginning to have roles outside of the hospital. Merging these two modes of preparation is proposed (see Chapter 18 for further discussion of this issue).

Combining CNS and practitioner programs would be cost-effective. The merger could also lead to stronger preparation at the master's level as resources could be combined. The combined programs would reduce confusion for the public concerning nurses with advanced preparation. McCarty (1986) suggested that the graduate of the com-bined program be titled "specialist in nursing." Such a title would not be site-specific and would allow graduates to function in the acute care setting as well as the community.

A curriculum for this program could consist of core courses in theory, research, and ethics. Options for specialization could include acute care and community, with subspecialties available in each area. Assessment courses, physiology courses, and other courses could like-wise be taken by students in both tracks.

Opposition to a merger of this nature would most likely occur because of the strong ties faculty have to one of the two programs. However, the need for clarity in what expertise and knowledge can be expected of nurses prepared at the master's level gives credence to consideration of this model.

## Preceptor Model

Cost-effectiveness is the name of the game in health care and in education. While it is difficult to uncover "real" costs of a specialty program, it must be acknowledged that a sizeable number of students are needed in a specialty area for the program to be cost-effective and to provide quality education. The author believes that a specialty area needs to admit at least 8 students a year for it to be cost-effective. Others believe that this number needs to be at least 15. Except in large metropolitan areas, it is difficult for a specialty area to secure this number of students each year.

An educational model for the CNS proposed by the author is to have the core courses and process elements of the curriculum taught by faculty members who have an academic appointment. Students would select clinical areas for specialization in which there are clinical specialists in the particular community. The school would hire a clinical specialist for a percentage of time (perhaps 25 per cent) to direct the study of the two or three students who have selected the specialist's area. Several students may wish to specialize in oncology, some in gerontology, and a third group in neuroscience nursing. The preceptors would be oriented to the curriculum and would work closely with the academic faculty. However, responsibility for selecting content in the specialty area for seminars and classes would rest with the preceptor. The preceptor CNS and the faculty member would be jointly responsible for the education of the students.

The preceptor model would allow schools to accept students for a number of specialty areas. Since geographical mobility is a problem for many nurses, graduating large numbers of students in one specialty within a region makes it very difficult for graduates to secure jobs. The proposed preceptor model would help to alleviate this problem. This model would also provide students with the opportunity to pursue the area of specialization in which they are interested.

Other advantages of such a model would be a closer working relationship between academia and service. Preceptors, depending upon the policies of particular institutions, would hold adjunct or clinical teaching appointments. The preceptor model would provide for specialization in newly developing specialties; in the current system, there is usually a lag between the identified need in the clinical area and the development of specialty programs to meet the need. Lastly, having a percentage of the CNS's salary paid by the educational institution would help support the CNS role in the clinical agency.

The author views this model as one that could be operationalized immediately. While the model would require considerable communication to guarantee success, the benefits seem to outweigh the time and effort that would need to be invested. The preceptor model could be used to advantage in merged CNS/practitioner programs.

## Doctoral Preparation for CNS Role

The previous two models looked at modifications of the present system of education for the CNS. Doctoral preparation would be a distinct shift in the traditional educational preparation. In 1971, Berge-son questioned whether it was possible to prepare a CNS at the master's level because of the vast amount of knowledge and skills required for this role. She stated, "expert knowledge implies a thorough understand-ing of the field of concentration. This level of understanding and clinical competence are hallmarks of a clinical specialist" (p. 24). The level of knowledge and skills necessary for the CNS to be an effective practitioner has continued to increase. A sound educational foundation for specialization requires in excess of two years. Nursing should, therefore, give serious consideration to doctoral preparation for the CNS role.

While the goal of Ph.D. programs is the preparation of nurse researchers/scholars, the Doctor of Nursing Science degree (D.N.S.) is aimed at producing scholars knowledgeable about clinical practice. However, current D.N.S. graduates are usually employed in faculty roles, rarely as clinical specialists. The three-year programs would provide students with in-depth knowledge concerning clinical problems and methods for solving these problems. Graduates would be more confident of their abilities and would thus function effectively in the clinical area. Preparation for specialization in nursing would be similar to the many other disciplines that require three years of preparation.

Graduates of D.N.S. programs would have more research prepa-ration. Thus, the CNS would be able to design and carry out research on identified clinical problems. Research on clinical problems is a high priority for nursing; nurses knowledgeable about both clinical problems and research methodology are needed to address these problems and improve patient care.

An argument against preparation of the CNS at the doctoral level is the added cost of an additional year of education. Opportunities to work as research or teaching assistants would provide students with an enriched learning experience in addition to financial remuneration. Although financial implications are important, more critical is the determination of what is needed to prepare competent specialists.

While preparation for the CNS at the doctoral level is most likely not in the immediate future for nursing, the model merits discussion. The author believes that the model is feasible and would contribute significantly to a more prominent role in the health care system for the nursing profession. Therefore, preparation at this level is recom-mended.

### References

Ahrens, W., and Norris, B.: Expanded roles in critical care: Nurse practitioner or clinical specialist? Dimen Crit Care Nurs 2(2):98–100, 1983.

Aiken, L.: Nursing's future: Public policies, private actions. Am J Nurs *83*:1440–1444, 1983.

American Association of Colleges of Nursing: Essentials of College and University Education for Professional Nursing. Washington, D.C., American Association of Colleges of Nursing, 1986.

American Nurses' Association: Facts about Nursing 86–87. Kansas City, ANA, 1987.

American Nurses' Association: Nursing: A Social Policy Statement. Kansas City, ANA, 1980.

American Nurses' Association Commission on Nursing Research: Guidelines for the Investigative Function of Nurses. Kansas City, ANA, 1981.

Benner, P.: From novice to expert. Am J Nurs *82*:402–407, 1982.

Bergesen, B.: Preparation for clinical specialization. J Nurs Educ *10*:21–26, 1971.

Brown, E.: Nursing for the Future. New York, Russell Sage Foundation, 1948.

Bulechek, G., and McCloskey, J.: Nursing Interventions: Treatment for Nursing Diagnoses. Philadelphia, W.B. Saunders Company, 1985.

Carrieri, V., Lindsey, A., and West, C. (eds): Pathophysiologic Phenomena in Nursing. Philadelphia, W.B. Saunders Company, 1986.

Cason, C., and Beck, C.: Clinical nurse specialist role development. Nurs Health Care *3*:25–26, 35–38, 1982.

Coleman, J., Dayani, E., and Simms, E.: Nursing careers in the emerging systems. Nurs Management *15*(1):19–27, 1984.

Crisham, P.: Resolving ethical and moral dilemmas of nursing interventions. In Snyder, M. (ed): Independent Nursing Interventions. New York, John Wiley & Sons, 1985, pp. 25–43.

Diers, D.: A combined basic-graduate program for college graduates. Nurs Outlook *24*:92–98, 1976.

Edlund, B., and Hodges, L.: Preparing and using the clinical nurse specialist. Nurs Clin North Am *18*:499 507, 1983.

Feild, L.: Current trends in education and implications for the future. In Hamric, A. B., and Spross, J. (eds): The Clinical Nurse Specialist in Theory and Practice. New York, Grune and Stratton, 1983, pp. 237–256.

Fenton, M.: Identifying competencies of clinical nurse specialists. J Nurs Admin *15*(12):31–37, 1985.

Fickeissen, J.: Getting certified. Am J Nurs *85*:265–269, 1985.

Goldmark, J.: Nursing and Nursing Education in the United States. Report of the Committee for the Study of Nursing Education and a Report of a Survey by Josephine Goldmark. New York, Macmillan, 1923.

Institute of Medicine: Nursing and Nursing Education: Public Policies and Private Actions. Washington, D.C., 1983.

Kelly, L.: Dimensions of Professional Nursing. New York, Macmillan, 1985.

Lewis, E.: The purposes and characteristics of master's education. In: (NLN #15-1840) Developing the Functional Role in Master's Education in Nursing. New York, National League for Nursing, 1980, pp. 1–11.

Lynaugh, J., Gerrity, P., and Hagopian, G.: Patterns of practice: Master's prepared nurse practitioners. J Nurs Educ *24*:291–295, 1985.

Lysaught, J.: Action in Nursing. New York, McGraw-Hill, 1974.

McCarty, P.: NPs, clinical specialists share nursing's cutting edge. Am Nurs *19*:24, 1986.

McCormick, K.: Preparing nurses for the technologic future. Nurs Health Care *4*:379–382, 1983.

McKevitt, R.: Trends in master's education in nursing. J Prof Nurs *2*:225–233, 1986.

McLane, A.: Core competencies of clinical nurse specialists. Nurs Res *27*:48–53, 1978.

Meleis, A.: Theoretical Nursing: Development and Progress. Philadelphia, J.B. Lippincott, 1985.

Murphy, J., and Hoeffer, B.: Role of the specialties in nursing science. Adv Nurs Sci *5*(4):31–39, 1983.

National League for Nursing: Characteristics of Graduate Education in Nursing Leading to the Master's Degree (#15-1759). New York, NLN, 1978.

National League for Nursing: Master's Education in Nursing: Route to Opportunities in
    Contemporary Nursing 1984-85. New York, NLN, 1984.
Powell, D.: Nurses—"High touch" entrepreneurs. Nurs Econ *2*:33–35, 1984.
Recommendations for clinical practice for the oncology clinical nurse specialist. Oncol
    Nurs Forum *12*:66–70, 1985.
Reed, S., and Hoffman, S.: The enigma of graduate nursing education: Advanced
    generalist? Specialist? Nurs Health Care *7*:43–49, 1986.
Sills, G.: The role and function of the clinical nurse specialist. *In* Chaska, N. (ed): The
    Nursing Profession: A Time to Speak. New York, McGraw-Hill, 1983, pp. 563–579.
Snyder, M.: Independent Nursing Interventions. New York, John Wiley & Sons, 1985.
Williamson, J.: Master's education: A need for nomenclature. Image *15*:99–101, 1983.

# Chapter 16

# The CNS in Collaborative Relationships Between Nursing Service and Nursing Education

*Lorry Gresham Kenton*

> Collaboration means true partnership, in which the power on both sides is valued by both, with recognition and acceptance of separate and combined spheres of activity and responsibility, mutual safeguarding of the legitimate interests of each party, and a commonality of goals that is recognized by both parties. This is a relationship based upon recognition that each is richer and more truly real because of the strength and uniqueness of the other.
>
> *(American Nurses' Association, 1980, p. 7)*

Collaboration between nursing service (NS) and nursing education (NE) is critical to the future of the profession. The CNS is in a logical position to develop collaborative relationships in which there are responsibilities for both service and education. This chapter will present incentives for and obstacles to NS/NE collaboration, discuss some models of collaboration, and present some examples of NS/NE relationships that currently exist. Strategies for successful NS/NE collaboration will be offered.

## HISTORICAL PERSPECTIVE

NS/NE collaborative efforts are not a recent phenomenon. Christy (1980), Grace (1981), and Mauksch (1980) have provided a history and description of the types of NS/NE relationships that have existed since 1900. These include the training school (in which the nurse training program was the responsibility of nursing administration within the hospital), nursing education within a hospital structure (in which NS and NE positions exist side by side under hospital administration), contractual arrangements, unification, collaboration, affiliation, and independent nursing practice by faculty. Unification models, such as those at Rush University, Case Western Reserve, and the University of Rochester, have been discussed in detail by Christman (1982), Gresham (1983), Nayer (1980), and Sovie (1981a, 1981b). Baker (1981), in summarizing past and present collaborative models between university nursing programs and health care agencies, arrived at several conclusions: there is a critical need for more voluntary collaboration between NS and NE; current efforts are not meeting the need to fully utilize professional resources; the principal obstacle to successful NS/NE collaboration is a longstanding commitment by nurses to either service or education; and the success of collaboration depends on the talents of faculty and the efficient use of consultants and leaders in nursing.

## FORCES AFFECTING COLLABORATIVE EFFORTS

### Driving Forces

Major market forces affecting NS and NE have been summarized by Whitney (1986; see Table 16–1). The author's major premise is that service and education can collaborate more effectively because many goals are similar. Table 16–2 compares long- and short-term goals of NS and NE. Although these goals are similar in many ways, Whitney (1986) noted that since different models have varying emphases on long- and short-term planning skills, a variety of strategies must be considered. Differences in organizational structures will also affect strategies.

There are additional factors that compel NS and NE to collaborate. The population of patients in hospitals is more acutely ill and the length of stay is shorter, which means that very efficient care is required. Discharge planning is complex since patients' needs are many and often require multiple community services. More clients in hospitals are aged or chronically ill, and they require specialized long-term follow-up ('Ten Trends," 1986). Given the complexity of patient needs after discharge, much home care should be delivered or at least coordinated by a CNS. Growth of community-based care also creates opportunities for inde-

**TABLE 16–1. Market Forces Affecting Service and Education**

| SETTING | | MAJOR MARKET FORCES | |
| --- | --- | --- | --- |
| | Financial Factors | Organizational Structures | Characteristics of Target Markets |
| Service | • Prospective reimbursement<br>• Shrinking budgets<br>• No direct reimbursement for general nursing services<br>• More copayment by patients<br>• Advances in medical technology requiring continual cost outlays | • Movement toward more acute care outside hospitals<br>• Changes in nursing care patterns<br>• Competitive arena<br>• High technology | • Better informed patients<br>• Increasing share of costs by patients<br>• Increased demand for provider choices by patients |
| Education | • Fewer scholarship/loan programs<br>• Higher tuitions<br>• Conservative economy<br>• Long-term investment<br>• Retooling of faculty necessary without concurrent increase in funding | • Increasing diversity of available programs<br>• Overbuilt for present population<br>• Slow to change<br>• Continuing education needed for faculty to upgrade skills and knowledge | • More diverse student population<br>• Diversity of coursework demanded by parents and students<br>• More emphasis on marketable output |

(From Whitney, F. W.: An economic view of collaboration between nursing service and education. ©1986 Anthony J. Jannetti, Inc., Publisher, *Nursing Economic$*. Reprinted with permission. Reprints of table available only from *Nursing Economic$*, North Woodbury Road/Box 56, Pitman, NJ, 08071.)

**TABLE 16–2. Comparison of Long- and Short-Term Goals in Nursing Education and Service Settings**

| Goals | Nursing Service | Nursing Education |
|---|---|---|
| *Short-term* | • Recruiting employees<br>• Retaining and promoting employees<br>• Managing budget<br>    costs<br>    revenues from service provided<br>    extramural grants<br>    development funds<br>• Managing physical plant and supplies<br>• Producing nursing service<br>    supervising safe, legal practice<br>    continuing education for current practice<br>    documenting services offered<br>    coordinating nursing services with other<br>    services in the setting and the community | • Recruiting faculty and students<br>• Retaining and promoting faculty<br>• Managing budget<br>    costs<br>    tuition<br>    extramural grants<br>    development funds<br>• Managing physical plant and supplies<br>• Producing educational programs<br>    supervising program development and<br>    classes<br>    teaching classes<br>    supervising teachers and students<br>    promoting faculty through academic<br>    channels<br>• Coordinating coursework within entire<br>    university<br>• Producing scholarly work<br>• Communicating with community |
| *Long-term* | • Providing continuous nursing service units<br>• Building cadre of nursing service employees<br>• Designing and creating employment markets<br>• Testing practice procedures and methods<br>• Sharing practice-based research studies with<br>    colleagues to enhance development of<br>    nursing theory and knowledge | • Educating students for productive employment<br>• Building cadre of educators with current skills<br>    and knowledge<br>• Designing and building future educational<br>    programs<br>• Adding to existing knowledge through<br>    research |

(From Whitney, F. W.: An economic view of collaboration between nursing service and education. ©1986 Anthony J. Jannetti, Inc., Publisher, *Nursing Economic$*. Reprinted with permission. Reprints of table available only from *Nursing Economic$*, North Woodbury Road/ Box 56, Pitman, NJ 08071.)

pendent nursing practice, which is ideal for faculty practice, research, and student learning.

The incentive for NS to collaborate with NE in this scenario is that service must have qualified staff to care for these individuals. NS must have some means of influencing the curriculum of students who will be future staff. The incentive for NE to collaborate with NS is that its faculty must maintain clinical competency in a rapidly changing care environment if they are to teach and produce practitioners who can function in current and future health care systems. Clinical practicum sites are also needed for students.

Faculty need research ideas and assistance as well as sites for data collection. All of these can be found in institutional, community, and ambulatory care NS agencies. In addition to faculty needing clinical resources, more students will also require them as the number of clinically oriented doctoral programs increase (Whitney, 1986).

NE can benefit from collaborating with NS in another way. If, as Ginzberg (1981) predicted, nursing student enrollment declines drastically in the near future, colleges and universities may have difficulty justifying some faculty positions. Retention of faculty could be aided by such strategies as sharing the cost of faculty salaries with NS. For NS, sharing salaries with NE or trading time and expertise without exchange of money would be an incentive to collaborate. Under pressure to contain costs, nursing service staff positions are at risk, especially CNS positions (Ginzberg, 1981; Joel, 1985; Whitney, 1986). NS can benefit from the expertise and knowledge of those in NE. NS needs more leaders who can participate fully and professionally in a challenging and rapidly changing health care system; it is up to NE to prepare these leaders. Service and education need each other. The CNS in a collaborative relationship with NS and NE is in a position to affect standards and delivery of care, curriculum, and student learning.

## Restraining Forces

A number of reasons have been offered to explain the lack of NS/NE collaboration. These include the fact that clinical practice usually does not contribute to promotion or tenure, time commitments are excessive, and monetary compensation is limited or nonexistent. The most significant obstacle to NS/NE collaboration is the lack of incentives for faculty to practice (Gresham, 1983; Holm, 1981; Joel, 1983; Mauksch, 1980; Sovie, 1981b). Organizational structures and the nature of the work that exist in academia inhibit collaboration with NS. Heavy teaching loads, committee work, and an emphasis on research and publication make it difficult to achieve the flexibility necessary for a joint-appointment CNS. It is often difficult even to recruit faculty who are willing to practice. Primary reasons for this include a lack of financial compensation and the fact that in most academic settings, practice, unlike research and publishing, is not viewed as a scholarly endeavor.

Another obstacle to developing collaborative relationships between NS and NE is related to growing economic constraints evident in the health care system since 1980. Increasingly, careful examination is being made of health care providers and their services. The more skilled individuals are being scrutinized more closely because of their higher salaries. CNSs face loss of jobs unless they can demonstrate a significant contribution to the financial status of the care setting (Joel, 1985). Without budgeted positions in NS for CNSs, it becomes more difficult, although not impossible, for NS to create a collaborative relationship with NE.

## Strategies for Dealing With Restraining Forces

Christman (1982) described the unification model as one way to build flexibility into a nursing budget. The unification of service and education can allow for an increase in the number of CNSs on the same academic budget. For example, if an academic salary exists for one CNS, four could actually be supported by allocating one-fourth the salaries to education and three-fourths to service. Unification allows greater flexibility in using salary dollars since there are ". . .many permutations and combinations that can be tailored to promote individual efforts and act as incentives to fuel the professional development of each member" (Christman, 1982, p. 95).

To prevent loss of CNS positions or to negotiate for additional ones, CNSs must prove their worth to the employing agency. "State-of-the-art nursing can significantly affect length of stay, avoid or minimize complications, and ensure documentation of complications of a borderline clinical nature" (Joel, 1985, p. 173). Such sophisticated nursing care is the purview of the CNS. Nursing must show its direct contribution to the fiscal viability of the agency by documenting CNS impact on individual cases, turning those that would have lost money into ones that save or make money for the agency (Joel, 1985). Such data are needed to establish the CNS as a significant participant in the changing health care environment. This work must be initiated by the CNS.

Academicians are more likely to consider including clinical practice into promotion/tenure criteria when contributions are specific and clearly documented. Evidence of scholarly practice must be defined and provided by the CNS. An example is clinical research or publications arising out of practice. Again, the burden to produce documented scholarly clinical work is on the CNS. Academicians must then be willing to consider CNS practice as a potential scholarly effort. Rigidity about what constitutes scholarly work will only stifle creativity and hold back progress in the profession. When practice is recognized as necessary for promotion or tenure, collaboration between NS and NE will be expedited.

## OUTCOMES/BENEFITS OF COLLABORATION

Whitney (1986) identified four areas in which NS/NE collaboration is beneficial. First, NS and NE need to collaborate in order to improve and document the cost-effectiveness and quality of nursing care, development and dissemination of new knowledge, and "the economic value of nursing research in practice" (Whitney, 1986, p. 40). Such joint research provides a wealth of opportunity to faculty and students and presents clinicians with opportunities for scholarly activity. Additionally, NS would benefit from data obtained, and the profession would benefit from new knowledge generated and new collaborative relationships established.

Whitney's second point was that nursing must take a leadership role in developing and implementing new health care delivery systems. "Through collaboration between service and education, services based on theory and research methods can be developed" (Whitney, 1986, p. 41). Such research can also provide a data base upon which to make recommendations for future health care policy. A third reason why NS and NE must collaborate is to prepare the nursing leaders of the future. NS and NE must work together to identify the knowledge and skill that will be needed in future health care delivery systems. Service settings provide practical experiences for knowledge testing and research by faculty and students.

Finally, joint research is needed to "develop new ways to measure indices of quality and evaluate performance. Research can develop a stronger empirical basis for nursing practice while examining the usefulness and effectiveness of interventions" (p. 42). Joint NS/NE research is necessary to promote and substantiate the goals of both. Joint projects provide more assurance that research will be practice-based and therefore incorporated into practice. Patients and staff, as well as the nursing profession, benefit from this type of collaboration.

While the obstacles are challenging, there are a number of successful collaborative NS/NE efforts around the country. A review of some of these models and some common elements can provide direction and stimulate creativity for those who want to develop such relationships.

In the first edition of this book, the discussion of joint appointment CNS role implementation was organized according to the following six keys for successful implementation:

- A supportive organizational structure
- A balance between personal and organizational goals
- Communication
- Regular clinical practice
- Economy of effort
- Defining realistic expectations.

For this second edition, these factors are best discussed as organizational or individual elements of success. The element of defining realistic expectations has been incorporated into a new section on role development for the CNS in a collaborative relationship.

## ELEMENTS OF SUCCESSFUL NS/NE COLLABORATION

The factors associated with successful NS/NE collaboration can be categorized as organizational or individual:

Organizational Elements
1. A supportive organizational structure
2. Communication

Individual Elements
1. Balance/congruence between personal and organizational goals
2. Communication
3. Regular clinical practice
4. Economy of effort.

### Organizational Elements

*Supportive Organizational Structure*

No one model of NS/NE collaboration will be appropriate for every organization. A variety of collaborative models are being tried. Styles' (1984) model may be very useful for those planning to develop a collaborative relationship, as it provides for degrees of collaboration ranging from no relationship to one of unified structure. Stages between the two extremes include communication, consultation, consent, and unified policy. Styles predicted that the future for nursing lies in the areas of communication and consultation, in which myriad possibilities exist for joint NS/NE ventures.

Barrell and Hamric (1986) described a collaborative model based on Styles' concept: a university school of nursing linked with a university hospital department of nursing. Formal lines of communication and areas of joint responsibility were identified between the dean of the school of nursing and director of nursing services, between two assistant deans and the hospital's assistant director for nursing education, between academic department chairpersons and clinical directors, and between faculty and unit leaders/CNSs on some clinical units. No money was exchanged in this arrangement. "Commitments are reciprocal and are designed to be negotiated for feasibility with the participants' supervisors and to be evaluated annually" (Barrell & Hamric, 1986, p. 498). Expectations have been identified in the areas of communication, consultation, and consent, three levels of Styles' model. This model has been evaluated favorably by both service and education.

A new collaborative relationship was begun in Denver, between the Children's Hospital and the School of Nursing at the University of Colorado Health Sciences Center. The senior vice president for nursing at Children's worked with the dean of the school to plan and implement the new relationship. (D.J. Biester, personal communication, June 20, 1986). Shared positions were established for a nurse researcher, the associate director for nursing research at Children's and assistant professor at the school of nursing. A practitioner teacher position (full-time with the hospital during the nonacademic year) was shared half-time with the school during the regular academic year. There were plans for shared positions in home health and education. All the individuals in shared positions had a faculty title and were unit-based within the hospital to facilitate the three missions of both settings: client care, education, and research. An advantage of this collaborative model is the opportunity for joint research, wherein a clinically based faculty member pursues grant proposals with faculty members at the school of nursing. One key to accomplishing effective working relationships between nursing service and nursing education was to ensure mutual goals of the leaders in both areas. Nursing leaders at Children's and the school of nursing believed that they were on their way to developing a high quality collaborative relationship.

Joel (1985) described the roles of CNSs who were part of the Rutgers University Teaching Nursing Home Project. In the formal link between the college of nursing and the nursing home, some CNSs held line positions as clinical directors of units in the home. Other CNSs held staff positions and provided tertiary care to residents on a referral basis. The nature of the CNS's specialization depended upon the needs of the nursing home's residents. The author speculated that CNSs "could even be contracted for independently and reimbursed on a fee-for-service basis or shared among several institutions" (Joel, 1985, p. 176).

Cox's (1985) constructive analysis of what went wrong with one joint appointment position can be beneficial to those seeking any type of collaborative relationship. She suggested that obvious internal and external support be established before a position is accepted. "For a practice position, external support refers to department head and university support; internal support refers to the agency's administration and staff" (p. 135). The author further clarified both kinds of support. It is important for the university department head to support the CNS's practice role by not diminishing time allocated for practice. The value of practice vis-à-vis research and teaching must also be communicated clearly. Further external support can be provided by clearly delineating how practice will contribute to university promotion and tenure. "Clinical practice outcome evaluation criteria on a par with teaching and research outcome criteria (such as course and student and peer evaluations, proposals written, grants received, and publications) must be developed, implemented, and respected" (p. 136). Cox noted that allowing clinical practice time to faculty and then ignoring clinical productivity as a part of evaluation discouraged development of joint practice-teaching roles.

Evidence of internal support requires that agency administration and staff be committed to making a joint position work. Cox (1985) emphasized that individual clinicians bring to an agency a variety of skills and problems that need to be defined and analyzed during the planning stages of a collaborative relationship. Cox's own experience provides an example. She offered the agency clinical and research skills at the doctoral level which, as it turned out, did not fit with the overall approach of the agency. Problems specific to a joint appointee, ". . .such as part-time availability, different approaches to clinical problems, and shared allegiances" (p. 136), must be anticipated and discussed at the beginning of a collaborative relationship.

Another structural factor important to success is the amount of time allocated to both the university and service agency. Cox (1985) suggested that a minimum of 40 per cent clinical time is necessary in order to maintain the CNS's interest, commitment, and loyalty. If less time is spent in clinical practice, the CNS's enthusiasm and impact could be diluted.

Algase (1985) recommended that persons planning faculty practice programs consider joint appointments, shared appointments (in which no money is exchanged), dual appointments (in which one person holds essentially two part-time positions, one in service and one in education), and faculty practice (usually a separate business).

### Communication

The CNS in a collaborative relationship with NS and NE should expect to frequently clarify the multiple responsibilities and activities involved in such a position. This must be a continuing effort since activities and time involvements may shift over the course of months. As educational commitments shift during an academic year, the CNS may have more or less time for practice. Staff, clients, and faculty to whom one is accountable must be made aware when responsibilities and time commitments have changed. Such communication need not be interpreted by the CNS as "reporting to" staff or others. Instead, it indicates respect for those whose primary or only focus may be clinical practice. Clinical staff and leadership personnel must understand and respect the different, equally important responsibility for educating students. It is the responsibility of the CNS in a collaborative relationship to keep others aware of the varied activities and time commitments negotiated (Gresham, 1976).

One useful approach is for the CNS to post a weekly (or monthly, as appropriate) schedule in both the clinical area and faculty office where clinical staff and faculty colleagues can see it. All regular meetings and activities should be reflected, including contact time with students (teaching, advising, office hours), class time, clinical practice, and lecture preparation time. In this way clinical staff and faculty peers will be easily reminded of the types of activities included in a collaborative relationship. This simple strategy can also prevent others from thinking that the CNS is "not working" when not in the clinical area or not visibly teaching. The CNS can strengthen the credibility of both NS and NE by demonstrating that both are important. Posting a current and complete schedule also makes it easier for others to contact the CNS should a clinical or educational need arise.

It is important to the overall success of the CNS in a collaborative relationship to receive regular communication from NS and NE about their respective goals and expectations. This is particularly important when there are changes in either objectives or expectations. Communication of this type of information may be accomplished via faculty or nursing service leadership meetings or periodic individual review sessions. However, experience shows that such communication may not always be initiated by those responsible. It is prudent then for the CNS to ask for specific feedback regarding changes in goals or expectations.

## Individual Elements

### Balance/Congruence of Personal with Organizational Goals

The CNS must have a set of personal and professional goals and be aware of the goals of the college of nursing and the service agency. CNSs should understand the organization's responsibilities for client care and student education. Based on this information it can be determined what is and is not negotiable for the CNS's time and activities. For example, if a clinical unit has overwhelming short-term needs for the CNS's time (due to an influx of new staff and an increase in patient acuity), negotiation or renegotiation of prior agreements may be necessary. This would appropriately involve leaders from both NS and NE as well as the CNS to ensure mutual agreement about goals and activities.

It is critical for CNSs to clarify and periodically (several times a year at least) reassess changing needs of both NS and NE because these can affect their own goals and expectations as well as anticipated timeframes for their accomplishment. Cox (1985) found through personal experience that when the CNS's personal and career goals are widely divergent from those of the agency or institution, success in a joint or shared position is in jeopardy. For example, Cox attempted to do some nursing clinical research in an agency when it was determined that the staff and administration were not ready for that level of nursing involvement. Everyone in the situation was frustrated.

A plan of action (individual goals translated into specific activities) for attaining goals must be carefully developed. For example, a CNS new to the faculty role may wish (as a long-term goal) to lecture effectively to groups of nursing students. To assist in reaching this goal, the CNS might use some clinical time to prepare a series of staff development programs and incorporate teaching/learning skills. Discriminating between the various options and activities available, bearing in mind the potential of each to be used in a variety of ways, then implementing the role on the basis of these decisions will enhance the potential for success and satisfaction. For example, both NS and NE usually have multiple committees that regularly need members. CNSs should be judicious in accepting committee memberships. Too much committee work can channel time and energy away from direct clinical or academic activities, which provide the true substance to the role of a CNS in a collaborative relationship.

Once goals and activities have been identified and agreed upon by those involved, a written contract or letter of agreement should be developed. This should include a time commitment specified per week or month for each of the activities and expectations. A written agreement should be viewed as something that can be renegotiated, especially in the early stages of a new collaborative relationship. However, it should be taken as a serious commitment, not to be disregarded. It may be necessary at times to refer to written commitments when others question how time is being spent or have different expectations.

### Communication

Communication of the elements of a negotiated contract or agreement must be ongoing with staff, students, peers, and (when appropriate) clients. If all necessary considerations were made prior to making the agreement, it should provide direction for implementation of the role.

### Regular Clinical Practice

Regular clinical practice in which the CNS can demonstrate clinical expertise is key to credibility in a collaborative relationship. Clinical practice is also the source for research questions, which, when explored, can improve the quality of care provided. The way the CNS intervenes with clients serves as a model for the staff nurses caring for other clients. Sutton (1973) summarized some benefits of clinical practice for the CNS: (1) direct care by the CNS provides an opportunity to observe staff delivering care, which facilitates identification of their strengths and weaknesses and allows for the planning of staff development programs; (2) the CNS is also available to staff when on the clinical unit with students; (3) because of the CNS's link with the clinical agency, changes in the environment which will enhance student learning are easier to make. For example, purchasing reference books for unit staff which would also benefit students could easily be facilitated by a CNS with responsibilities for NS and NE. The CNS will be aware of resources available to students in the clinical area and therefore may facilitate the students' use of those resources to improve care. Student ideas for improving care are more acceptable to staff when the CNS has established clinical credibility and is seen as an integral part of the unit. Finally, staff can often assist in evaluation of students when they are familiar with evaluation criteria.

Felder (1983) noted additional benefits when CNSs provide direct clinical care: patients who are part of the CNS's caseload receive high quality care; the CNS will experience the frustrations and obstacles that the staff do and is thus in a good position to problem-solve solutions; the visibility and accessibility of the CNS provide more opportunities to act as an advocate for nursing; interdisciplinary efforts are improved as is the awareness by others of nursing's role; classroom teaching is enhanced; the CNS's own skills and knowledge are kept current; and autonomous nursing practice is enhanced.

An example of individual collaboration between nursing service and nursing education can be found in the work done by Dr. Carolyn Webster-Stratton (personal communication, April 16, 1986) at the University of Washington School of Nursing in Seattle. Although her appointment was in the school of nursing as an associate professor and was not a joint appointment, Dr. Webster-Stratton, a nurse and psychologist, managed to do clinical practice, research, and education. Dr. Webster-Stratton had support from two grants, one focusing on education and one emphasizing clinical research. Over the course of a year, her time was allocated as approximately one-third education and two-thirds clinical research. There were both advantages and disadvantages with this arrangement. Not all the nursing faculty practiced. For those who did have clinical responsibilities, there might have been evening hours or crises with clients that became priorities for the clinician. This may have interfered with some academic expectations (such as faculty committee meetings) and caused friction.

This example demonstrates a creative approach to NS/NE collaboration through one person's activities. Rather than use an existing nursing service agency, the faculty member developed her own practice setting with the support of research funds.

Smith (1981) discussed obstacles to faculty practice and made some specific suggestions for overcoming them. The first and most important suggestion was to rearrange priorities so that nursing practice was of prime consideration. Once this was done it was easier to adjust time schedules to allow for practice. Independent nursing knowledge and skills must be identified and practiced. All aspects of the health care system (community- and institution-based) must be explored and considered as potential ways to provide faculty access to clients and improve nursing practice. Nursing roles must be re-examined to include "ownership" of clients, authority to admit clients to illness institutions, contracts between hospitals and individual/group nursing practice, and fee-for-service arrangements.

### Economy of Effort

Christman (1979) suggested that economy of effort was basic to successful implementation of the complete professional nursing role, which he described in terms of the practitioner/teacher model. The concept of economy of effort, simply stated, means making the most out of every professional activity. It is extremely helpful to the CNS who must constantly juggle activities and make decisions about priorities. The CNS in a collaborative relationship must look at every activity with this question in mind: How can I make the most out of this activity?

In the first edition of this book, a number of questions were offered as helpful in economizing efforts and maximizing their effects (Table 16–3). To further clarify and explain economy of effort, examples can be helpful. Clinical practice offers myriad opportunities for learning since every client situation is unique. The CNS is in a position to use clinical situations for staff and student education and can bring advanced skills and knowledge to every clinical situation. Staff and students can learn and clients can benefit from a CNS who can incorporate the latest skills and research into practice. The CNS can use clinical and academic resources to assist staff or students in solving difficult situations.

The CNS has the expertise and responsibility to identify and analyze facts, issues, relationships, and feelings in clinical situations. For the CNS, this can involve clients, staff, students, self, and perhaps peers. An especially unique or difficult patient situation could be written up as a case study for the education of staff, students, or peers. Research questions arise out of such situations. A case study might be used for peer review, publication, or as an example of scholarly clinical practice. Referring again to the work done by Dr. Webster-Stratton at the University of Washington, she met both educational and clinical interests by obtaining grants, which also contributed to the goals of the school of nursing. Including graduate students in clinical research and using the research in teaching are examples of economy of effort. Dr. Webster-Stratton will use her clinical research as a basis for publication in the future. This is one excellent way to deal with the "publish or

**TABLE 16–3. Questions Focusing Economy of Effort**

Regarding clinical activities:
- What can be learned from each clinical situation?
- What can the CNS bring to the situation that is different?
- How can students and staff or clients and their families learn from the situation?
- Can a clinical situation be used again? If so, how and for whom?
- Can significantly rewarding or disappointing clinical situations be identified and lessons learned from them?

Regarding any other activity or project CNSs are involved in:
- Is it a publishable idea?
- Would it serve as an alternate teaching/learning strategy for staff, students, or peers?
- Could it be adapted for client teaching? How?
- Could the CNS contribute to the development of staff, students, or peers by involving them in or delegating to them the activity, instead of doing it oneself?
- Could it be used for continuing education inside or outside one's place of employment? How?
- Could it help to develop or strengthen one's own professional consultation? How?

perish" issue. (C. Webster-Stratton, personal communication, April 16, 1986).

Because time is precious to a CNS, any project or activity must be carefully scrutinized for multiple use. A CNS's own position and role in a collaborative relationship or a model of practice might be a publishable idea. A CNS who developed a research project could include staff or students as data gatherers; this provides practical experience with research and may assist students with course objectives or staff with promotion criteria. For example, audiovisual productions of nursing grand rounds were initiated and directed by a CNS. These productions were subsequently used as part of periodic staff development and as an adjunct to student clinical learning experiences. A unit project to develop standardized care plans was benefitted by a CNS who asked for student input into the project. The care plans, once approved, were adapted for client teaching by including scientific rationale and applying teaching/learning strategies to specific parts of the care plans.

CNSs have opportunities to develop staff and students by involving them in or delegating to them a project, instead of doing it themselves. Identifying research questions, participating in literature review, and data gathering and analysis are all activities that can be shared or delegated. Projects will certainly take longer to complete when others are involved. But the long-term benefits make the wait worthwhile. Staff on one unit worked together to write an article for publication. CNSs could encourage staff or students to test or define a nursing diagnosis and contribute findings to the national professional endeavor.

Often the CNS can use aspects of clinical projects as examples for student learning, whether they are clinical examples in lectures or case studies in seminars. A literature review done for a clinical research project might also be used for a class lecture, clinical staff development, or in consultation. The CNS who maximizes every effort will find that time can be saved and knowledge, skill, and productivity enhanced.

## ROLE DEVELOPMENT OF THE CNS IN A COLLABORATIVE RELATIONSHIP

Many CNSs in collaborative relationships do not give themselves a chance to succeed because they expect to fulfill all aspects of their role right from the beginning. It takes a minimum of one full year to experience interaction among all components of the role and to begin to feel comfortable with them. Clinical specialists who will be providing direct client care should allow themselves a minimum of three months to become familiar with care delivery systems and other health team members. For those who are new to teaching, becoming familiar with the educational system, admission and progression criteria, curriculum, individual courses, and faculty/student resources takes at least one academic period (quarter or semester). CNSs who will be teaching for the first time, or for the first time in a new system, will need more time in the beginning to develop lectures, examinations, and teaching plans. These allowances for time in clinical and education should be factored into the initial written agreement regarding the CNS's activities and time commitments.

At one large medical center employing many CNSs, those who were new to teaching or to the clinical area were given a six-month adjustment period. For the first three months, nearly all the new CNS's time was spent on the clinical unit caring for patients and working with staff. During this time the CNS became familiar with staff and patient care on the unit. For the second three months the new CNS was assigned a group of students for clinical teaching and perhaps a seminar to co-lead with an experienced CNS. During the second three months, the CNS spent a majority (60 to 70 per cent) of the time involved with educational activities, becoming familiar with the curriculum, and student teaching. These first six months' activities were spent under the close supervision and guidance of an experienced CNS. The last six months of the first year was defined by the developing strengths, interests, and goals of the new CNS and by the needs of both the clinical and academic arenas.

Such a situation may be called a luxury by some or impossible by others. However, for a CNS new to a collaborative relationship, this type of "easing into" the role may be critical to success in the position. This author has seen numerous CNSs, new to joint appointment positions, leave by or before 12 months because they felt they could not meet the multiple expectations placed upon them. Part of the responsibility belongs to the new CNS who must negotiate for an adjustment period. It is the opinion of this author that collaborative or joint positions may not be appropriate for new CNSs. The skills required for negotiation, time management, leadership of others, self-discipline, and self-confidence may not be adequately developed in the new CNS. The one possible exception to this may be a situation at a large university/medical center where there are many CNSs employed who can offer support and guidance.

During the first year, the CNS in a collaborative relationship will probably need (and should seek out and accept) assistance in setting priorities. Some trade-offs should be anticipated. This becomes most evident in the process of negotiating time and activities when the balance between personal and organizational goals must be reached.

Several of the CNS's own goals may have to be changed to become closer to what is possible within the organization, or the timeframe for accomplishing a goal may have to be altered.

For example, an experienced CNS who was new to a particular joint position wanted to develop a psychiatric consultative role on adult medical units. In looking at the needs of her own unit and those of the school of nursing, both of which had great need for her expertise, a compromise was reached. For the first six months the CNS would spend the majority of her time on a particular unit and in clinical student teaching. This would meet the immediate needs of the unit and school as well as allow the CNS to establish a base for consultation and an opportunity to get to know other staff and faculty. The last six months of the first year the CNS negotiated to emphasize the consultative aspect of her role, which would also meet a goal of the clinical institution: to improve the psycho-emotional care on adult medical units. It is very important, however, for the CNS to plan ways of achieving individual success. This means planning some goals that are easily achievable and planning intermediate steps to be used in reaching longer-term or more complex goals. Individual priorities and interests need to be communicated to the appropriate people within the organization. (One must take time to find out who these are). Specific activities and suggestions can then be offered. One must also be prepared to renegotiate an agreement at any time if experience shows it is not working or if needs are changing.

Closely associated with making reasonable expectations of oneself is identifying sources of support. The CNS should anticipate some ambiguity and frustration initially and should plan to deal with these. Expert clinicians know the value of anticipatory planning for potential problems. We teach this to clients and to students, and we should practice it more on ourselves. Counseling services if available in one's place of employment, nursing administrative personnel, and others outside the place of work (such as spouse or friends) can all be sources of support. For the CNS in a joint or collaborative role, peers in similar positions are the best sources of support (see Chapter 14). Others who are managing or have managed dual NS/NE responsibilities know the unique pressures of time, feelings of split allegiances, and the challenges of dual responsibility. Experienced CNSs can provide structure, guidance, and assurance to the new CNS during the first critical year. This support is so important that it is a factor one must look for when seeking a joint NS/NE position: Are others in similar positions employed and do opportunities exist, formal or informal, for support, supervision, or guidance? For new CNSs it is probably wise to consider only situations in which there are other CNSs in collaborative relationships. The professional support and experience available will be necessary. If possible for the first six to nine months, the new CNS should limit the number of different activities. For example, clinical teaching of students and maintaining a strong clinical base rather than becoming heavily involved in a special project will help prevent the new CNS from feeling (and being) frazzled.

## SUMMARY

As the economic base of health care continues to change, nursing will be forced to consider new models and methods that will keep the profession in an influential leadership position. Models of collaboration discussed in this chapter exemplify the numerous models being developed. Inherent in developing new collaborative models is the willingness on the part of leaders in NS and NE to take the risks necessary to create new structures. One has to see beyond the traditional in order to be creative. During these cost-constraining times, administrators may be afraid to take risks, a factor that may threaten collaboration. Risk-taking is at the heart of innovation, and innovation is essential to developing collaborative models (A.B. Hamric, personal communication, March 24, 1987).

Collaboration is required for the viability and growth of both nursing service and education. Collaborative relationships between NS and NE will keep education relevant and service theory-based. The CNS must take a leadership role in the development and implementation of NS/NE collaboration.

*References*

Algase, D. L.: Financing faculty practice: Elements of a strategic plan. Nurs Econ *3*:328–331, 356, 1985.
American Nurses' Association: Nursing: A Social Policy Statement. Kansas City, ANA, 1980.
Baker, C. M.: Moving toward independence: Strategies for collaboration. J Nurs Admin *11*:34–39, 1981.
Barrell, L. M., & Hamric, A. B.: Education and service: A collaborative model to improve patient care. Nurs Health Care 7:497–503, 1986.
Christman, L.: The practitioner-teacher. Nurs Educ *4*:8–11, 1979.
Christman, L.: The unification model. *In* Marriner, A. (ed): Contemporary Nursing Management. St. Louis, C. V. Mosby Company, 1982, pp. 91–95.
Christy, T.: Clinical practice as a function of nursing education: An historical analysis. Nurs Outlook *28*:493–497, 1980.
Cox, C. L.: Nursing practice in action: Diary of a casualty. *In* Barnard, K. E., & Smith, G. R. (eds): Faculty Practice in Action. Kansas City, American Academy of Nursing, 1985, pp. 130–138.
Felder, L. A.: Direct patient care and independent practice. *In* Hamric, A. B., & Spross,

J. (eds): The Clinical Nurse Specialist in Theory and Practice. New York, Grune and Stratton, 1983, pp. 59–71.

Ginzberg, E.: The economics of health care and the future of nursing. J Nurs Admin *11*:28–32, 1981.

Grace, H. K.: Unification, re-unification; reconciliation or collaboration—bridging the education/service gap. *In* McClosky, J. C., & Grace, H. K. (eds): Current Issues in Nursing. Boston, Blackwell Scientific Publications, 1981, pp. 626–643.

Gresham, M. L.: Conflict or collaboration: A head nurse's view. *In* Chamings, P., & Markel, R. (eds): Symposium on the Clinical Nurse Specialist. Indianapolis, Sigma Theta Tau, 1976.

Gresham, M. L.: Joint appointments. *In* Hamric, A. B., & Spross, J. (eds): The Clinical Nurse Specialist in Theory and Practice. New York, Grune and Stratton, 1983, pp. 129–148.

Holm, K.: Faculty practice—noble intentions gone awry? Nurs Outlook *29*:655–657, 1981.

Joel, L. A.: Stepchildren in the family: Aiming toward synergy between nursing education and service—from the faculty perspective. *In* Barnard, K. E. (ed): Structure to Outcome: Making it Work. Kansas City, American Academy of Nursing, 1983.

Joel, L. A.: Preparing clinical specialists for prospective payment. *In* National League for Nursing (ed): Patterns in Education: The Unfolding of Nursing. New York, NLN, 1985, pp. 171–178.

Mauksch, I. G.: Faculty practice: A professional imperative. Nurs Educ *5*:21–24, 1980.

Nayer, D. D.: Unification: Bringing nursing service and nursing education together. Am J Nurs *80*:1110–1114, 1980.

Smith, G. R.: Faculty practice plans: Latent obstacles to success. *In* McClosky, J. C., & Grace, H. K. (eds): Current Issues in Nursing. Boston, Blackwell Scientific Publications, 1981, pp. 551–557.

Sovie, M. D.: Unifying education and practice: One medical center's design. Part 1. J Nurs Admin *11*:41–49, 1981a.

Sovie, M. D.: Unifying education and practice: One medical center's design. Part 2. J Nurs Admin *11*:30–32, 1981b.

Styles, M. M.: Reflections on collaboration and unification. Image *16*:21–23, 1984.

Sutton, L.: The clinical nurse specialist in a dual role. *In* Riehl, J. P., & McVay, J. W. (eds): The Clinical Nurse Specialist: Interpretations. New York, Appleton-Century-Crofts, 1973.

Ten trends to watch. Nurs Health Care *7*:17–19, 1986.

Whitney, F. W.: An economic view of collaboration between nursing service and education. Nurs Econ *4*:37–42, 1986.

# Health Policy: Implications for the CNS

Shirley A. Girouard

## INTRODUCTION

The role of the clinical nurse specialist (CNS) has been discussed in the preceding chapters from a variety of perspectives. Throughout appears the theme of leadership, requiring the CNS to apply specialized knowledge and skills to influence the quality of health care. This leadership role must include activities that influence policy decisions affecting nursing education, practice, and research. Such decisions take place within individual organizations and at the level of local, state, and federal government. Policy decisions, wherever they are made, influence CNS practice and the quality of patient care. "Policy sets directions and determines goals or other principles" (Diers, 1985).

Health care is influenced by the directions, goals, and principles of institutions and units of government. Within organizations, policies are developed that direct how nursing will be practiced. Similarly, governmental units make decisions that affect the role nurses will play in the health care system. The following illustrates how policy decisions can influence nursing practice:

> Mr. C. had surgery for prostatic cancer and was recovering in the hospital without complications. He was discharged from the hospital, although he was not ready to assume self-care and had no one at home to assist him. A referral was made for home nursing care, which continued for two months until Medicare denied further payment for services. He was not able to receive Medicaid or local welfare support, and due to a deterioration in his condition, was readmitted to the hospital.

Although the scenario depicted here is hypothetical, it reflects a commonly occurring phenomenon. As illustrated in Table 17–1, Mr. C's care was influenced by a number of policies. It is clear that the way

**TABLE 17–1. Patient Care Needs and Public Policy—An Illustration**

| CARE NEED | RELATED POLICY |
|---|---|
| Hospital care for surgery | Medicare for payment of services<br>DRG/Prospective payment |
| Home care | No hospital policy for follow-up<br>Skilled nursing care/Medicare benefits |
| Continued home care | Denial of Medicare benefits (home bound rule)<br>Medicaid ineligible<br>Welfare ineligible |
| Rehospitalization | Medicare coverage |

in which a CNS practices in a hospital or community and the quality of care patients receive are influenced by institutional and governmental policies. The impact of health care funding policies illustrated here is just one example of the effect of policy decisions on nursing and health.

The primary focus of this chapter will be on the role of the CNS in relation to public policy. It is also important to note that the same processes and principles apply to the role of the CNS in relation to organizational policies. Included in this chapter are an overview of United States health policy, a discussion of the roles of the profession and the CNS in health policy, definitions and descriptions of policy and politics, and suggestions for political involvement.

## OVERVIEW OF UNITED STATES HEALTH POLICY

In a little more than 100 years, the health care system has changed and grown dramatically. As described by Torrens (1984), three major periods in the history of health care have preceded the present: the era prior to the introduction of hospitals, the introduction of science and technology as major forces in health care, and the introduction of new mechanisms for funding health care.

Prior to the 1850s, health care consisted of a loose combination of personal services without any organizational framework. Then health care began to move to hospital settings and was influenced by the introduction of new scientific methods. After World War II, significant scientific and technological advances continued and were accompanied by greater public attention to the social and organizational aspects of health care.

Health care insurance, introduced in the 1930s, continued to grow during the 1940s and 1950s. The introduction of Medicare and Medicaid in the mid-1960s had a significant impact, contributing to a major period of expansion in the health care sector as well as increasing the involvement of government in the health care system.

The present health care climate can be characterized by changes in relation to competition, cost containment, the financing of health care, the organization of health care, and the role of government in the health care system.

The Department of Health and Human Services reported (*Medical Benefits*, 1986) that, in 1985, $425 billion were spent on health care. This represents 10.7 per cent of the gross national product, the highest ever for health care. With a general inflation rate of 3.9 per cent, the 8.9 per cent increase in spending for health care from 1984 indicates that the present cost-containment measures are not totally effective. This escalation of health care costs has resulted in attempts at cost savings and efficiency, including prospective payment, deregulation, and the promotion of competition.

Competition in the health care system has been fostered by concerns about the inflationary costs of health care, ever-increasing technological changes, and changing attitudes about the role government should play in health care. All have contributed to the present situation (Sapolsky & Altman, 1981). Cost-containment efforts, the most obvious result of these changes, have created a competitive climate influencing nurses. Nurses must compete with physicians and other providers for third-party reimbursement and access to research and education dollars.

Patients/clients are also affected by the competitive health care climate. For example, consumers presently have a number of options available for receiving and financing health care. Thus, consumers must be knowledgeable about what health care services they need and what they can expect from these services. Ethical dilemmas are also created by cost-containment efforts when resources are not sufficient to meet all needs in a quality manner. Difficult decisions need to be made in allocating resources.

Although most Americans have some sort of coverage for their health care expenses, it is estimated that 10 to 20 million Americans are uninsured or underinsured. Employers provide the majority of health insurance coverage through Blue Cross/Blue Shield or one of the commercial agencies. The federal government, another major purchaser of health care, funds Medicare, Medicaid, Veterans Administration health services, health care for the armed services, and other specific health care programs such as those for maternal-child health. State governments are involved in the administration of the Medicaid program. They also provide services for the mentally ill and developmentally disabled and, with much variation from state to state, provide or finance other health care programs.

Today, there is concern about the government's role in health care, particularly that of the federal government as a major funding source for health care needs. Federal funding for health care is being questioned and in some cases reduced. Since this movement is primarily at the federal level, increasing demands are being put on state governments to fill the void. Local governments are also being asked to provide funds for a greater number of health service agencies because of decreasing federal funds and changes such as the DRG/prospective payment program.

Given the importance of policy decisions, the CNS needs to apply expert knowledge and skill to influence policy at whatever level it is being formulated. The unique role of CNSs as both care providers and leaders allows them to assess the impact various policy alternatives will have on clients and on the nursing profession. Policy makers at all levels need this type of input if they are to make decisions in the best interests of health care consumers.

## PAST AND PRESENT ROLE OF NURSING IN HEALTH CARE POLICY

The overview of United States health policy demonstrates the relationship between policy and a rapidly changing health care system. It is not surprising that nurses are more aware of the implications of policy on practice. This concern has led nurses to become more involved with the policy process. From 1976 to 1982 there has been an increase in the number of articles in the nursing literature dealing with legislative and political processes (Lake & Lamper-Linden, 1983). Lake and Lamper-Linden also pointed out that prior to the 1960s, there was not a "legislation" heading in the nursing index. Similarly, it was not until 1976 that the heading "politics" was introduced.

Nursing's role in the policy process is apparent in *The American Nurse,* the *American Journal of Nursing, Nursing Economic$,* and other professional nursing journals. In fact, it is rare to review any nursing journal in which there is not some attention given to a public policy issue and/or the implications of a public policy change. One only needs to review the "Newscaps" section of recent issues of the *American Journal of Nursing* to realize the importance of health policy for the nursing profession. The November 1986 issue lists the following "headlines":

- New bill would launch community nursing centers
- Medicare "quality" bill survives AMA attack
- Two states OK "prescribing" (by any other name)

- Deficit dims hope for bigger boost in DRG rates
- Hospitals hurting under HHS's payment policies

Nurses are also becoming familiar figures at state houses and on Capitol Hill. Nurses' involvement in the policy process is becoming increasingly important as allocation decisions are being made about funding for nursing education, research, and health care. Nursing's unique and important contributions to the health care system will depend upon its ability to influence how these decisions are made and what the outcomes will be.

The potential for nursing to influence health care is great. Milio (1981) provided a framework for considering what health care policy might be like if the values of the nursing profession were to be the prominent guiding force. She indicated that health policy could be approached from the perspective of the relationship between illnesses and their origin. Using this nursing model, attention would focus on illnesses that originate in the environment and in personal behavior. Funding and systems for the prevention of illness and disability would be more likely to receive attention on the political agenda than those that focus on an illness/medical model.

## HEALTH POLICY AND THE CNS

The above discussion has implications for the nursing profession and indicates that the CNS as a leader in the profession and as an expert in clinical practice can and should assist in affecting public health policies that are being developed at all levels of government. The CNS has the opportunity to contribute to this trend of greater political influence and, thus, to fulfill some of the obligations of the role as outlined in the AMA's *Nursing: A Social Policy Statement* (1980). According-ing to this document, the CNS has responsibilities related to the advancement of the profession, working with others to plan and evaluate health programs for people at risk and to address health care trends. These areas of responsibility are, to a large extent, the focus of public policies. Thus, if the CNS is to fulfill the role obligation, it will be necessary to become involved with the public policy process.

The importance of political involvement to influence the making of policy is perhaps best illustrated by providing some examples of legislative decisions that have importance to the CNS. The examples that follow represent only a few of the many state and federal policy decisions that affect clients, the nursing profession, CNS practice, and society in general.

## Clients

Health-related outcomes and health behaviors are both influenced by public policy. An example of how policy affects health-related outcomes is the prospective payment system legislation enacted by Congress in 1984. With the introduction of this change in Medicare reimbursement, patients are more likely to be discharged "quicker and sicker" than previously. Shorter lengths of stay have been documented in the literature (Hartley, 1986). Although not as well documented, there is indication that shorter lengths of stay mean that the outcomes the CNS expects for certain groups of patients by the time of discharge will be different and that the requirement for home care will, in many cases, be increased. MacMillan-Scattergood (1986) stated that the demand for home health services may raise ethical dilemmas associated with the allocation of resources and produce conflicts between institutional and professional values. By providing testimony and lobbying, the CNS can inform policy makers about these issues and the effects they have on health care.

## Profession

A major way policy influences practice is through the regulation of the profession. State nurse practice acts control entry into practice and govern the basic elements of who may do what within nursing and in relation to other provider groups. Nursing is also influenced by the level of funding allocated to education. For example, the decrease in federal monies for undergraduate and graduate education has contributed to the nursing shortage. State allocations for colleges and universities are also important considerations for the future of nursing education.

The impact of legislation on nursing research activities provides yet another example of policy that should be of concern to the CNS. The establishment of the National Center for Nursing Research (NCNR) illustrates this point as well as the interrelationship between issues of importance to nursing and the public policy arena. Larson (1984) described the importance of government recognition of nursing as an important health care resource. The establishment of NCNR is an excellent example of how nurses can influence public policy decisions and produce positive changes for the profession (White & Hamel, 1986). Similarly, trends in funding for CNS programs in mental health and oncology parallel government interest in specialty areas of health care.

### CNS

One of the major roles of state government is to regulate the practice of health care providers, including nurses. As Peplau (1985) pointed out, control over the profession of nursing is an issue being debated within and outside the nursing profession. One question the CNS must face is that of who should regulate advanced practice. Should certification be controlled by government agencies or by the profession? The CNS can share with legislators the profession's view that nursing practice should be regulated by the profession.

Another government role is the regulation of the insurance industry. State and federal governments frequently make decisions about who will be compensated for providing health care services. This matter is of particular importance to the CNS wishing to engage in private practice. Twenty-five states (Griffith, 1986) have legislation related to third-party reimbursement for nursing practice. Another example of legislation that may have an impact on the way in which the CNS practices is the Medicare Community Nursing and Ambulatory Care Act (HR 5457). Adoption of this federal legislation would provide the CNS access to reimbursement and a practice setting that is currently not widely available.

### Society

The unique perspective of the nursing profession can provide an added dimension to health policy debates. As described in the ANA social policy document (1980), nursing is involved with human responses to health problems. Nurses, as the largest group of health care providers, possess a wide range of experience and a unique understanding of the implications of health policy decisions on consumers. The nurse advocate role can be carried into the political arena. Perhaps more than any other group, nurses see the impact of policy decisions at the level of the individual health care consumer. Unfortunately, the perspective of nurses is not always shared with policy makers.

## POLICY AND POLITICS: DEFINITIONS AND PROCESS

If CNSs are to become involved with policy making, it is important to have an understanding of the process and the context in which it occurs. For example, if the CNS wishes to help shape a state government's policies regarding radiation exposure in the workplace, it is not enough to know the substance of the issue. The CNS needs to understand how decisions are made and how to intervene to achieve desired outcomes.

An example may help to illustrate the link between policy, politics, and political action. The mental health division of one state government had identified a problem of not having enough licensed persons to provide medications to patients in the state psychiatric hospital. In an attempt to resolve this problem, the division proposed to the legislature a policy that would allow unlicensed persons (to be called medication specialists) to give medications following a brief course of instruction. Although there were a number of alternatives to the proposed policy, such as increasing the salaries of licensed persons, changing the working conditions for licensed persons, or otherwise altering the system to attract and retain nurses, the legislature proposed to allocate its fiscal (valued and scarce) resources in the manner described in the division's proposal. Having determined that the proposed policy change will compromise safety and quality of care, the state nurses' association and others concerned about the issue used political action to prevent passage of the law.

The term *policy* is used in health policy and nursing literature in a number of ways. Anderson (1979) provided the following basic definition of policy: "A purposive course of action followed by an actor or set of actors in dealing with a problem or matter of concern." This definition indicates that policies have a purpose, direction, or goal and consist of a series of actions aimed toward achieving a specific outcome. Bullock, Anderson, and Brady (1983) described public policy as policy "developed by governmental institutions and officials through the political process (politics)."

Public policy also refers to what governments do to meet certain needs. Local, state, and federal governments provide direct and indirect funding for health care services. Funding is provided through programs such as Medicare and Medicaid and through contributions made to support local hospice activities. The provision of direct services by the government is exemplified in the establishment of psychiatric care in state hospitals and programs such as the Indian Health Service.

Public policy may be either positive or negative. Positive public policies are those developed to address a problem. Negative policies are reflected in situations in which a problem has been identified, but government does not act to resolve the problem. Examples of positive policies are the DRG/prospective payment policies established in an attempt to reduce the costs of Medicare. The identification of the need to provide funding for home health care and the government's failure to do this illustrate a negative policy. Public policy is further described as "based on law and is authoritative" (Bullock, Anderson, and Brady, 1983). This implies that governments can intervene to impose penalties when laws are not obeyed.

As shown in Table 17–2, the policy process includes six basic steps that are similar to the steps of the nursing process. The policy process begins with the identification of a problem. Someone or some group perceives a need that they believe could be addressed through government intervention. This step in the process requires that the person or group get the attention of the government in relation to the problem. Once recognized by government, the problem needs to become part of the policy agenda. From all of the many problems that are brought to the attention of the government, only a few are selected for inclusion on the legislative agenda.

Once the problem is recognized and becomes part of the legislative agenda, solutions to the problems need to be proposed and presented as alternatives. This step is referred to as *policy formulation*. *Policy adoption* refers to the phase of the policy process which involves convincing the government to support a particular solution to the problem. Public hearings, votes by each of the legislative bodies, and the signing of the bill by the governor are involved in the adoption process.

Acceptance of the policy, i.e., the passage of legislation, is followed by its implementation—the way in which the bureaucratic structure operationalizes the policy decision. The policy process concludes with the evaluation of the policy: did the policy work? Although an often neglected part of the policy process, evaluation is important to determine whether or not the policy is effective.

## Context of Policy Process

The CNS wishing to provide care to a patient or group of patients always assesses the context in which the proposed care will be given. Similarly, the CNS wishing to influence the policy process must under-

**TABLE 17–2. Steps in the Policy Process**

| POLICY PROCESS | NURSING PROCESS |
|---|---|
| 1. Problem identification/formation | 1. Assessment/nursing diagnosis |
| 2. Set the policy agenda | 2. Determine goals |
| 3. Formulate policy | 3. Develop care plan |
| 4. Adopt policy | 4. Adopt plan with input from patient and others |
| 5. Implement policy | 5. Implement care plan |
| 6. Evaluate policy | 6. Evaluate outcomes |

(Adapted from Bullock, C., Anderson, J., and Brady, D.: Public Policy in the Eighties. Monterey, CA, Brooks/Cole, 1983.)

stand the context in which policy formulation takes place. Although the context in which particular policy decisions are made varies, there are some critical areas of focus. Bullock, Anderson, and Brady (1983) identified three major elements of the policy context: history, environmental factors, and the political system. Past policies will influence future policy changes; thus, the history of similar types of policy decisions should be evaluated.

These authors also stated the need to assess environmental factors that influence policy making: "From the environment come demands for policy action, support for the political system, and limitations and constraints on what can be done by policy makers." Environmental factors include the political culture, public opinion, the social system, and the economic system. Political culture refers to the values and beliefs that society has about political power and how it is exercised. The last element of policy context for the CNS to understand is the political system itself. The structure and process of policy making include how bills become law, what the rules of the process are, and how implementation occurs.

Politics is a major force shaping public policy decisions. Simply defined, politics influences others to behave or think in a particular way. Most commonly, politics is described as the authoritative allocation of scarce resources such as money, health, prestige, power, and status. Scarcity relates to the fact that all of society's resources are not available in sufficient quantities for all citizens (Kalisch & Kalisch, 1982). In our society, governments often have the legitimate power (authority) to allocate resources. Political actions, which will be discussed in greater detail later, are the efforts made by individuals and groups to influence persons in authority to allocate resources in a particular way.

## INFLUENCING THE POLICY PROCESS

As indicated in the discussion above, public policy decisions related to health care have a significant impact on nurses, clients, and society. The CNS, as a nursing leader and clinical expert, should become involved with actions that will benefit the nursing profession and health care. Former ANA President Eunice Cole (1985) stated:

> As a profession inherently responsive to people, nursing cannot separate itself from politics and public policy. We understand in human terms what, to policy makers, appears as flat abstractions on paper. Only by being willing to enter into the political arena can we insure that our elected representatives legislate in the interests of the health needs of their constituents.

The knowledge and skills the CNS acquires through graduate education and nursing practice can be readily applied to the political arena. Clinical knowledge provides the substance or information needed to influence policy decisions. Research knowledge and skills are similar to those required for policy analysis. Written and verbal communication skills can be used to disseminate policy information. Leadership and organizational abilities are helpful to CNSs when they wish to direct others to influence policy decisions. CNSs come to the political arena with a wealth of knowledge and skills!

Although well prepared to participate in political action, CNSs may need to learn more about the structure and process of government. There are a number of ways to obtain the needed information. Organized nursing groups such as the American Nurses' Association, state nurses' associations, the American Association of Colleges of Nursing, and specialty nursing organizations are obvious sources. Political parties, health groups, and government agencies are other possibilities. It is unlikely that CNSs would not be informed about current health care issues, since they read the professional literature and attend professional meetings. Finally, the well-informed CNS will use public media as a source of information about health policy and political issues.

Prepared with the necessary knowledge and skills, CNSs can participate in the political process in a number of ways. Table 17–3 suggests possible levels of involvement and relates them to the steps of the policy process. Recognizing that there are multiple demands made on the CNS, it is important to note that there are effective, yet quick, actions that even the busiest CNS can take.

At the first level of political action, the CNS would function in a supportive political role: contributing to political action committees and working with other more involved nurses who deal with the analysis, organization, and direction of political efforts. The CNS could be on a legislative mailing list and/or could participate in a telephone tree to be kept informed and to assist with lobbying efforts.

The second level of political action reflects greater involvement by the CNS. Through nursing and other health care forums, the CNS helps to identify health care issues in need of government intervention. Once identified, efforts would be made to have the issue become part of the policy agenda and to assist others in exploring policy options. By providing expert testimony and input into the implementation and evaluation phases of the policy process, CNSs increase their sphere of influence. For example, gerontology clinical specialists in New Hampshire recognized the need for "living will" legislation. In discussions with their colleagues in other specialty areas, interested community groups, and legislators, they developed a policy that was introduced as

**TABLE 17–3. CNS Involvement in Political Action**

| Level | Policy Step | CNS Activities |
|---|---|---|
| I | Problem identification | Contact nursing and other groups |
| | Set agenda | Write letters to editor |
| | Formulation | Talk to government officials |
| | Adoption | Call/write legislators; inform public; inform nurses |
| | Implementation | Set procedures for own setting |
| | Evaluation | Assess outcomes in own setting/inform others |
| II | Problem identification | Identify problems needing legislative action |
| | Set agenda | With others, contact key legislators for support |
| | Formulation | |
| | Adoption | Provide expert testimony; lobby/assist other nurses to do same |
| | Implementation | Provide consultation |
| | Evaluation | Work with others to plan evaluation/report results |
| III | Problem identification | Identify programs for government action |
| | Set agenda | Act as advocate/consultant |
| | Formulation | Provide policy analysis |
| | Adoption | Organize and direct lobbying efforts |
| | Implementation | Consult with government agencies |
| | Evaluation | Report/disseminate results |

a bill. Working with the state nurses' association's lobbyist, the CNSs provided testimony at House and Senate hearings and mobilized other nurses to help with lobbying efforts. After the bill became law, they worked with nursing, legal, and institutional representatives to disseminate information about the new law to the public. To evaluate the effect of the law and to identify problems, these CNSs acted as a resource for problem-solving.

The third level of political involvement moves the CNS to a greater focus on the policy aspects of health care. At this level nurses are becoming increasingly visible to elected officials, campaign and legislative staff, lobbyists, and appointed government employees. When involved at this level, the CNS would play a major role in all aspects of the policy process. For example, a CNS might advise the lobbyist for a state nurses' association to assist in establishing legislative priorities for nursing, prepare other nurses for political involvement, organize and direct lobbying efforts, and provide a voice for nursing at the level of state government.

Other political action options available to the CNS relate to the elective process. Having elected officials supportive of the nursing profession and of health care issues of interest to nurses facilitates achieving valued outcomes. The CNS might consider one or all of the following: contributing to campaigns, volunteering for campaign work, becoming involved with local and state political parties, and participating in political action committees.

With whatever activities CNSs choose to become involved, the expertise they bring can have an impact on policy decisions made through the political process. CNS involvement also helps to enhance the image of the profession through visibility and communication about the role of nursing and that of the CNS. The impact of public policy decisions on health care and the nursing profession cannot be ignored. As recognized nursing leaders, CNSs must become involved in the political process and assist other nurses to do the same. The personal and professional rewards are great and our health depends on it!

## INFLUENCING POLICY: AN ILLUSTRATION

Health policy and legislative issues associated with acquired immunodeficiency syndrome (AIDS) can be used to illustrate the role CNSs can play in the political arena. Growing concern about AIDS has prompted state and federal officials to respond with numerous legislative and administrative proposals. The example presented here, although hypothetical, will describe a scenario similar to that which is occurring in many states across the country.

Responding to the problem of AIDS, the state department of public health explored a number of possible efforts that could be used to address the problem. Preventive measures, treatment, funding, and changes in insurance laws are some of the general areas under consideration to determine which policy proposal to bring to the legislature. The department of public health is also concerned about protecting civil liberties and has debated which approaches would least interfere with these rights. In discussing the issue with legislators interested in sponsoring the bill, the policy formulated for the bill would establish a program for public education and for screening of high-risk groups.

The public health department knew that public awareness of the AIDS problem was growing. Thus, it was not difficult to have this issue become part of the policy agenda for the upcoming legislative session. In this case, the adoption of the policy requires the state house, senate, and governor to accept the proposed bill supporting AIDS education and screening so that it could become law. In this example, upon passage of the bill, the division of public health would design public educational programs related to the prevention of AIDS and would develop mechanisms for seeing that these programs were made available in schools, to health care providers, and so forth. The screening aspect of the program would require the department to establish blood screening and counseling programs throughout the state in accordance with the provisions of the law. Evaluation might include long-term monitoring to establish whether or not the incidence of the disease was reduced and to determine the level of knowledge people in the state have about the illness and its prevention.

As mentioned earlier, some CNSs wish to influence policy decisions because they know that such decisions affect health-related behaviors. One major component of the proposed legislation is public education about AIDS and its prevention. As a provider concerned with and responsible for health education, the CNS should welcome this legislation. Government resources available to provide AIDS education would increase the likelihood of knowledge dissemination and, thus, would foster preventive health behaviors.

To effectively influence policy decisions concerning AIDS, the CNS would need to be aware of the policy context including public attitudes about the disease and the role of government as a force in addressing the problem. In this instance, media attention indicates that AIDS is seen as a major public health issue requiring governmental intervention. An assessment of the social system revealed which groups might become involved in the expected debate when the proposed legislation was introduced. Religious groups, the gay community, health care organizations, and civil libertarians would be expected to participate in the process. Allocation of the state's fiscal resources, part of the economic context, would need to be considered. In a state with a strong economy, it is more likely that funds could be provided for AIDS education and screening.

The CNS would also look at the political culture of the state from the perspective of how the proposed AIDS education and screening program would be perceived. In a state where health education is seen as a proper role for government, the CNS would expect a proposal for AIDS education to be better received than in a state where public health education is not the norm.

It would be necessary to know the components of the legislature and how they operate. For example, CNSs would need to determine what processes enable a policy idea to become law. These processes include the committees, the hearings, the voting process, and the amendment process. To be involved in preparing the policy proposal, CNSs would need to know which agencies of government would carry out the policy and be responsible for its implementation.

The role of CNSs in the policy process relates to their practice focus. For example, CNSs employed by the division of public health would analyze how previous infectious disease policies were handled.

The attitudes of various agencies of government about similar decisions and how they have been addressed would be the focus of attention. Questions to be asked might include: what agencies have been involved? What fiscal resources were made available? What types of regulations were employed?

CNSs employed by the department of public health would be involved with all phases of the policy process. CNSs in a community health setting or involved with the treatment of AIDS patients in hospitals would be more likely to be directly involved in the first four steps of the process. For example, these CNSs could have brought the problem to the attention of the department of public health and worked with them to get the issue on the agenda, formulate the policy, and lobby for the adoption of the policy. Other CNSs, when alerted to the proposed legislation, could contact legislators, send letters to the editors of their local newspapers in support of the bill, and encourage other nurses to assist in the lobbying effort.

Once the bill became law, community health and hospital-based CNSs could play a major role in planning how their agencies would work with the department of public health to implement and evaluate the AIDS education and screening program.

## SUMMARY

This chapter has provided the CNS with an overview of the policy process and the rationale for CNS involvement through political action. As indicated by the examples given, the CNS is in a position to provide expert clinical knowledge about many health policy issues. Furthermore, the CNS's skills can be readily applied to influence outcomes that affect health care directly and indirectly. Some suggestions have been provided as to how CNSs can put their unique contributions to work influencing this process. As indicated by the levels of political action, there is something for all CNSs to do, whatever the level of interest or availability. The challenge and the opportunity are there. If CNSs are to fulfill the social obligations of the role, they must become involved.

The views expressed in this chapter are solely those of the author, and official endorsement by The Robert Wood Johnson Foundation is not intended and should not be inferred.

## References

American Journal of Nursing (ed): Newscaps. Am J Nurs *11*:1288, 1986.
American Nurses' Association: Nursing: A Social Policy Statement (Publ. No. NP-63). Kansas City, ANA, 1980.
Anderson, J.: Public Policy Making: Decisions and Their Implications (2nd ed). New York, Holt, Rinehart & Winston, 1979.
Bullock, C., Anderson, J., and Brady, D.: Public Policy in the Eighties. Monterey, CA, Brooks/Cole Publishing Co., 1983.
Cole, E.: Introduction. *In* Mason, D., and Talbott, S. (eds): Political Action Handbook for Nurses. Menlo Park, CA, Addison-Wesley, 1985.
Department of Health and Human Services: Health care spending's share of GNP reaches a new high. Medical Benefits *16*:1–2, 1986.
Diers, D.: Policy and politics. *In* Mason, D., and Talbott, S. (eds): Political Action Handbook for Nurses. Menlo Park, CA, Addison-Wesley, 1985.
Griffith, H.: Implementation of direct 3rd party reimbursement legislation for nursing services. Nurs Econ *6*:299–304, 1986.
Hartley, S.: Effects of prospective pricing on nursing. Nurs Econ *1*:16–18, 1986.
Kalisch, B., & Kalisch, P.: Politics and Nursing. Philadelphia, JB Lippincott, 1982.
Lake, R., & Lamper-Linden, C.: A subject bibliography on legislative and political action. Nurs Health Care *6*:334–337, 1983.
Larson, E.: Health policy and NIH: Implications for nursing research. Nurs Res *6*:352–356, 1984.
MacMillan-Scattergood, D.: Ethical conflicts in a prospective payment home health environment. Nurs Econ *4*:165–169, 1986.
Milio, N.: Promoting Health Through Public Policy. Philadelphia, FA Davis Co., 1981.
Peplau, H.: Is nursing's self-regulatory power being eroded? Am J Nurs *2*:141–145, 1985.
Sapolsky, H., & Altman, S.: Federal health programs: An overview. *In* Altman, S., and Sapolsky, H. (eds): Federal Health Programs. Lexington, MA, Lexington Books, 1981.
Torrens, P.: Historical evolution and overview of health services in the United States. *In* Williams, S., & Torrens, P. (eds): Introduction to Health Services (2nd ed). New York, John Wiley & Sons, 1984.
White, D., & Hamel, P.: National center for nursing research: How it came to be. Nurs Econ *1*:19–22, 1986.

# The CNS and
# The Nurse
# Practitioner

*Harriet J. Kitzman*

## INTRODUCTION

The 1980s have brought extensive changes to the health care industry and important challenges to the health care professions. Concomitant with those changes and challenges has come the maturation of the role of the master's-prepared nursing specialist in the delivery of health care. Specialists in nursing with advanced degrees have been classified in a general way as either nurse practitioners (NPs) or clinical nurse specialists (CNSs). Elsewhere, individual histories describing the development of the CNS role and that of the NP role have been compiled (Kitzman, 1983; Sparacino, 1986), and descriptions of educational programs to prepare nurses for those roles have been set forth. Certification programs for NP and CNS role encumbents are available. All this is evidence of the evolving institutionalization of these roles.

While extensive histories of CNS and NP role development are available, many questions remain. Among these are questions having to do with the contributions of each role as well as their similarities and differences. It has been difficult, in general, to identify which group has been responsible for specific advances in the practice of nursing. Developing concurrently, CNSs and NPs have contributed significantly to the evolution of each other's role. It might be argued that CNSs, being first on the health care scene, created the climate necessary for the full recognition of the existence of an advanced body of clinical nursing knowledge and skills, identified the need to keep clinical practice central in the advanced study of the discipline, and provided the opportunity to demonstrate the impact of professional practice autonomy within the structure of nursing. The CNS was not a staff nurse or a supervisor but was recognized within the structure of nursing for clinical expertise.

Similarly, it might be argued that NPs established a new practice role for nursing which required new skills, new understanding, and particularly new behaviors, a role that acknowledged and demonstrated a more complete contribution of nursing to health care (Mauksch, 1968). NPs also demonstrated the impact of professional role autonomy within the structure of interdisciplinary practice. The NP became recognized within the interdisciplinary structure as the physician's colleague instead of the physician's nurse. In short, while strides had been made by CNSs in the direction of new attitudes and behaviors in clinical practice long before NPs appeared (Fagin, 1986), the NP movement hastened the CNS's development.

Some of the lack of clarity in the differentiation between CNS and NP contributions has to do with different conceptualizations of the roles. For example, a decade ago Ford (1979b) described the NP as a nurse for all settings: "The nurse practitioner is fast becoming the norm for qualified professional nurses regardless of setting in which they find themselves" (p. 516). The ANA's scope of practice statement, however, described the NP as a provider of primary care (1976). If these two statements are considered simultaneously, the implication is that all care by well-qualified nurses is primary care, regardless of the services provided. This is a statement few would accept, at least when primary care is considered ambulatory care. Such statements appear to represent different fundamental conceptualizations of the two roles.

Until recently, the differences and similarities of the NP and the CNS had not been fully described. Thus, there has emerged no common understanding of their interrelationships. What can be said individually about the CNS or the NP? Have the histories of these two groups been sufficiently separate as to expose the members to different professional socialization? What has been the impact of the changing health care system on roles, and what can be expected in the future? The discussion that follows will build upon the schema provided in the first edition (Kitzman, 1983) for examining these differences and similarities. In so doing, the events that have precipitated changes in the interrelationships between NPs and CNSs will be identified, and the consequences these changes are likely to have for the master's-prepared specialist in nursing will be proposed.

# CHARACTERISTICS OF THE NP AND CNS ROLES

## Professionalism

The quality of professional socialization is a central concern. When considering professionalism as marked by professional character, spirit, or methods, CNSs are not distinguishable from NPs. The NP was seen as being able to create a new image for the nurse, demonstrating the health services that can be offered by a nurse prepared with increased professional knowledge and skills as well as with new attitudes about role autonomy, responsibility, and accountability within the organization of health services. The CNS has been professionally socialized to project the same image. In order to be effective in professional practice and in interdisciplinary health care planning, implementation, and evaluation, both NPs and CNSs "use sophisticated clinical knowledge . . . demonstrate a high level of accountability to persons served and to teammates, and . . . assume roles commensurate with professional nursing preparation" (Ford, 1979a, p. 113).

Since level of education is often considered a measure of professionalism, it is important to examine the educational programs of each group. One finds that the length and level of professional education for NPs and CNSs are, with some exceptions, comparable. CNSs have historically been prepared at the master's level. While the majority of early NP programs led to certificates of completion, this trend was reversed and by fiscal 1985, 81 per cent of the NP programs funded by the Division of Nursing, Public Health Service, U.S. Department of Health and Human Services led to a master's degree (Geolot, 1987).

Since CNS and NP educational programs with their accompanying professional socialization are becoming comparable with regard to level and length, one might expect professional recognition and accountability to also be comparable. Recognition for advanced practice competence is established for both NP and CNS through the profession's certification programs. Such recognition is taking on increased importance for the populations served.

An important component of professionalism is recognition of the need for continued learning and for updating skills and information. While continuing education is not a substitute for a formal advanced program, it is part of the professional's responsibility. As knowledge expands and the scope of nursing practice changes, the professional will have the skills required to continue to learn and to practice using current knowledge and technology. Both NPs and CNSs are taking advantage of the continuing education opportunities currently available.

## Range of Knowledge and Skills

Range of knowledge and skills can be considered in two dimensions: breadth versus depth and assessment versus intervention. Although both NPs and CNSs have a range of knowledge and skills that enable them to retain a holistic approach to patient care, differences have existed with regard to the depth and application of knowledge and skills. NPs have been expected to possess and utilize a broad range of physical, psychosocial, and environmental assessment skills; they have been expected to respond to the full spectrum of common health and illness problems of the population for which they provide care. The NP's assessments and interventions have been expected to be broad and complete mental, psychosocial, and physical health assessments aimed at total well-being.

CNSs, while retaining a holistic approach to the patient, have been able to be more selective in competencies developed. They have focused on aspects of care of specific populations that generally are characterized by both age and already identified health care problems. As a result, the CNS has had a narrower range of advanced assessment skills and has intervened in greater depth with a narrower spectrum of problems within the defined population served.

In general, it might be argued that systematic assessment skills and high-level clinical judgment and intervention skills have been required of both the CNS and the NP. The differences have come in the range and depth of both of these activities.

The arguments about breadth versus depth and generalist versus specialist continue. Some regard the NP as a generalist and the CNS as a specialist. Others regard them both as specialists. As nurses obtain advanced education and practice within a defined population, they develop expertise for responding to the needs of that population. That is true whether the population is one found in a health promotion clinic or in an intensive care unit. A true generalist at the advanced level with equal skills across all populations is not to be found. Nursing is too broad, and the knowledge and skill base is too advanced. It is not possible to obtain or maintain the level of expertise required for advanced practice with all populations. NPs and CNSs are both specialists because of their advanced practice expertise. The question now becomes, specialist in what?

## Practice Domain: Primary Versus Secondary and Tertiary Care

Practice domain is frequently used in defining the NP role, since this specialist was orginally seen as fulfilling health care needs in primary care. The CNS role, in contrast, developed originally in tertiary care settings, and much of the literature on the role has continued to emphasize secondary and tertiary care.

While practice domain differentiation is relevant from a historical perspective, inconsistencies based on primary care versus secondary and tertiary care services have increased. Nurses prepared in NP programs have chosen to provide specialty, nonprimary care services, and CNSs have practiced and continue to practice in primary care settings.

Curriculum experts have grappled with the issue, but no consensus has evolved. Some graduate programs have incorporated preparation for ambulatory care into existing CNS programs, while others have developed a separate primary care specialty NP program. Expansion of knowledge and clinical skills through research in all levels of care is occurring. NPs may have expanded their knowledge and clinical practice skill first in primary care settings, while CNSs may have expanded primarily in secondary and tertiary care settings; however, that distinction is no longer clear.

Will practice domain be used in the differentiation of NPs and CNSs in the future? Is primary care a specialty in its own right, or is it the core of all nursing specialties? In a thorough exposition of the NP's primary care domain of practice, Mezey (1986b) described the confusion and suggested that it originates in the different meanings of primary care. Differentiating between primary care as a mode of ambulatory care services and primary care as a concept, she proposed that the term "primary care" be reserved to describe a mode of practice delivered in ambulatory settings and that the concept of primary care—"coordinated, comprehensive care delivered throughout a course of illness, inclusion of health promotion as well as illness treatment, and the emphasis on education" (1986b, p. 41)—be considered integral to the nursing role regardless of setting. Mezey noted that it is time to "differentiate between the terms *practitioner* and *primary care*" (1986a, p. 113).

## Professional Autonomy

Because NPs carry out some medical/technical functions traditionally found in medical practice, the early development of the role found education and practice to be somewhat dependent upon the physician. CNSs, in contrast, have traditionally been prepared and have practiced exclusively within the tradition of nursing. Of all the areas of role definition, interprofessional alignment has probably produced the most conflict; from it, challenges have arisen concerning professional role identity, value systems, and allegiances.

In addition to medical/technical functions, many factors are responsible for the perception that NPs were aligned with physicians; most of these have changed since the inception of the role. Early NP programs were often co-directed by a physician and a nurse; physicians often taught a portion of the classes, particularly physical examination and history taking. This is no longer the situation, and nurse faculty are more in control of the curriculum (Geolot, 1987). In addition, in the past, many states that recognized practice of NPs have required physician sanction. Along with the increased recognition of NPs as specialists in nursing has come the recognition that nursing should govern its own practice. The recent development in Oregon, where prescriptive authority has been placed in the hands of the Board of Nursing, demonstrates the progress that has been made in this area. Early regulations in regard to NP-physician alignment that developed to govern NP practice have fallen behind actual practice and are being challenged. In this regard NP practice is becoming more similar to CNS practice, which has not required the utilization of regulations requiring a relationship with a physician.

Economic independence from physicians has been among the factors considered when determining professional autonomy. Some NPs have worked in private physicians' practices or have received their salary from the medical budget of an institution. While some NPs have had full economic and legal partnership arrangements, others have been employees of the physician's practice. In contrast, CNSs have historically been assumed under the nursing practice budget of institutions and have not received direct reimbursement from a physician or a medical budget.

Despite these considerations, the literature abounds with descriptions of well-qualified NPs and CNSs practicing with significant professional autonomy. In addition, that autonomy is being recognized through legislation. An example is the recent legislation that permits both the NP and the CNS, in collaboration with a physician, to certify and recertify the need for patient care in nursing homes (Nickels, 1987). As one examines the complex nature of health care, it becomes clear that the NP and the CNS both require professional autonomy.

## Interdisciplinary Collaboration

While nursing struggles for increased professional autonomy, the demands of health care suggest the need for greater collaboration in practice. As Mechanic and Aiken (1986) have suggested, "teamwork is no longer rhetoric about desired objectives but a reality in carrying out the technical procedures in caring for the more seriously ill hospital patients who require a greater complexity and intensity of care, and the growing numbers of patients in the community who depend on the successful coordination of medical, nursing, and social services, and rehabilitative approaches allied with other maintenance services" (p. 8).

How can the competing forces of the professional's need for autonomy, often thought to be implemented through independent practice, and the health care system's expectation of collaboration be reconciled? In order for reconciliation, it is necessary to acknowledge that professional autonomy does not require independent practice but rather can be exercised while collaborating. The need for recognition of professional autonomy, for purposes of designation of professional competence, is not inconsistent with the need for collaborative work. Indeed, as professional autonomy increases, resulting in fewer constraints on practice, barriers to interdisciplinary collaborative practice can be expected to decrease.

While to practice independently is often considered the highest level of professional competence, when it comes to health care, the highest level may in fact be collaboration. Implicit in collaborative practice is accountability for one's own practice as well as accountability to interdisciplinary colleagues for joint decision-making. In collaborative practice, the professional's expertise affects not only one's own services but also the services provided by others. In independent practice, the professional's influence is limited to those areas that are affected by independent actions. Parsons (1986) has gone so far as to challenge autonomy as a criterion of professionalism, suggesting that "nurses may decide to redefine the old prescribed norms for professional autonomy and be forthright rather than self-conscious about a preference for collaboration and consultation" (p. 274).

As one examines the complex nature of health care, it becomes clear that both the NP and the CNS require professional autonomy and colleagial relationships with physicians if the communication required to plan, implement, and evaluate clinical services is to be effective. Experience suggests that as competence increases, both NPs and CNSs are given the opportunity to demonstrate their professional autonomy while practicing collaboratively.

## Directness of Service

Historically, NPs have defined their goal generally as "to provide patient care" (Ford & Silver, 1967), while CNSs have defined their goal as "to improve patient care" (Crabtree, 1979; Holt, 1984). While these statements are oversimplifications, they do reveal the unidimensional focus of the role of the NP—to provide direct services—and the multidimensional role of the CNS—to provide both direct and indirect services. They also reveal the greater amount of time spent by the CNS in consultation, education, and general development of others who are providing direct care (Starck, 1987).

In reality, as NPs have been prepared in master's programs to carry out multiple leadership functions, they have increasingly found themselves responsible for many indirect services. In turn, as practices have advanced, many CNSs have come to hold positions in which they spend the majority of their time providing direct services. These direct care functions will be increasingly important as issues of reimbursement for nursing services come to the forefront. For example, which services will be reimbursible, and from which budget? Some scheme for making the distinction will be required.

Prior to the 1960s, advancement in nursing meant leaving direct care and becoming a supervisor or an educator. In many ways, this notion has been slow to change. Advancement through supervisory responsibilities was embedded in the structure of health care institutions, leaving no place for the advanced, clinically prepared expert who wished to provide direct services and to be recognized both structurally and financially for those direct services. Nevertheless, it has now become possible for nurses with advanced degrees to provide direct care and to achieve professional advancement through practice.

Inherent in master's preparation, whether NP or CNS, is specialization in clinical nursing, which forms the base for the expertise that is demonstrated through multiple direct and indirect care and leadership roles. These include practitioner, teacher, consultant, planner, evaluator, researcher, staff educator, patient advocate, and collaborative practitioner. The expertise in clinical nursing provides the content through which these activities are undertaken.

## SPECIALTIES IN ADVANCED PRACTICE

Part of the confusion that has come from the effort in nursing to differentiate role functions of the CNS and the NP has its foundation in the confusion regarding specialty designations. Do CNSs and NPs use the same nursing specialty classification? If not, why not? An exploration of the current specialty classification may be useful.

There has been general agreement since the early 1960s that

master's preparation in nursing should have clinical nursing as its focus, and that specialization should occur at the master's level (Williamson, 1983). Despite this agreement about specialization, however, programs have been diverse (Holt, 1984; Lash, 1987), and areas of specialization have been inconsistently defined. This inconsistency suggests that the natural divisions that form specialties have not been stable. Williamson (1983), in reviewing the National League for Nursing (NLN) brochure on graduate programs in nursing, found the nomenclature of graduate programs confusing. She found over 20 different titles in the general heading of curricula offered and over 125 different titles of specific areas of study in nursing. From this she questioned "the nature of graduate education in nursing" (p. 101).

Williamson argued that "graduate education in a discipline is conceptualized from the structure of the discipline. Indepth knowledge of a specialty area and the new skills required for practice form the basis of a graduate program" (p. 101). Following Williamson's premise that the structure of the discipline guides the division of specialties, one might then ask why nursing specialty divisions have been inconsistently defined. Have there been changes in the structure of the knowledge of the discipline which have resulted in changing specialties and the lack of consensus about specialty areas? Or, have changes in specialty divisions been driven by the changing divisions of clinical practice? Why has there been such instability in nursing's nomenclature?

There would appear to be at least three major reasons why nursing has had difficulty in the development of specialty designations. The first has to do with the development of nursing knowledge; the second involves the changing expectations produced as a result of changing needs and health care delivery modalities; the third relates to the nature of nursing itself.

The continued development of theory used to explain the phenomena of interest in nursing is apparent. Knowledge is expanding rapidly. The knowledge generated is, however, often not specific to populations that form current practice specializations. For example, using Williamson's framework, the basic knowledge of the discipline might suggest that coping with loss of function may be an area of specialization within nursing. While that may be considered the specialty of rehabilitation nursing, such knowledge is not limited in usefulness to rehabilitation nurses.

Many specialty divisions have been classified according to the medical division of care and/or the place of care. Specialization along medical divisions has its advantages in practice. Among them are the interdisciplinary interaction that is encouraged by common arrangements and the greater understanding of the disease entities, treatment regimens, and specific responses to particular diseases and treatments. One disadvantage is that many of the problems for which nursing is developing specialty expertise cut across traditional medical specialty divisions.

Place of care—institution or community—no longer provides the natural boundaries for specialty divisions of nursing care. Vertical integration of health care and the increased role of nursing in ambulatory and home care have created new demands and opportunities. For example, at one time biomedical technology was thought appropriate primarily to hospitalized patients. Today, technical supports such as ventilators are managed in the home by the patient, the family, and the nurse. Although technology still develops in acute care settings, it is rapidly moving into home care. At one time, nurses providing home care had limited responsibility for patients requiring ventilator support or complex intravenous therapy; today, such responsibility is commonplace.

The third reason for difficulty in designating specialties has to do with the nature of nursing practice. While nurses traditionally define specialty by population, such as pediatric pulmonary nursing, within that population, nurses are holistic in their approach. For example, the specialized nurse would care not only for the patient's pulmonary needs. It could be argued that a portion of the success of the NP can be attributed to the breadth of preparation that has facilitated overall clinical decision-making and the development of holistic nursing practice. As Reed and Hoffman (1986) identified, with "the introduction of the phrase comprehensive health care, the highly specialized individual may not be able to address the interaction of an individual's subsystems within the complex physical, psychological and social environment" (p. 44). The knowledge and skills that allow nurses to address this interaction are not always population-specific but are instead applicable to many populations. Although specialization at the advanced level is necessary, breadth sufficient to support holistic care needs to be retained.

While there are multiple factors interfering with the stabilization of nursing specialty nomenclature, specialization remains necessary for advanced practice, whether NP or CNS. Are the clinical specialties different for the NP and CNS? The answer seems likely to be no, although there may be different demands for direct care and leadership role functions in different settings.

In summary, specialization appropriately comes from the designation of areas of clinical expertise. This specialization should not be confused with role functions such as provider, educator, consultant, or administrator.

## CORE IN ADVANCED PRACTICE

This leads to questions for the NP and CNS about core knowledge and skills for advanced practice, regardless of specialty. Are there within graduate programs "commonalities in content, skills, and practices that apply no matter what the specialized area of preparation?" (Dumas, 1986, p. 30). It can be argued that a significant portion of the knowledge expansion that is occurring in nursing is core knowledge— knowledge that can be used in understanding the nursing needs of multiple populations. If this is true, the amount of core knowledge and skills can be expected to increase with continued theory development and clinical research.

Regardless of title, when nurses in advanced practice are involved in the direct delivery of care that is comprehensive, holistic, and continuing, they will need to draw upon core knowledge that will permit them to address the interaction of an individual patient's subsystems. While they may have knowledge specific to that patient population and can consider themselves specialists, the broader perspective from which they draw will be apparent.

The more complete the delineation of the core, the greater will be the understanding of the commonalities and differences of the specialties and the role functions. Also, greater will be the public's understanding of the competencies that can be expected of nurses in advanced practice.

## MERGING THE CNS AND NP ROLES

Kitzman (1983) called for greater clarity in specialization based on natural divisions that emerge out of practice. She noted that previous NP and CNS role distinctions were blurring. Spross and Hamric (1983) moved further and described a generic master's-prepared nurse specialist.

Mezey (1986a) recommended that the term nurse practitioner be used to designate a "specialist prepared at the masters level who delivers direct nursing services to patients irregardless of setting. The scope of practice of these practitioners derived from a blend of knowledge and skills which originated in both primary care and clinical specialist practice" (p. 113).

Support for the merging of roles can be found in *Characteristics of Master's Education in Nursing* adopted by the NLN in 1987. This document advocates a blend of advanced clinical practice and role preparation for graduates of master's programs. This blend is expected to produce "outcomes of leadership, management, teaching, research, intellectual curiosity, creative inquiry, collaborative and consultative skills, and professionalism" (Starck, 1987, p. 20).

Acceptance of a common understanding of the characteristics of a master's prepared specialist in clinical nursing who delivers direct nursing services would seem an appropriate place to begin. As core content and skills are better delineated and the areas of clinical specialization which make use of this core are more commonly understood, the competencies of the master's prepared nurse in advanced practice will be clarified. The competencies will not need to be designated by two roles, NP and CNS, but can be designated by one (practitioner/ specialist or some acceptable title). The role functions of consultant, educator, and so forth, which may be carried out by the master's-prepared nurse with specialization in an area of clinical practice, can then be separated from the direct provider role and identified by the function itself. Designation according to function will aid in the identification of the multiple services of master's-prepared nurses which need to be reimbursed as well as the potential sources of reimbursement for these functions.

## TITLING

In February 1987, members of the executive committees of the Council of Clinical Nurse Specialists and the Council of Primary Health Care Nurse Practitioners met at ANA headquarters to discuss common issues ("Advanced nursing practitioners," 1987). With agreement among the members that earlier distinctions between NPs and CNSs were fading, members asked the questions: "Should nurse practitioners and clinical nurse specialists carry the same title? If so, what should that title be?" (p. 19). These questions were not surprising; the differences between NPs and CNSs had become less clear and a call for singular titling had already been made (Kitzman, 1983; Spross and Hamric, 1983; and Mezey, 1986a), as noted above.

Titling is of greatest consequence during periods of transition, and the challenges to singular titling which have been generated following the ANA Council's report could well have been expected. For singular titling to occur, some or all must give up something. Currently, some master's-prepared nurses call themselves CNSs when interacting with some populations and NPs when interacting with others; even they are uneasy about giving up either title or accepting yet another. The titles hold different meanings to the different populations, and the individual nurses involved have a desire to match the title to the meaning they wish to convey.

Acceptance of a single title will undoubtedly be slow in coming. While titles are important for many reasons, it is easy to argue that nursing should be guided by societal needs and that the greatest importance of the title lies with the message that it conveys to the population served. One argument that might be put forth for a single title of "nurse practitioner" has to do with the fact that the NP has been legally recognized in most states. Thus, to retain that title would facilitate the public's continued understanding and recognition of advanced practice competency.

Nursing might concentrate on the emerging health care needs and make a decision on a title that would most accurately reflect the characteristics required to respond to those needs.

## Nurse Administrator and Nurse Practitioner/Specialist

Friedson (1986) identified three major factors that have contributed to changes in the profession of medicine. These are: (1) the method of financing health care, including the introduction of Medicaid and Medicare; (2) the advancement of technology, including limits to its appropriateness; and (3) the growth of competition. Just as these factors have precipitated changes in the medical profession, so have they precipitated changes in nursing. The changes have the potential to significantly affect the roles of master's-prepared nurses.

It might be proposed that the impact of these factors falls into two main categories: delivery of services and administration of services. With these changes the best prepared nurses are being given the opportunity to demonstrate the impact of quality nursing care on total health care utilization and costs. Once reimbursement is conceptualized through a capitated system as opposed to a fee-for-service system, the challenge to provide services that constrain the growth of overall health care expenditures becomes evident. Nursing now has the opportunity to define more completely the work of professional nursing in terms of patient outcome. Nursing can demonstrate the impact of its orientation to health; to skilled, compassionate care; and to optimal patient functioning on overall health care costs.

This opportunity cannot be actualized, however, without the leadership of nurses with highly developed administrative and managerial skills who can deal with the challenges precipitated by new methods of competition and financing. Nurses have important knowledge of the needs of patients and the resources required to meet those needs. Through assuming leadership in the health care system, nurses can use that knowledge in shaping policy and creating the opportunity to demonstrate patient outcomes that are associated with quality nursing care.

The nursing supervisor of the past has been replaced by a large cadre of well-prepared nurse administrators with staff who concentrate on the development of systems, methods, and procedures, documentation of quality, staff development, resource utilization, and so forth. Just as the physician administrator-executive has emerged, so has the nurse executive (Butts, Berger, and Brooten, 1986).

The differences between the NP and CNS today will likely be shifted to the differences between the nurse practitioner/specialist and the nurse administrator. Just as there have been commonalities in competencies of the NP and CNS, so will there be commonalities between the practitioner/specialist and the nurse administrator. Overlap will come in their common socialization to the discipline and to the practice of nursing at the advanced level and in leadership that can be expected from the professional nurse with an advanced degree. The practitioner/specialist would concentrate on the planning, provision, and evaluation of care, however, and the nurse administrator would concentrate on the development and maintenance of those systems that support care.

Nursing will not have the opportunity to demonstrate its potential in health care without careful attention to the development of systems that facilitate high-quality practice. In a prepaid system, one's contribution must be measured or it does not exist (Light, 1986). The new nurse administrators will have the capacity to understand the practitioner/specialists' potential and to develop systems that ensure that their contribution will be possible and can be measured. Innovation in nursing care delivery can be the hallmark as competencies for high-quality practice emerge from the combined NP/CNS competencies and are supported by well-prepared nurse administrators who can creatively shape the systems for practice.

## SUMMARY

The primary goal of NPs and CNSs is the same—to make available to the population served the highest quality of nursing care possible. That goal is met through creation of an environment that recognizes and facilitates excellent patient care, the provision of that care, and the continuing understanding and development of care processes. Research is needed to develop an understanding of the potential and the limits of nursing care provided by master's-prepared specialists in clinical nursing; it is also needed to disentangle the effects of economic and sociopolitical factors from those of clinical nursing expertise.

The distinctions between the CNS and NP are historical in nature, and many differences that once existed are no longer evident. The advanced clinical practice competencies of the master's-prepared nurse, whether NP or CNS, should be the continued focus.

As the shortage of nurses threatens, specialists may be considered a luxury; many may argue that the emphasis needs to be placed upon getting more nurses into the profession. This is short-sighted, however, since many of the factors that are currently thought to keep young people out of nursing (lack of professional autonomy, low status, and so forth) are just those that can be most readily countered by the nurse in advanced practice who functions in a system in which opportunities have been facilitated by the work of skilled nurse administrators. As more nurses at the advanced level demonstrate nursing's potential, nursing will become more attractive as a profession.

The challenges of the advanced practitioner of clinical nursing have never been greater. Demonstration of patient outcomes from nursing practice today has the potential to open up new opportunities for nursing, even as advanced care has the potential to improve the health and quality of life of its recipients. As Light (1986) has identified, "capitated systems will seek clinicians with the ability to minimize hospitalization, to ration ambulatory care wisely, to teach patients how to manage their problems themselves and to use fewer services, and to know how to manage a clinical team effectively" (p. 531). Are not these the skills that nursing has been striving to develop in its advanced practitioners, albeit at times indirectly?

Creating a clear understanding of the expected competencies of the master's-prepared advanced practitioner will be useful in our intraprofessional relationships, interprofessional relationships, and nurse/consumer relationships.

## References

Advanced nursing practitioners discuss common destiny. Am Nurs April p. 19, 1987.

American Nurses' Association: The Scope of Nursing Practice. Kansas City, American Nurses' Association, 1976.

Butts, P., Berger, B., Brooten, D.: Tracking down the right degree for the job. Nurs Health Care, 7:91–95, 1986.

Crabtree, M.: Effective utilization of clinical specialists within the organizational structure of hospital nursing services. Nurs Admin Q 4:1–10, 1979.

Dumas, R.: Challenging the curriculum: The future of specialization. *In* National League for Nursing (ed): Patterns in Specialization: Challenge to the Curriculum. New York, National League for Nursing, 1986, pp. 27–37.

Fagin, C. M.: Primary care as an academic discipline. *In* Mezey, M., and McGivern, D.

394  Harriet J. Kitzman

(eds): Nurses, Nurse Practitioners: The Evolution of Primary Care. Boston, Little, Brown and Company, 1986, pp. 29–36.
Ford, L.: The future of pediatric nurse practitioners. Pediatrics 64:113–114, 1979a.
Ford, L.: A nurse for all settings: The nurse practitioner. Nurs Outlook 27:516–521, 1979b.
Ford, L., and Silver, H.: Expanded role of the nurse in child care. Nurs Outlook 15:43–45, 1967.
Friedson, E.: The medical profession in transition. In Aiken, L., and Mechanic, D. (eds): Applications of Social Science to Clinical Medicine and Health Policy. New Brunswick, NJ, Rutgers University Press, 1986, pp. 63–79.
Geolot, D.: NP education: Observations from a national perspective. Nurs Outlook 35:132–135, 1987.
Holt, F.: A theoretical model for clinical specialist practice. Nurs Health Care 5:445–449, 1984.
Kitzman, H.: The CNS and the nurse practitioner. In Hamric, A., and Spross, J. (eds): The Clinical Nurse Specialist in Theory and Practice. New York, Grune and Stratton, 1983, pp. 275–290.
Lash, A.: Rival conceptions in doctoral education in nursing and their outcomes: An update. J Nurs Educ 26:221–227, 1987.
Light, D.: (1986). Surplus versus cost containment: The changing context for health providers. In Aiken, L., and Mechanic, D. (eds): Applications of Social Science to Clinical Medicine and Health Policy. New Brunswick, NJ, Rutgers University Press, 1986, pp. 519–542.
Mauksch, I.: The nurse practitioner movement: Where does it go from here? Am J Public Health 68:1074–1075, 1978.
Mechanic, D., and Aiken, L.: Social science, medicine, and health policy. In Aiken, L., and Mechanic, D. (eds): Applications of Social Science to Clinical Medicine and Health Policy. New Brunswick, NJ, Rutgers University Press, 1986, pp. 1–13.
Mezey, M.: Issues in graduate education. In Mezey, M., and McGivern, D. (eds): Nurses, Nurse Practitioners: The Evolution of Primary Care. Boston, Little, Brown and Company, 1986a, pp. 101–119.
Mezey, M.: The future of primary care and nurse practitioners. In Mezey, M., and McGivern, D. (eds): Nurses, Nurse Practitioners: The Evolution of Primary Care. Boston, Little, Brown and Company, 1986b, pp. 37–51.
Nickels, P.: Hundredth congress faces difficult issues in 87. Am Nurs 19:7, 10, Feb., 1987.
Parsons, M.: The profession in a class by itself. Nurs Outlook 34:270–275, 1986.
Reed, S., and Hoffman, S.: The enigma of graduate nursing education: Advanced generalist? Specialist? Nurs Health Care 7:43–49, 1986.
Sparacino, P.: The clinical nurse specialist. Nurs Pract 1(4):215–228, 1986.
Sparacino, P., & Durand, B.: Editorial on specialization in advanced nursing practice. Momentum 4(2):2–3, 1986.
Spross, J., and Hamric, A.: A model for future clinical specialist practice. In Hamric, A., and Spross, J. (eds): The Clinical Nurse Specialist in Theory and Practice. New York: Grune and Stratton, 1983, pp. 291–306.
Starck, P.: The master's prepared nurse in the market place; What do master's prepared nurses do? What should they do? In Hunt, S. (ed): Issues in Graduate Nursing Education. New York, National League for Nursing, 1987, pp. 3–23.
Williamson, J. A.: Master's education: A need for nomenclature. Image 15:99–101, 1983.

# PART V

# INNOVATIVE PRACTICE MODELS

Chapter
# The CNS in a Consultation Department

## 19

*Beverly L. Malone*

## INTRODUCTION

The future of the CNS is inventible, not inevitable. For this statement to be actualized, the CNS and administrator need to develop successful models of organization and work which protect the viability of the CNS role in the delivery of health care services. The purpose of this chapter is to provide CNSs and administrators with a model taken from a department that was successful in maintaining and supporting a CNS role while responding to cost-containment concerns. This was accomplished by helping CNSs become consultants and revenue generators. The effective application of this model is highly dependent upon the extent of the collaboration between the CNS and the administrator.*

Through the collaborative efforts of the CNSs and administrator, in a three-year period a consultation department of 17 members grew to a department of 25 members. Beginning with only a budget for personnel, no secretarial support, and limited office space, the department acquired a budget of $100,000, three secretaries, a business manager, statistician, research director, and first floor administrative office space for the department.

Productivity increased from approximately four published articles per year for the institution to 22 per year. Over the three years, income generation moved from zero to $450,000 per year. This income resulted from internal and external consulting contracts with private industry and community health care institutions and from research grants with local, state, and federal agencies. Five of the original 17 CNSs in the

---

*Nursing administrator will be referred to as administrator.

department returned to school to acquire doctoral preparation with the identified goal of returning and further expanding the CNS role.

## CONSULTATION: THE ORGANIZING FRAMEWORK

The most frequently used concept of consultation can be described as the purchase of expert information or an expert service. There is usually a basic assumption that the purchaser is clear about what kind of information or service is needed. The CNS often works under this type of contract with the head nurse, the nursing unit, or the nursing department. The consultation model to be described in this text incorporates this fundamental description while broadening the concept to include situations in which the purchaser is unclear about the need or service required. This model involves joint assessment, diagnosis, problem-solving, and evaluation by the purchaser and the consultant. Schein (1969) refers to these aspects as process consultation.

With this model of consultation as a framework, there is room to consider who the purchasers might be. In the most traditional use of the model, the purchasers of CNS services are nursing departments and sometimes physicians. However, the present consultation model extends the purchasers to include health care administrators, private industries, research and development units, nursing homes, other health care agencies, and the community-at-large. With the definition of purchaser expanded, there is simultaneous expansion of the marketing targets and thereby an increased possibility of income generation from sources outside nursing. The income generated can serve to offset the cost of the CNS to the nursing department and to the overall hospital budget.

In an article published in 1973, Newton described the role of a group therapist. He highlighted the demand characteristic for the therapist to simultaneously manage the internal and external boundaries of the group. This task is not a simple process. The CNS is in a similar position. CNSs cannot affort to focus solely on the internal workings of their patients, units, and self-defined areas of responsibility. CNSs who have assumed that they had this option have found their positions at risk from an administrative, budgetary perspective. It is therefore safe to conclude that CNSs must manage their internal responsibilities while monitoring and intervening in a positive way in the external suprasystems of the health care organization in which they work. The use of a consultation model provides the option for income generation through clinical practice, education, and research. Within this framework the internal and external boundaries and demands become manageable.

Historically, consultation has always been part of the CNS's role. However, until now CNSs consulted only internally. The benefits of their services were frequently lost within the nursing bureaucracy due to a lack of supervision, clear evaluation strategies, or the inability of the nursing department to quantify in dollars the quality of the CNS's work. The CNS must take the next step and develop skills and techniques for consulting for a fee outside the nursing department.

At this point, the reader may be puzzled about the exclusive focus on the consultative role component of the CNS. The entire structure of the income-generating, hospital-based, consultation department was built on strengthening the consultative aspect of the CNS's role. Admittedly, there are other critical components of the CNS role: clinician, educator, researcher, and, some might add, administrator. However, it is a basic tenet of the model that all other components, excluding administration, could be incorporated under consultation. (The characteristic of legitimate authority to hire and fire prevents the administration role component from inclusion under the umbrella of consultation.)

The following example might be helpful in illustrating the overriding theme of consultation within the established model. In a hospital setting, a CNS is providing ostomy care to a patient. The CNS is gentle, highly competent, and teaches naturally as the service is provided to the patient. There is no witness to this expert one-on-one care, but the patient's expression of comfort and ease with his changed body image is reflective of the quality interchange that occurs daily between him and the CNS. The CNS experiences great internal satisfaction from the interaction and caregiving process. The CNS considers the possibility of an article or research project about some aspect of the interaction.

What is wrong with this encounter from a consultation prespective? In situations such as hospitals, in which the CNS is not the 24-hour primary provider of nursing care, there has to be an emphasis on the skill and ability of the primary nurse provider. This provider is usually a staff nurse. The expertise of the CNS must be shared with the 24-hour nurse provider to ensure consistency and availability of quality nursing care for the patient. Therefore, if one reviews the previous example, the absence of a staff nurse as a learner, observer, and participant mitigates the lasting positive effect of the interaction between the CNS and the patient. From a budgetary and administrative perspective, the CNS whose expertise is shared with the 24-hour nurse provider is a better investment than the CNS whose expert care disappears from the setting at the end of the day or during periods of illness, workshops, and vacations.

In terms of publication and research aspects of the CNS and patient interaction example, the addition of a staff nurse to the equation represents a giant leap for the nursing profession. Through the facilitative and consultative efforts of the CNS, a staff nurse can become involved in publishing and research. This would represent an exemplary model of applying theory to practice and of having education and service meet at the patient's bedside. There is also the increased possibility that the staff nurse who is stimulated by publishing and research will be the staff nurse who will pursue higher education.

There is another major benefit to the consultation model proposed in this chapter. When the CNS functions in a consultative role, there are clear boundaries between the roles of the CNS and the role of the primary nurse provider. The staff nurse and the nurse managers responsible for the area of care are the purchasers of the CNS's expert services. The patient is a client of the primary nurse provider who coordinates all aspects of the patient's care. In this model, "all aspects of the patient's care" include medical to housekeeping needs. The CNS and the primary nurse provider jointly assess, diagnose, problem-solve, and evaluate the patient's care. With clear boundaries and expert consultation, the patient is more consistently assured of holistic and cost-effective quality care on a 24-hour basis.

## CONSULTATION MODEL

The goals of the consultation model were to: (1) enhance the delivery of patient care by providing expert information and learning to primary nurse providers; (2) become revenue generators through actualizing the role of the CNS in the areas of clinical expertise, education, and research; and (3) survive the "downsizing" of health care institutions while moving to an innovative stage for developing the CNS role.

With an emphasis on a consulting model, the following corresponding concepts must be addressed: contracting for or purchasing services, fees for service, time management, marketing, and evaluation.

Once the goals of the model had been identified, it became essential to create an organizational structure to facilitate the implementation of the model. This was accomplished through centralizing the CNSs under one department head. This department head was doctorally prepared, had previously been a CNS, and was presently responsible for staff development and education. There were advantages and disadvantages to the centralized structure. The advantages were all related to future goals: implementation of the consultation model, resulting in more consistent delivery of quality patient care; improved supervision and development of the individual CNS in the role; increased research and publication efforts by the CNS; and increased revenue generation.

The disadvantages were more related to the here and now. Roles and functions developed over time would be disrupted, which could result in the decrease of CNS direct patient care contact. Reporting relationships to administrators, who were also responsible for the nurse managers and the day-to-day operation of the institution, would be disrupted. This could lead to reduced CNS information and reduced power to act and intervene. The CNS role would be lost due to the replacement of staff development and education activities. If centralization was the preliminary step to eliminating the CNS role by wiping out one targeted cost center, there was potential loss of a job. Perhaps the greatest disadvantage was that the initial proposal for a consultation department was introduced by the nursing administration without the collaboration or input from the CNS. Once the implications of this mistake were recognized, a more collaborative process of joint meetings and discussions began. However, the lack of jointly beginning such an innovative proposal produced anger and added validity to the aforementioned disadvantages. Due to this imperfect beginning, an administrative decision to initiate the consultation model was made. This decision was based on the threat to the budgetary survival and growth of the CNS role.

## Contracting for Service

The consultation model incorporated the concept of contracting from two major perspectives: internal contracting and external contracting. The internal contracting process frequently involved the primary nurse provider, nurse managers at various levels of administration, physicians, and any other individuals or groups under the umbrella of the overall institution. For example, in the original model, the College of Nursing and Health was identified as a prospective internal contractor since the college and the hospital were both part of the medical center complex under the umbrella of the university.

### Internal Contracting

The implementation of contracting began with an assessment of what the department members were doing, internally and externally, and equally important, exactly what services were being given away. This meant renegotiating previously established relationships in which CNS time was expected and demanded as a free service. CNSs reviewed their relationships with the College of Nursing and assessed at what point their contribution to the students' training should become a joint appointment arrangement, with parts of their salaries covered. They also reviewed their relationships with physicians, especially those situations in which private work was being performed without reimbursement. The following is an example of internal contracting.

The diabetes CNS, a born entrepreneur, took very seriously the series of discussions that focused on the fact that nursing services could no longer be given away. She approached her physician colleagues. For several years, twice a week, she had conducted classes for the private patients of her physician colleagues. It had not occurred to her to suggest reimbursement even though she knew the importance of the information she regularly shared with her patients. She felt a great deal of internal satisfaction. Yet, these private patients were charged for her teaching time, and the money was placed in the physicians' coffers, known as the Faculty Practice Plan. The CNS's concern about reimbursement was greeted with shock and disbelief by the physicians. She requested that her administrator intervene.

The physician and his business manager met with the administrator and the CNS. The administrator's argument was logical. With budgets tightening and hospital reimbursement patterns changing, the CNS's role was in jeopardy. Although nursing would be pleased to give away free service to physicians, there was no longer a choice. Hours of CNS service had to be monitored and appropriately charged to the users, or the expert service of CNS would cease to exist. Both physician and business manager reluctantly acknowledged the validity of the argument, and a verbal agreement was reached. The meeting ended successfully.

Within 15 minutes of the close of the meeting, the physician was on the phone to the administrator disclaiming the validity of the agreement and angrily lamenting nursing's absence of compassion for patients and the excessive costs of health care. The administrator's response was that this nursing service would stop until an agreement was reached.

Two weeks later, the medical department had purchased one-fifth of the diabetes CNS's time. This small victory inspired the CNSs to continue to develop the department, for they had witnessed the impossible become the possible. At this point, it must be noted that the chief nursing executive agreed and supported the administrator's withdrawal of services. Without this support, the issue could have ended in nursing's defeat. This represented a major breakthrough with physician colleagues.

A different aspect of internal contracting, one that did not involve reimbursement, was the contracts between the CNS and the clinical administrator. These contracts were part of nursing administration's insurance package to guarantee that the CNS would remain involved with individual clinical areas. The detailed content of the contract was worked out with the first line nurse managers (head nurses) and their immediate supervisors, who were called directors. The CNS would then negotiate with the nursing administrator responsible for those clinical areas which goals were most important and needed immediate attention. Through this process, targeted goals for the year were identified and mutually agreed upon by the CNS and the clinical administrator. Also included in the contract was the method of evaluation to be used by the nursing administrator (Table 19–1).

### External Contracting

External contracting (Table 19–2) simply involves anyone outside of the overall institution. One of the major tasks for implementing the model was the clear identification of prospective clientele in the external contracting arena. Four major groupings emerged: community health care institutions, private industry, local and state government, and federal government.

Internal contracts, regardless of amounts, never had the appeal of the first external contract. For example, the general medicine CNS had been working on obtaining funds to study hypothermia blankets from a nursing care perspective. She had selected a chief manufacturer of the product, had attempted to stimulate interest in the research, and was repeatedly stonewalled. Phone calls were randomly returned, and when contact was made, double messages were frequently communicated from the sales representative. In a remarkable collaborative move, the College of Nursing's associate dean for research, who also had an appointment in the department of nursing, suggested the luncheon strategy. She and the CNS took the indecisive sales representatives to lunch and convinced them to visit the institution. The sales representatives, who brought along their director of research, were impressed with the technology and resources within a major medical center. Furthermore, they were impressed with the breadth and depth of the CNS's knowledge of the utility, scientific basis, and practicality of their products. As a result an agreement was reached. For the year, a $10,000 retainer fee was established to secure the services of the consultation department. The services included review and feedback on new prod-

**TABLE 19–1. Consultation Department Internal Contract: Enterostomal Therapy CNS**

**Sign and date to indicate agreement with contract:**

(signature) _____ (date) _____

| GOAL | ACTION | EVALUATION |
|---|---|---|
| Increase the nursing staff's skills in the technique of pouching. | 1. Evaluate staff's pouching techniques by clinical observation and demonstration and informal staff meetings during daily patient care rounds on the units.<br>2. Offer inservices on pouching techniques when a need has been identified and/or provide inservice upon request by staff or head nurse.<br>3. Keep staff updated on new approaches to pouching and changes in equipment through memos, inservices, and demonstrations.<br>4. Encourage clinical nurses to assume responsibility of pouch changes and maintenance of adequate pouching supplies for individual patients. Be available to demonstrate, assist, and support the staff upon request by page.<br>5. Consult with the staff regarding difficult pouching situations. Facilitate problem-solving, development of a plan, and evaluation of results upon request.<br>6. Introduce staff to innovative uses of pouching (i.e., fecal incontinence, draining wounds, and fistula) in response to patient care needs by inservice and/or demonstration.<br>7. Continue with the development of E.T. resource nurses. | 1. Available by page.<br>2. Daily record sheet will reflect number of referrals, areas from which referrals were received, reason for referral, and total number of E.T. nurse visits.<br>3. Bimonthly report of activities submitted to director of the consultation department.<br>4. Monthly time log will reflect total amount of time spent in the various clinical areas.<br>5. Staff and head nurse feedback.<br>6. Annual workshop for new E.T. resource nurses. Continued development of present E.T. resource nurses during regular follow-up meetings and one-on-one development on the units. |

Developed at the University Hospital, University of Cincinnati.

ucts from various perspectives: cardiac, neurological, diabetes, home health, and so forth. The nursing administrator guaranteed that, with a three-day notice, feedback on the utility of new products would occur. The feedback sessions involved deciding which CNSs needed to be and could be present to collectively discuss a new potential product. The CNSs were consistently impressive and informative, not only to the company but also to one another. Their confidence in their own consultative abilities grew.

A second client service was gathering background information or data about an unfamiliar piece of equipment to help a sales representative prepare a presentation. Such service may require access to extensive medical literature. The third type of service most frequently requested was bringing together a panel of experts, e.g., anesthesiologist, microbiologist, and pharmacist. The consultation department would play a coordinator role, providing the experts, the space, and the refreshments. The experts would be paid as subcontractors with the consultation department. It was most cost-effective for the company to work with the consultation department rather than attempt to do the job themselves. The department had the space and established communication networks and was dedicated to making the process simple and smooth, yet productive for the company. The department also had reliable knowledge about which physicians, microbiologists, and pharmacists to interview. The company worked with only one department but had access to the medical center's full range of expertise without any additional negotiations. This initial contract was extended for a three-year period until the company moved to a new West Coast location. At this time they still need the services of the consultation department and fly their staff and department members back to the medical center to achieve the results that had been previously established.

## Fees for Service

To establish a fee-for-service scale, the hospital finance department was consulted. Using the highest CNS salary, they calculated an hourly figure that included fringe benefits and overhead. This figure, $25 per hour, represented the minimum the department would have to charge to break even. In the city, in 1983, the average acceptable rate for various types of consultation was $50 per hour. The administrator established $50 as the hourly fee for consultation from the department. This fee did not include travel-related expenses.

The establishment of an hourly fee was not a difficult task. The difficulty involved overcoming the resistance of the CNS to charging a

## TABLE 19–2. Consultation Agreement

This agreement between [name], located at [city], [state] (hereinafter referred to as "the Company"), and the University of Cincinnati, on behalf of the University Hospital (hereinafter referred to as the University Hospital) is entered into this _____ day of December 1985.

*Consultation Services*

The scope of this agreement shall be the testing by the Nursing Consultation Department of the University Hospital of the two products manufactured by the Company as identified in and in accordance with the Company's protocol in effect as of the date of this agreement.

*Confidential Matters*

As the Company will be providing the University Hospital with confidential information concerning its products which may relate to such areas as marketing strategy, sales potential, and technical and scientific information, such information will be kept strictly confidential. The University Hospital agrees not to disclose any information provided by the Company to any party except those directly participating in the testing of the Company's products as described herein. Further, the University Hospital agrees to keep the results of any consulting and/or testing efforts confidential and agrees not to divulge or communicate to any person, firm, or company such information other than to the Company.

The University Hospital will submit to the Company for review all proposed papers, abstracts, and drafts dealing with work undertaken in consultation and/or testing pursuant to this agreement prior to submission to any publication or editor, including but not limited to in-house publications of the University Hospital. The Company shall have thirty working days from receipt of any proposed paper, abstract, or draft for any opportunity to review such material to determine whether any of the information contained therein may be deemed proprietary in nature, discloses an invention or discovery which might be patentable, or communicates any other information or data which may be deemed confidential pursuant to the provisions of this agreement. The Company agrees to advise the University Hospital in writing within this thirty-day period as to any objections to the publication of any part of the material submitted.

*Reporting*

Reporting as to the consultation services and testing provided by the University Hospital to the Company shall be coordinated through [name, titles], clinical monitor or such other coordinating representatives as may be designated by the Company.

*Payments*

The Company hereby agrees to pay the University Hospital for the above services the sum of [amount] per patient tested, for a maximum of [service rendered]. Payment is to be made upon completion of testing and receipt by the Company of the required reports, photographs, and other supporting data for a minimum of [number] patients.

*Travel and Living Expenses*

The University Hospital shall submit a written estimate of any reasonable travel and living expenses deemed necessary to be incurred by the University Hospital for the performance of the consulting services and testing which may take place away from the normal place of work or residence of the University Hospital representatives involved in the consulting and testing described herein. Such expenses shall be reimbursed by the Company only in such circumstances wherein prior approval from the Company for expenses has been obtained.

*Term*

The consulting and testing pursuant to this agreement is to be completed by the University Hospital within [time frame] of receipt of the testing supplies.

*Independent Contractor*

The University Hospital shall perform all services under this Agreement as an independent contractor and neither it nor its employees, servants, officers, or agents shall be deemed to be employees, servants, officers, or agents of the Company.

*Indemnification*

The Company will indemnify the University Hospital against any payments which the University Hospital would be required to make on account of liability imposed upon the University Hospital by law for damages because of personal injury (including death) sustained by any person because of the testing and consulting done pursuant to this Agreement at the University Hospital utilizing the Company's products if said injury occurred while the Company's protocols and package insert instructions for use were being followed with respect to the product. The Company will further indemnify the University Hospital against any payments made to settle any claim for such an injury provided the Company concurs in the settlement. The Company will either defend any such claim on behalf of the University Hospital or pay the University legal fees and other expenses of defending said claim.

The company will not indemnify the University Hospital against claims that are not related to use of the Company's investigational product, or against claims that arise as a result of any failure to follow the Company's protocols, or against claims that arise from negligence on the part of the University Hospital's staff.

The University Hospital must contact the Company promptly in writing of any claim of injury for which the Company might be responsible, and the Company reserves the right to control the defense or disposition of such claims.

For the University

For the Company

_____

_____

Date

Date

Developed at the University Hospital, University of Cincinnati.

fee. This is not an isolated CNS problem. The nursing profession has knowingly and, at times, unknowingly sponsored an attitude of reluctance for its professional members to be reimbursed for their services. In the consultation department, CNSs reacted with indignation that they were being asked to charge for services that they had routinely given away. An effective intervention was to remind the CNSs who had served on a panel that they were the only professionals who were not paid for their time. As a result of many discussions concerning philosophy, mission, and the purpose of nursing, a mutually agreed-upon approach was established.

The CNSs were not expected to set a fee for every service delivered, but they were expected to make a clear, conscious decision in each transaction as to whether to charge a fee. Cognitive restructuring techniques were used as department members practiced saying "I charge" before a mirror, into a tape recorder, and to one another. As time progressed, department members could teach other nurses to say, "I charge." There were a variety of fee options, ranging from hourly service to yearly retainer fees. Fee setting was centralized, and the administrator approved all negotiated fees.

Early in the growth of the department, the department head contacted the director of the hospital finance department. As a revenue-producing department, there was the need to stay within the prescribed guidelines established by our accountant colleagues. They had stated very clearly that managing the billing and collecting the revenue of several thousand dollars was an inefficient use of their time and, in addition, that nurses were not revenue generators. As a result, the administrator's personal secretary managed the accounts for the consultation department until a major nationally recognized university hospital decided to explore using the department's consultation model, not only for their nursing department but also for the entire hospital. The consultation department decided to use this occasion to approach the finance department once again to overcome their initial resistance. The timing was good. The finance department decided to take over all accounting functions. The finance department made a presentation to the visiting university's financial officers, at which time the administrator for the consultation department mentioned how supportive the finance department had been. The collaboration involved in preparing for the visitors was very predictive of the future relationship between the consultation and finance departments.

## Time Management

During the first year of the new department, the CNSs were extraordinarily anxious about meeting the various performance expectations that they and the administrator had developed. How should their time be appropriated? The administrator devised a percentage breakdown—the 50/20/20/10 model. At least 50 per cent of the CNSs time had to remain clinical for the role to be accurately represented. Twenty per cent of their time was allocated to building and developing the structure and processes for the consultation department. Another 20 per cent was dedicated to external consultation and money-making activities. The final 10 per cent was for their own professional development with a heavy emphasis on publishing and an even greater emphasis on publishing with a staff nurse.

There were some (e.g., critical care and cardiac CNSs) who spent 70 per cent of their time in the clinical areas but exemplified the blending of clinical nursing research, publishing, income generation, and clinical hands-on care. For example, the critical care and cardiac CNSs identified a clinical problem involving nosocomial infection rates with disposable and nondisposable transducers. Along with a master's-prepared nurse in infection control, they decided to study the problem. At the same time, they surmised that a company that produced the transducers might have some interest in the findings. A company was approached by the CNSs and administrator. A breakfast meeting was held and funds for the study were obtained. The critical care CNS won the Research Award from the National Critical Care Association, which included travel monies. In addition, their research has been published. This time management example is a win for the CNS, a win for research, a win for the consultation department, but most importantly a win for patient care.

The 50/20/20/10 model is only a rule of thumb to guide CNSs in allocating their time in portions instead of having them attempt to give 100 per cent in all areas. In the first year of the department's existence, there were frequent discussions concerning frustrations and doubts. However, the more successful the department became, the more revenue was generated, the more articles were published, the more comfortable the CNSs became with their own consultative skills, the less frequently the 50/20/20/10 model was discussed.

## Marketing

In the business literature, there is the basic concept of the marketing mix that, if properly identified, will assist business in identifying its marketing strategies (Kotler, 1980). The marketing mix is composed of four Ps: Product, Price, Place, and Promotion. Too frequently, it is mistakenly assumed that marketing is only promotion. The product is simply the entity that one has to sell. There is a clear danger in being unfamiliar or unsure about one's product. In the case of the consultation department, CNS services were a viable product. The administrator was very familiar and very sure about the product. The price is the fee assigned to preparing, delivering, and evaluating the product plus a margin of profit. The price included the opportunity cost of the CNS delivering a particular service to a contractor instead of working in the normal setting for regular pay. Obviously, indirect costs such as fringe benefits, heat, light, space, and telephone service must be represented in the fee to determine a margin of profit.

The place is really another word for the distribution—who wants the product. The consultation department easily identified nursing homes, home health care, and other health care agencies. The more difficult area to identify was industry. As mentioned before, the one-on-one sales rep campaign proved to be productive for the department. In identifying specific interested companies, promotion became important.

The department had no funds for promotion. Fortunately, networking with nurses and others is a productive endeavor. For example, there was a nurse who managed her own production company. She was searching for sites to produce and film health care training programs. The consultation department was searching for promotional material at no charge. A trade was made. The consultation department acquired sophisticated brochures and business cards, and the production company used medical center locations to film their programs. This barter relationship continued for the first two years of the department's development. The production company realized that a CNS guide or liaison would facilitate their filming in the complex University Hospital setting. A consultation contract was arranged. After working with the CNS who became the production company's liaison, the company decided to hire her as an actor in the training films and as a consultant to the writing of the script. The trade-offs provided funding for other promotional activities or the department. After the first two years, the two entities began to exchange dollars for services.

The product evolved, and targeted services expanded. One of the psychiatric CNSs developed an employee assistance program for the hospital. She now consults with other institutions in organizing and implementing employee assistance programs. A CNS midwife was hired to start a midwifery program under the auspices of the nursing department. There are now four CNS midwives and physicians who are hired to consult with them. This program is profitable to the hospital and the consultation department. Another CNS had a special interest in intravenous therapy and particularly chemotherapy. There is now a subdepartment of intravenous therapy. The clinicians report to the CNS and run an outpatient intravenous therapy program that is very profitable. All of these programs and subdepartments are part of the consultation department. At this point, even without any external consultation with industry, the consultation department would be income-generating. However, industry has continued to respond positively.

## Rewards and Evaluation

One of the primary questions asked about the revenue-generating consultative model is what motivates the CNS to work in this broad and demanding context. The major motivator seems to be actualizing the full extent of the CNS role, which most master's-prepared nurses are taught in their graduate programs to expect. A second motivator is the learning opportunity that safely prepares the CNS for future professional entrepreneurial activities that will not have the safety net of salary and institution. A third motivator is the survival and growth of the CNS role.

With many contracts, the CNS had the option to accept consultation on behalf of the department or to take vacation time and personally accept the consultation and any revenue generated. Due to the basic survival orientation and the peer pressure to generate revenue, the CNSs most frequently consulted on behalf of the department. One must consider that many of the consultation projects required the participation of more than one CNS and access to medical center resources. The administrator did not question the CNSs about their individual decisions. The fact that revenue continued to grow satisfied all curiosity.

### Elements of Evaluation

BIMONTHLY REPORTS. These described the clinical, educational, consultative, and research activities of the CNS. This tool was used to quantify the number of patients and patient contact hours, the number of educational activities and nurses affected, the types of consultation and research activities, and the dollars derived from these activities.

INTERNAL AND EXTERNAL CONTRACT REVIEWS. Each CNS internally contracted with the administrators of each division of the nursing department. These individual contracts specified the CNSs' goals and action plans. External contract reviews simply involved whether the purchaser had adequately and professionally received the contracted services.

PEER REVIEW. This involved formal meetings of three to five CNSs to discuss the process of *how* they met their goals. The group focused on issues of CNS availability and follow-through, interpersonal style, and approach to working with the primary care providers. The content of these process-oriented peer review sessions was not reported to the administrator; only attendance and frequency of peer review meetings were part of the formal administrative review.

SELF-ASSESSMENT. Finally, a self-assessment method was prepared by the CNS. With this battery of evaluation tools, the administrator independently prepared the final evaluation. The administrator and CNS met and discussed the evaluation. Merit increases were directly related to the outcome of these evaluation sessions.

It is often difficult for the independent CNS to receive focused and structured evaluation. However, it is the responsibility of an administrator to mold and refine the CNS role to become a productive and viable one that is clearly essential to the mission of the institution.

## SUMMARY

The CNS and administrator must align their forces and collaboratively establish CNS activities that are visibly recognized as critical to the delivery of patient care and the survival and growth of the health care institution. This can be achieved by CNSs using a consultative model and working with the primary care provider (the staff nurse) as the consultee. Entrepreneurs and revenue generators are valuable assets in all health care facilities. The CNS is educationally and experientially well prepared to become a revenue-producing professional. Yet, the CNS needs the commitment and organizational skills of the administrator to create, develop, and sustain the structure that will support and sustain this innovative role.

### Acknowledgments

A special note of recognition is given to the nurse clinicians, resource nurses, primary care nurses, and all others at University Hospital of the University of Cincinnati who contributed to the development of this model.

### References

Girouard, S.: The role of the clinical specialist as change agent: An experiment in preoperative teaching. Int J Nurs Studies *15*:57–65, 1978.
Kotler, P.: Marketing Management: Analysis, Planning and Control (4th ed). Englewood Cliffs, N.J., Prentice-Hall, Inc., 1980.

Luciano, K., & Darling, L.: The physician as a nursing service consumer. J Nurs Admin 15:17–20, 1985.

Malone, B. L.: Evaluating the clinical nurse specialist. Am J Nurs 12:1375–1377, 1986.

Newton, P.: Social structure and process in psychotherapy. Int J Psychiatry 2:480–525, 1973.

O'Connor, P., & Malone, B. L.: A consultation model for nurse specialist practice. Nurs Econ 2:107–111, 1983.

Schein, E.: Process Consultation: Its Role in Organizational Development. Reading, MA, Addison-Wesley Publishing Co., 1969.

# The CNS in
# a Nurse-Managed
# Center

*Susan E. Davis Doughty*

## HISTORICAL ASPECTS OF
## NURSE-MANAGED CENTERS

Nurse-managed centers (NMCs) are thriving examples of innovative practice models. Master's-prepared RNs in advanced practice are in control of the organization, practice, and environment of nursing in NMCs throughout the country and are modeling the core of autonomous practice as defined by Mundinger (1980): ". . . being able to offer a unique therapy . . . [with the] freedom to provide that service without interference or permission . . . not a nurse providing medical care without medical supervision . . . [but] a nurse providing nursing therapy that complements and often overlaps medical care."

The roots of this activity can be found in the Frontier Nursing Service (FNS) of the 1920s. The nurses of the FNS have provided family health care for the mountain people of Kentucky for the past 60 years. They are most remembered through Mary Breckinridge and the nurse midwives who travelled by horseback and cared for mothers and babies. FNS outcomes are impressive: a Metropolitan Life Insurance study shows that of the first 10,000 births at the FNS between 1925 and 1954, 60 per cent were home births under adverse conditions with only 11 maternal deaths (2 not attributed to obstetrical cause), compared with the national mortality of 36.3 per 10,000 live births (Warner, 1978). Mountain people respected the nurses of the FNS but would not follow through with instructions unless they also trusted their nurse. That trust had to be earned through time, knowledge, honesty, understanding, and respect (Warner, 1978).

In the 1930s, Hildegard Peplau (1979) modeled autonomous nursing practice by describing and applying processes and outcomes of therapeutic interaction in psychiatric nursing. She emphasized the need

**415**

for proper academic preparation to adequately respond to patient needs and worked to provide appropriate curricula for nursing students at the undergraduate and graduate levels. Psychiatric nursing services were among the first to develop specialty practice standards and to receive direct third-party reimbursement.

In the 1950s, community public health departments established "well baby" clinics to fill a need that continues today. Out of this public health clinic movement, the first nurse practitioner (NP) demonstration project was developed in 1965 at the University of Colorado under the leadership of Loretta Ford, RN, EdD, and Henry Silver, MD. Their objective was to develop a new nursing role designed to deliver improved health care to well children and their families. Such a role expanded the nurse's scope of practice and served as a model for NP programs that followed (Ford, 1967).

In her practice in the 1970s, Lucille Kinlein crystallized notions of autonomy with the hanging of a "shingle" outside her private office in Maryland. Her controversial techniques, which some say bordered on the practice of medicine, forced the nursing community to re-examine the scope of nursing practice and nursing's commitment to society. She focused on client health care needs that nurses can meet and successfully sought direct reimbursement for nursing services. Documenting the results of her services, she demonstrated cost-effective care and led the way toward advanced "specialist" practice described in the American Nurses' Association's (ANA) *Nursing: A Social Policy Statement* in 1980.

Although the CNS was originally prepared for tertiary care, the CNS is the optimal nurse to direct an NMC. Training and education for the role of advanced practice in a graduate clinical program equip the CNS to take in a great deal of information and to quickly sift the relevant variables that give meaning to the situation. CNSs must have a keen ability to assess, diagnose, and develop practical alternatives with their patients, teaching them what they need to know, taking in new data, and refocusing as indicated. A high-level commitment to quality patient care motivates the CNS to evaluate practice according to criteria and standards and to change practice according to outcomes. The CNS is educated to be a change-agent, a risk-taker responsive to patient needs and societal expectations. As a researcher, the CNS tests theories and gathers data to better clarify practice; as a leader, the CNS stimulates optimal performance from others working toward measurable goals. Professional development is a priority and often comes through networking and peer review, as well as through attendance at national workshops for advanced practitioners.

The roles of the CNS and NP that evolved to keep pace with society's needs and the nursing profession's expanding knowledge base are discussed earlier in this book (Chapter 18). Kitzman has concluded that the restorative and rehabilitative skills of both roles must be combined to effectively address health care needs, regardless of the setting. The NMC provides an optimal opportunity for such client-centered practice and arises from deep and broad roots of society's needs for diagnosis and treatment of responses to actual or potential health care problems as well as from nursing's response to those needs. Studies recently conducted by the Health Care Finance Administration, Kaiser-Permanente, and the Federal Office of Technical Assistance indicate that "between 60 and 80 per cent of primary care activities previously considered an exclusive part of the physician's role can be assumed by professional nurses with advanced education in primary care without a decrease in quality; and that people cared for by nurses are more satisfied with their care, resulting in improved patient compliance and superior patient outcomes" (Lundeen, 1985).

## ESTABLISHING A NURSE-MANAGED CENTER

### Definition

For an unknown reason, the nursing profession had difficulty clearly stating in the literature a generally accepted definition of an NMC. When the American Nurses' Association worked with Senators Inouye (D-HI) and Packwood (R-OR) to introduce the Community Nursing Centers bill (S.410) in February, 1983, they defined an NMC as an "independent, organized setting providing both on-site and off-site services, with the administration, supervision and coordination of care by registered nurses, and with formal protocols assuring the arrangement for necessary consultation or referral" (*American Nurse*, March 1983).

Lundeen, an RN who directed an NMC in Chicago, writes that NMCs are more than clinics managed by nurses. They are "centers where the scope of services surpasses the usual delivery of direct medical services to include wellness activities provided by and directed by nurses [using] expanded skills . . . [which] in no way excludes physicians or other members of the interdisciplinary team" (Lundeen, 1985). She listed three criteria essential to an NMC: support for nurses to explore the limits of their practice, research on nursing process and patient outcomes, and focus on needs of the consumer. Lang proposed that education and research components must be built into the NMC and that nurses do more than "manage" care; they would be wise to control care through the political process, peer review, and implementation of practice standards. She added that the term "center" may limit nurse-managed services to a physical location and provide too narrow a concept (Lang, 1983).

## Current Perspectives on NMCs

This author concurs with Spross and Hamric's description of future advanced nursing practice and submits that the model NMC be defined and based on their assumptions, which are:

- Direct reimbursement for nursing services is available.
- Mechanisms for granting the CNS practice privileges in various settings exist.
- Consumers clearly understand services and can contract directly.
- Mechanism for certification exists and is the standard for practice.
- Mechanisms for consultation, referral, and teamwork exist among professional groups and within nursing (Spross & Hamric, 1983).

Spross and Hamric indicate the importance of the CNS not being confined to one setting, although being based primarily in one setting is acceptable. With the client as central focus, the CNS "will move freely into various settings to consult, coordinate, facilitate or deliver direct care" (Spross and Hamric, 1983).

Profiles of NMCs may vary, but their hallmark is professional nurses in advanced practice who are in control of organization, practice, and environment (Lang, 1983). Examples of NMCs cited in the literature or known to the author are depicted in Table 20–1. Each of these examples gives evidence of nurses in advanced practice providing the leadership for the center.

# CONTRIBUTION OF NURSE-MANAGED CENTERS TO THE NURSING PROFESSION

## Nursing Education

Since nursing is an applied discipline, a long-standing criticism of nursing school faculties has been that they lack involvement in nursing practice. Christman advocated that "when the best prepared nurses—nurse faculty members—practice regularly and consistently, the quality of clinical practice will leap forward" (Christman, 1980). NMCs provide an unparalleled opportunity for faculty practice. Over one hundred schools of nursing in the United States have set up centers that offer

**TABLE 20–1. Current NMC Models**

| MODEL | NURSING SERVICE FOCUS | EXAMPLES |
|---|---|---|
| 1. University nursing faculty | Community and/or campus; model of practice for students; opportunity for practice and research for faculty | (over 100 nationally) Center for Nursing, University of Southern Mississippi (Kinlein, 1977). |
| | | Nursing Center for Family Health, Purdue University (Lang, 1983). |
| | | Nursing and Health Information Center, Herbert Lehman College, City University of New York (Lang, 1983). |
| | | Community Health Services, College of Nursing, Arizona State University (Lang, 1983). |
| | | The Nursing Center, University of Wisconsin-Milwaukee School of Nursing (Lang, 1983). |
| | | Women's Health Exchange, College of Nursing, University of Illinois (Lang, 1983). |
| | | Clinical Practice Unit, Pace University (Culbert-Hinthorn, et al., 1985). |
| 2. Community low income family health center | Primary care to low income families and/or the elderly | Community Health Projects, Inc., West Covina, CA (Tennant, 1980). |
| | | Eric Family Health Center, Inc., Chicago, IL (Lang, 1983). |
| | | Childbearing Center, New York City (Lubic, 1983). |
| | | Chronic Disease Care Program, Henry Ford Hospital, Detroit (Clementino, 1981). |
| | | The Wellness Center, Mansfield, CT (Lang, 1983). |
| | | Decentralized Clinics, Memphis, TN (Miller, 1980). |

*Table continued on following page*

**TABLE 20–1. Current NMC Models** *Continued*

| MODEL | NURSING SERVICE FOCUS | EXAMPLES |
|---|---|---|
| 3. Ambulatory care facility/specialty clinic | | |
| A. Adult day hospital | Nonsurgical acute oncology treatment (medications, diagnostic procedures) | Memorial-Sloan Kettering Hospital, New York City (Onischuck, 1984). |
| B. Community hospital, chronic care program | Primary care of the chronically ill | Pacemaker Clinics, Methodist Hospital and St. Mary's Hospital, Madison, WI. |
| | | Chronic Care Clinic, DeWitt Army Hospital, Ft. Belvoir, VA (Bystran, 1974). |
| C. Veterans' hospitals | Primary care of the chronically ill veteran | Multiple Sclerosis Clinic, West Haven, Veterans' Administration Medical Center, West Haven, CT (Wahlquist, 1984). |
| | | Tuberculosis Clinic, Miami Veterans' Administration Hospital, Miami, FL (Peterson, 1977). |
| | | Epilepsy Center, West Haven Veterans' Administration Medical Center, West Haven, CT (Shope, 1974). |
| | | Congestive Heart Failure Clinic, Hines Veterans' Administration Hospital, Hines, IL. |
| | | Pacemaker Clinic, Veterans' Administration Hospital, Hines, IL. |
| D. Medical center | Primary care of the acute or chronically ill | Premature Clinic, Los Angeles County, USC Medical Center, Los Angeles, CA (Teberg, 1980). |
| | | Cardiac Nurse-Managed Clinics, Johns Hopkins Hospital, Baltimore, MD (Crews, 1972). |
| | | Pacemaker Clinic, St. Mary's Hospital/Mayo Clinic, Rochester, MN. |
| 4. Rural clinic | Primary care in low population areas | Darrington Nurse Clinic, Darrington, WA (Weinstein, 1974). |
| | | Community Hypertension Clinic, Wabasha, MN (Brennan, 1979). |

nursing services to the community and at the same time offer students the opportunity to observe, learn, and test the best of nursing practice (Lang, 1983). An NMC is a way of demonstrating a philosophy of autonomy. When traditional clinical sites are used, nursing students may become confused because some hospital environments, or the "medical model" of nursing practice, limit their ability to practice. Faculty must be wary, however, of developing practice sites on the basis of the needs of students and clinicians rather than of the needs of the client population served.

## Nursing Practice

Clinical practice implies application of theory and content of fundamental sciences to the health care of patients to reach desired health goals. Christman labeled this "a complex process that demands an orderly method and requires vigorous adherence to the methods of science" (Christman, 1980). Thinking and behaving, he wrote, are intertwined completely so as to be automatic, and the clinician uses knowledge of the sciences according to the role practiced. Society's demands on health care professionals in the past 15 years have led to an increased depth in training of health professionals and a greater overlap of mutually shared competencies and tasks. NMCs have provided an organizational model that encourages the competencies of each practitioner to be used freely without compromising standards of care for patients.

Practice standards and criteria used to evaluate nursing interventions in NMCs are currently being developed across the country. Generic and specialty standards are available from ANA and specialty nursing organizations, but these generally serve as a guide to nurses as they develop their own standards based on the needs of the population served and the resources available. Monitoring of practice to determine if care is appropriate has yet to be developed in practice to the extent that it is in the literature. Lang (1983) advocated peer review through district nurses' associations as one option. Without some consistent method of quality assurance, legislation or other mechanisms to reimburse nursing services are less likely.

It is an obligation of the CNS practicing in an NMC to create a common view for the public regarding the level of professional responsibility and accountability that can be expected of such a nurse. Currently, all types of educationally prepared RNs—diploma, AD, BSN, and graduate students—practice in NMCs. The ANA's *Social Policy Statement* affirms the BSN as entry level for professional practice and the graduate nursing degree for specialty practice. The specialist's practice in an NMC meets the demands of advanced or specialty practice, regardless of the title of CNS or NP, and requires graduate-level preparation in the area of practice along with eligibility for certification in the area of specialty.

## Nursing Research

NMCs offer a unique environment to conduct two types of nursing research: one that will more clearly define nursing practice, and one that will substantiate the quality and value of the service of the center itself. Some centers such as the Wellness Center in Mansfield, Connecticut, were created precisely for research with the provision of nursing care as a means to that end (Lang, 1983). Research evaluation of NMCs as a whole will be discussed later in this chapter. Research that adds to the clarity of practice and contributes to the profession will be addressed at this point.

Nursing research is necessary to test current and proposed theories in nursing as well as to generate data about nursing diagnoses, interventions, and outcomes of those interventions. Pace University's Clinical Practice Unit has supported studies appropriate to an NMC: "the effectiveness of imagery, identification of individuals at high risk for the development of alcoholism, client and nurse practitioner perception of the empathy of other nurse practitioners, the effect of trigenerational life events on family health, and health needs in a university community" (Culbert-Hinthorn, et al., 1985). The faculty at Pace are currently incorporating theory development into the center to promote less "activity-oriented" and more "goal-oriented" practice.

The NMC provides a setting for comprehensive health care to promote positive health behaviors and prevent recurrence of health problems. For the center to be viable, the CNS must maintain a client-focused rather than a research-focused practice. Such client-focused nursing practice, supported by theory and evaluated by outcomes, allows for testing of data that arise from the nurse-client interface that occurs in NMCs, through formal nursing research. A more mature nursing science with a better understanding of the phenomena of nursing will inevitably follow.

# ASSESSMENT OF NEED/VIABILITY OF NURSE-MANAGED CENTERS

Certain factors contribute to the success of an NMC. Assessment of the nurses' knowledge and skills in management and business as well as in clinical areas, of the community's needs and influencing forces, and of financial options is important before initiating such a center. In addition to the traditional role-based skills most graduate clinical programs provide for the CNS, a working knowledge of marketing and business management is helpful to the CNS who operates an NMC. Many graduate programs encourage students to take elective credits in these areas, since these skills are becoming more essential to health care providers of the future. Extensive clinical experience with the population to be served contributes to the success of an NMC.

Assessing the community's (or population's) needs and the influencing forces can be a complex process. There is much in the literature to substantiate the provision of primary care by nurses through NMCs (Lundeen, 1985; Clementino, 1981; Bystran, et al., 1974; Lubic, 1983; Tennant, et al., 1980; Lewis, et al., 1969; Weinstein, 1974; Brennan, et al., 1979; Vander Zwaag, et al., 1980), but specific needs and forces must be considered carefully (Table 20–2).

A financial assessment is critical to the survival of the clinic and the CNS's sanity. Gone are the days when the nurse expects to work for nothing, but the first year the center is in operation will be the most financially fragile. Grant monies, such as the $1,000,000 received by the Adult Day Hospital in New York City (Onischuck, 1984), help to launch an NMC. Developing a list of needs is a crucial first step, e.g., rent, utilities, salaries, taxes, equipment, advertising, stationery, insurance, and professional incorporation costs. Other expenses that need to be considered include moving costs, automobile use, education, consultation, and other miscellaneous costs.

Establishing financial resources is the next step. Such resources include patients who are able to pay; third party insurance; school of nursing budgets; grants (many foundations are currently funding cost-effective means for providing health care, such as Robert Wood Johnson, Henry J. Kaiser, and so forth); private or business donations; hospital budgets (as a cost-saving maneuver to compete with other agencies); federal block grants; or contracts with unions, health depart-

---

**TABLE 20–2. Influencing Forces to Be Considered in Establishing an NMC**

Current mechanisms in place for care of the patients to be served
Perceived need by patients
Setting needed (university, hospital, free-standing)
Access to patients
Available health resources for the patients to be served
Political climate toward nurses providing autonomous care
Financial support needed
Financial options available
Local/state corporate law regarding professional centers

ments, industry, and Health Maintenance Organizations (HMOs). Over 37 states provide some legislation for expanded nursing practice, and many provide direct reimbursement to nurses (Mezey, 1983). In Maryland, the first state to achieve direct reimbursement for nursing services, insurance companies have established mechanisms for review of "reasonable rates of reimbursement" (Mezey, 1983). In Washington, ANA-certified nurses are eligible for reimbursement from the State Medical Assistance program. CHAMPUS (Civilian Health and Medical Program for the Uniformed Services) reimburses nurses with either ANA or state certification without referral or supervision of a physician. Third-party reimbursement is directly available to certified psychiatric master's-prepared nurses in Maine, Wisconsin, Vermont, and other states. A current listing of reimbursement specifications in each state is available from ANA headquarters in Kansas City, MO (ANA Publication No. D-76).

The Community Nursing Centers bill (S.410), introduced by Senators Inouye and Packwood in February 1983, would have provided community nursing centers with reimbursement by Medicare and Medicaid for health maintenance and preventive services for infants, children, recently discharged psychiatric hospital patients, and long-term care patients. Nursing faculty, visiting nurse services, and other community nursing services would have been involved in providing care. At that time, the government was trying to cut expenditures for health care, and the bill died after one hearing. With ANA help, a new proposal was written similar to a nursing HMO model or prepaid home health services of Medicare, which would save the government 5 per cent across the board. This bill would offer nursing services to the general public through a prepaid model (along with physical and occupational therapy and speech and language therapy). In October 1986, the congressional budget office estimator prepared a budget for the proposal which was significantly less than the previous bill: $10 million the first year, $50 million over three years. Congressman Gephardt (D-MO) introduced it as H.R. 5457, the "Community Nursing and Ambulatory Care Act," but Congress recessed before action was taken. Modifications were made through Ways and Means and Energy and Commerce hearings, and the bill was reintroduced as H.R. 1161 on February 19, 1987. A companion bill was also introduced in the Senate by Senator J. Chaffee (R-RI) in mid-May 1987 as S.B. 1010. As a result of that process, the Community Nursing Act legislation became an amendment to the Omnibus Budget Reconciliation Act of 1987 (Public Law 100-203). Four demonstration projects are to be in operation by July 1, 1989, and the Health Care Finance Administration is processing requests for proposals for these demonstration projects.

The Community Nursing Centers legislation has the potential to convince legislators to fund nursing care and promote the emerging awareness that nurses can usually provide primary care of equal or better quality than physician care at a reduced cost. This fact is well-established in the literature (Lundeen, 1985; Lubic, 1983; Tennant, et al., 1980; Lewis & Resnick, 1967; Vander Zwaag, et al., 1980). Regardless of current obstacles to the establishment of NMCs, Table 20–3 lists certain forces that indicate great promise for the future of this model of health care.

With the passage of a bill such as this, CNSs will be in a position to influence individual state and local governments in deciding how to spend limited Medicare and Medicaid monies. CNSs may be able to persuade them to invest in an NMC that will provide cost-effective health care and prevention programs at the same or lower costs as other care providers. The CNS must verify that the NMC will make a difference that will justify the investment. The process of seeking reimbursement assists the CNS in clarifying critical outcomes or indicators of success.

## IMPLEMENTATION OF A NURSE-MANAGED CENTER

Principles for establishing a private practice and an NMC are quite similar. The advantage that a CNS in an NMC has is support through colleagues and resources (university, hospital, community health agency, and so forth). An individual developing a private practice must often seek out and request such support. The peer support that is available from such alliances is vital to the CNS in an NMC. It provides an advantage over the professional isolation that can occur in private practice (see Chapter 21).

Once a CNS posesses the necessary skills (including principles of business and management) and experience to entertain the idea of

**TABLE 20–3. Forces Influencing Viability of NMCs**

Trend for early discharge from hospitalization
Continued hampered access to health care; 10% of US population do not have source
Changes in third-party reimbursement
Deinstitutionalization of mental health services
Continuation of scientific advances increasing survival and incidence of chronic illness
Need for measured cost-efficiency
Increased consumer awareness of options
Emphasis on prevention, self-care
Development of distinct nursing frameworks, separate but complementary to medicine, emphasizing restorative and rehabilitative skills

establishing an NMC, the first step is to survey the need of the community or population for the particular service to be offered. Using both formal and informal consultation, the CNS can seek information about the needs of the community while informing possible referral sources of a service. Consultation takes time and energy, but if the CNS's presentation through consultation is professional, credible, and capable, individuals will eventually seek out the NMC, and the CNS will be able to make informed judgments about the client population. The costs of consultation should be factored into start-up costs. Suggested sources for consultation include other nurses, physicians, lawyers, nursing schools, local nursing associations, local community groups, pharmacists, and health care delivery agencies.

Once the need is established, mechanisms for marketing the service and establishing a referral base are important. Fees for services which are realistic and encompass all expenses, yet remain competitive, need to be established. Fee schedules in the community help the CNS establish what the client is accustomed to paying, but the CNS must compute time with each patient, service provided, responsibility assumed, overhead costs, and third-party reimbursement rate and come to a conclusion about a fee schedule for the NMC. It would be wise to consult with other providers in the area regarding the climate for fee-for-service versus contract or health maintenance model, since the concept of fee for service is being challenged as a viable mechanism for future reimbursement.

Decisions about location, acquiring supplies, record-keeping, billing, and organizing care must be made. The Small Business Administration can be quite helpful in providing written material or workshops to assist in business decisions if the NMC is to be a free-standing facility. If the CNS is to be self-employed in the NMC, it is wise to maintain another position until the center becomes viable and practice is economically supportive. A network of successful nurses in NMCs can help solve problems and validate decisions as well as offer support during difficult times.

## EVALUATION OF NURSE-MANAGED CENTERS

If NMCs are to focus on patient care as their reason for existence, then successful patient outcomes along with growth of practice and economic viability can be used to determine success. Research studies established to measure the attainment of individual clinic objectives are frequently designed by the CNS in an NMC. Variables studied include patient care outcomes (Clementino, 1981; Hoeffer & Murphy, 1985), patient satisfaction (Bystran, et al., 1974; Clementino, 1981; Brown, et al., 1979; Culbert-Hinthorn, et al., 1985), practice growth (Culbert-Hinthorn, et al., 1985; Bystran, et al., 1974; Brown, et al., 1979; Wahlquist, 1984), and time-motion studies (Bystran, et al., 1974; Lewis, et al., 1969). Quality assurance studies and peer review of practice are also ways to determine whether objectives have been successfully met.

Amid forces influencing the establishment of NMCs, their viability in the future will be measured by their ability to reduce economic costs of disability at all levels while providing top quality care and offering broader access to health care services (see Table 20–3).

Part of the reason for nurse midwives' success is the quality of data from which they can justify changes in existing care and reimbursement. Nurse midwives at childbirthing centers in New York have dramatically reduced the cost of child-bearing while reducing infant mortality and morbidity. Lubic, a pioneer in the development of free-standing child-birthing centers in New York, was cited as a *Ms.* magazine "woman of the year" for her contribution. She hopes the creative response to the needs of childbearing families will not only "reduce cost to families, but also motivate nurses in other settings to use more fully their remarkable potential" (Lubic, 1983).

Nurse midwifery studies clearly demonstrate success. Other studies verifying nursing practice as cost-effective compared with medical practice are paving the way for third-party reimbursement but remain inconclusive in that the activities of nurses differ somewhat from physicians. Nurses are usually more concerned with supporting role functions, physicians with technical aspects of diagnosis and treatment of disease (Brown, et al., 1979; Bystran, et al., 1974; Brennan, et al., 1979; Lundeen, 1985; Lewis, 1967, 1969).

In order for the impact of NMCs to be consistent, formal evaluation research must continue and reach the literature. Wahlquist (1984), who manages a multiple sclerosis clinic, wrote of the importance of evaluation processes and outcome measures and of using these results in formulating objectives and scope of service to be provided by the CNS. She measured morbidity as an index of nursing intervention effectiveness: the contribution the nurse makes to keeping MS patients out of the hospital through managing the interdisciplinary effort and providing consistent care needed through a rehabilitative approach. She found a significant decrease in febrile urinary tract infections, medical complications (excluding pneumonia), and family crises during the year of intervention, demonstrating decreased morbidity as an index of CNS intervention effectiveness.

At a time when the consumer is wary about the way health and illness care are managed, it is of utmost importance for the CNS in an NMC to address quality assurance so that patients can identify the actions of individual nurses in the same way that they can identify those of their personal physicians (Christman, 1980). From this effort, a base of support will begin and the perception of the nursing profession will improve.

## ESTABLISHING A NURSE-MANAGED CENTER: A CASE STUDY

As a graduate student, the author had the opportunity to assist her CNS preceptor to establish a federally funded nurse-managed hypertension center in the ambulatory care division of the University of Wisconsin-Madison Clinical Science Center. For her graduate research, she interviewed patients who had cardiac pacemakers and noted the obvious need for consistent nursing care among yet another population. Once graduate work was completed, the author sent a short questionnaire to all patients who had had cardiac pacemakers inserted at the community hospital that had employed her as a CNS in critical care. The need and desire for a nurse-managed cardiac pacemaker center was established. The hospital funded it as an opportunity for outreach and referral (the 150 patients came from a 90 + mile radius) as well as a revenue center, since Medicare and Medicaid were both reimbursing for pacemaker follow-up. Average age of eligible patients was 79.

The author established a partnership with the nursing director who managed cardiovascular ambulatory services; the business of the clinic was handled by this nurse administrator, while standards of practice and delivery of care were handled by the author. Schedules for telephone contacts and visits were set according to American Heart Association (AHA) standards, which were less frequent than the maximum allocated by third-party providers. Fees were set by what seemed appropriate, since there were no other clinics in the area. They also were below the maximum reimbursed charges. Fees were applied consistently, even though some patients did not pay. Medicare and Medicaid were billed for the services with the hospital provider number for those who qualified; third-party payers were billed for those who did not qualify (at that time not all third-party payers covered this service); and patients who did not qualify for reimbursement of some sort received the service without charge. Even with start-up costs for monitoring equipment, office space, and office equipment, the clinic was a revenue generator for the hospital from the start, since the salaries for the nurses were under a separate cost center due to other institutional responsibilities. The physician consultant was also salaried by the hospital. Other than salaries and initial equipment, the biggest cost was in long distance phone rates, and the hospital WATTS line helped cut these costs.

Setting standards of practice was not difficult. The more experience the CNS has with the population served, the easier it is to practice. The author worked with patients who had cardiac pacemakers for nine years prior to assessing the need for and developing the NMC. Knowledge about cardiovascular physiology and pacemaker technology and how to keep this knowledge current was second nature. Additional content in the area of nursing care of the aged population was obtained through the adult/aging NP track at a local university, which allowed the author to practice with more sophistication in physician-nurse interchanges, differential diagnosis and case finding, and support for grieving losses in the patient population. The author used ANA and AHA standards as a guide but then developed individual standards and used peer review for monitoring practice. Other CNSs in the Madison-Milwaukee area agreed to participate in peer review informally as a professional courtesy.

Standards were developed around nursing diagnoses, and the author acted as a case manager in case finding and referral to physicians, physical therapists, dieticians, clergy people, mental health nurses in private practice, and community health nurses. The effectiveness of nursing interventions was based on outcomes measured by the author, patient, and family. Nursing care plans were kept in a Kardex and notes were kept in a chart for each patient.

The pacemaker clinic offered a unique environment to test the author's hypotheses about adjusting to life with a pacemaker. For patients who used denial as a coping mechanism, data for unpublished studies were gathered on internal versus external locus of control of patients and on the influence of frequency of telephone contact. The proximity of a university faculty also allowed the author to use doctorally prepared nursing resources for research design.

The clinic is in operation today, 13 years later, and continues to be nurse-managed with other health professionals providing consultation. Educating the physicians as to the difference between providing nursing care and practicing medicine continues to be a challenge. Patients call the nurses with symptoms needing medical intervention such as chest pain, pocket infection, or dyspnea, and appropriate referrals to the patient's local internist, cardiologist, or cardiovascular surgeon are made.

As the NMC developed, the scopes of practice for medicine and nursing became less clear, which fostered a subtle, underlying tension in the clinic between the hospital cardiologists and the nurses. The nurses became so adept at the technology of pacing with the three different brands of pacemakers used that they frequently schooled the physicians on fine points. One of the nurses assisted in the catheterization lab with all insertions, and the other met weekly in conference with the physicians, clarifying nursing interventions and diagnoses regarding coping and adjusting to life with a pacemaker. Both nurses made rounds on hospitalized patients, assisting staff with nursing care and physicians with reprogramming. Gradually, the service provided became distinct enough for the physicians not to want to perform it themselves or to hire a less prepared health care worker in their private practice. Given the growing preponderance of physicians, the clinic is not as vulnerable to MD takeover because the nurses have established a valuable practice that is finer in technological assistance and broader in service (with coping and support through aging) than physicians are usually willing to provide. In fact, in the author's pacemaker clinic practice, several medical students caring for clinic patients considered applying for the school of nursing, since their medical practice seemed to be rather hurried and "cut and dried" compared with the less hurried pace and creativity in problem-solving that the CNS enjoyed with her patients.

Patients with pacemakers in the area around Madison frequently asked to be followed by the NMC. Physicians in competing practices asked that clinics be formed in their facilities. This pacemaker clinic has provided a model for at least two other pacemaker clinics in Madison as well as several others in surrounding midwestern cities and states. Services provided in the clinic include a formal assessment of the functioning of the pacemaker by telephone transmission in an established schedule that meets AHA standards, and annual physical assessment, medication review, pacemaker program evaluation, nursing consultation, and 24-hour access to a pacemaker clinic nurse for assistance.

Some cardiologists in the country still do not provide formal follow-up for paced patients, even though it is a standard articulated by the AHA and all patients receive a telephone transmitter as part of their pacemaker package. Other cardiologists use national technical computer services or technicians in their offices to provide follow-up. Formal nurse-managed care provides patients with feedback about their pacemakers and cardiac status. In addition, because the pacemaker patients are often elderly and have other chronic health problems, the NMC offers a perfect opportunity to provide comprehensive nursing care for health maintenance and illness prevention.

Physicians in Madison have come to depend on the NMCs and refer patients for nursing care as well as pacemaker follow-up. Physician back-up remains as a consultant service in each clinic, and the revenue generated supports the viability of the centers in the hospitals.

## ISSUES CONCERNING NURSE-MANAGED CENTERS

Several issues have evolved out of the development of NMCs which remain worthy of thought and analysis. Such issues include establishing appropriate fees and adequate time to pay fees, practicing within the realm of nursing, delegating to appropriately prepared individuals, providing for adequate care in the CNS's absence, maintaining confidentiality, and advertising appropriately. Nursing is a profession in transition, and the CNS's constant awareness of professional behavior will strengthen ethical as well as legal practice. The ANA code for nurses can provide guidance but using a network of peers in similar practice provides the opportunity to work through the difficult process of coming to conclusions about ethical dilemmas. Including those well versed in nursing ethics in such a network is recommended, since objectivity is difficult when one's own practice is being examined, and solutions to ethical dilemmas require seasoned judgment.

NMCs may strengthen future collegiality between physicians and nurses. In graduate programs with university-based clinics, specific behaviors congruent with the expanded role are built into the curriculum. The professional socialization of students includes theory and clinical experiences that emphasize nurses' contributions to patient outcomes and effective collaboration with other health care providers.

Legislative issues that arise include examining what is necessary for support of a NMC in each state. As nurses practicing in NMCs develop a patient constituency, a political base for support will evolve. Changing the nurse practice act may be necessary, and the CNS can help monitor input to prevent unintentional restrictions on practice. Third-party reimbursement for nurses is often included in such political activity, and the CNS can speak to standards of care and credentials of care providers in such efforts. For a further discussion of the CNS and health policy, see Chapter 17.

## FUTURE OF NURSE-MANAGED CENTERS

The health care system is rapidly changing in response to political, economic, and technological changes. As nursing evolves over the next 50 years, factors in place today will influence its development. Examples of efforts to attain professional autonomy while serving the needs of clients are clearly woven through contemporary nursing practice: primary nursing in the hospital, clinical decision-making by nurses along with physicians in critical care units, the work of nurse midwives in communities and hospitals, and the existence of NMCs in all settings.

Major forces influencing the role of the CNS in an NMC include growth of the medical profession, concerns with rising costs, changes in patterns of illness, increased client participation, and increased use of computers. Predictions for supply and demand of professional nurses made as recently as 1984 are proving inaccurate with the declining enrollment in colleges of nursing. Using forecasts made by Eli Ginzberg, Bezold and Carlson suggest that other health professionals including physicians will compete with nurses even more in the coming years, especially in areas of primary care (1986).

Reasons for office visits to physicians were recently identified by the National Ambulatory Care Survey (Bezold & Carlson, 1986). These reasons include general medical exams, prenatal exams, postoperative visits, throat symptoms, back symptoms, earache or ear infection, headache, and abdominal pain. Factors that may affect clients' responses to these conditions include self-care computer software, less surgery, less extra weight, more exercise, meditation, and autonomic control. Many of these variables fall within the scope of nursing practice. Given the self-limiting nature of these conditions, coupled with better capability to self-diagnose and treat, primary care interventions may well change dramatically over the next 20 years (Bezold & Carlson, 1986). Currently, 50 to 80 per cent of primary care complaints can be handled by protocols, and CNSs may find more need for their services in case-management activities (Andrews, 1986).

A projected reduction in cancer and heart disease will make way for debilitating neuromuscular, trauma, infectious (AIDS), or psychiatric conditions that demand management better provided by the CNS. "To deal with chronic illness, clients need information and instruction about self-monitoring and self-treatment as well as the concerned attention of a practitioner prepared in the social as well as medical sciences, who is willing to spend time and whose services are not so expensive that the agency or third party provider cannot afford that time. Nurses are particularly well-suited to fit that bill" (Andrews, 1986). Studies show that advanced practice nurses do better than physicans in areas such as continuity of care and emphasis on prevention, amount of advice offered, amount of time spent listening to patients, and communication skills and support. Patients of nurses in primary care rank higher on knowledge about appropriate exercise and activity than patients of physicians (Andrews, 1986).

Entry level for advanced practice at the master's or doctoral level must be endorsed by the profession as a whole in order for the future of nursing and NMCs to be secure. Professional credentialing and certification procedures to regulate CNS practice will allow for a consistent standard of care that the public can expect and insurance carriers can support. Areas of specialization will arise out of nursing needs, breaking away from the medical model and evolving to nursing models, such as those based on developmental needs and health maintenance needs, or to other models consistent with human responses to health and illness. Nurses *will* practice collaboratively with physicians using a distinct practice that is complementary to medicine but further refined and articulated by research arising from NMCs. Such research will also reveal the necessity of these clinics because they offer competent providers, productive and efficient care, and services that are accessible, affordable, and preferred.

A sound strategic plan on the part of the nursing profession as a whole, as well as individual nurses in advanced practice, is essential to prevent or remove obstacles to enhanced responsibility and practice in the NMC.

## Acknowledgment

The author wishes to acknowledge the contribution of Leslie Rohde-Katzman, MSN, RN, in the establishment of the nurse-managed pacemaker clinic at Methodist Hospital, Wisconsin, in 1975.

## References

American Nurses' Association: The Regulation of Advanced Nursing Practice as Provided for in Nursing Practice Acts and Administrative Rules (Publ. No. D-76). Kansas City, American Nurses' Association, 1983.

American Nurses' Association: Nursing: A Social Policy Statement (Publ. No. NP-63). Kansas City, American Nurses' Association, 1980.

Andrews, L. B.: Health care providers: The future marketplace and regulations. J Prof Nurs 2:51–63, 1986.

Bezold, C., & Carlson, R.: Nursing in the twenty-first century: An introduction. J Prof Nurs 2:2–9, 1986.

Brennan, L., et al.: The Mayo three-community hypertension control program: III. Outcome in a community-based hypertension clinic. Mayo Clin Proc 54:307–312, 1979.

Brown, J., et al.: Evaluation of a nurse practitioner–staffed preventive medicine program in a fee-for-service multispecialty clinic. Prev Med 8:53–64, 1979.

Bystran, S., et al.: An evaluation of nurse practitioners in chronic care clinics. Int J Nurs Stud 11:185–194, 1974.

Christman, L.: Leadership in practice. Image 12:31–33, 1980.

Clementino, D. A.: Henry Ford Hospital clinics manage physician-referred chronic disease patients. Urban Health 10:33–35, 1981.

Crews, J.: Nurse-managed cardiac clinics. Cardiovasc Nurs 8:15–18, 1972.

Culbert-Hinthorn, P., et al.: A nurse managed clinical practice unit: Part I—the positives. Nurs Health Care 6:97–100, 1985.

Detmer, S. S.: The future of health care delivery systems and settings. J Prof Nurs 2:20–27, 1986.

Ford, L., & Silver, H.: Expanded role of the nurse in child care. Nurs Outlook 15:43–45, 1967.

Hoeffer, B., & Murphy, S.: Specialization in nursing practice. In American Nurses' Association (ed): Issues in Professional Practice, #2. Kansas City, American Nurses' Association, 1985.

Kinlein, M. L.: Independent Nursing Practice with Clients. Philadelphia, J. B. Lippincott Co., 1977.

Kitzman, H.: The CNS and the nurse practitioner. In Hamric, A., and Spross, J. (eds): The Clinical Nurse Specialist in Theory and Practice. New York, Grune and Stratton, 1983, pp. 275–290.

Koltz, C. J.: Private Practice in Nursing. Rockville, MD, Aspen Publishing, 1979, pp. 55, 93–95, 146–147.

Lang, N.: Nurse-managed centers: Will they thrive? Am Nurs 83:1290–1296, 1983.

Lewis, C., & Resnick, B.: Nursing clinics and progressive ambulatory care. N Engl J Med 277:1236–1241, 1967.

Lewis, C., Resnick, B., et al.: Activities, events and outcome in ambulatory patient care. N Engl J Med 280:645–659, 1969.

Lubic, R. W.: Childbirthing centers: Delivering more for less. Am J Nurs 83:1053–1056, 1983.

Lundeen, S.: Nurse-managed centers offer more to patients, nurses (editorial). Am Nurs 17:4, 22, 1985.

Mezey, M.: Nurse-managed centers: Securing a financial base. Am J Nurs 83:1297–1298, 1983.

Miller, R., ANA Lobbyist, Washington, D.C. Personal communication.

Mundinger, M.: Autonomy in Nursing. Germantown, MD, Aspen, 1980.

Onischuck, M.: Role of nursing in the adult day hospital. 1984, unpublished manuscript.

Peterson, L., & Green, J.: Nurse-managed tuberculosis clinic. Am J Nurs 77:433–435, 1977.

Peplau, H.: Power: Nursing's challenge for change. In Sills, G. M. (ed): Hildegard E. Peplau: Leader, Practitioner, Academician, Scholar, and Theorist (Publ. No. 9–135). Kansas City, American Nurses' Association, 1979, pp. 169–78.

Riccardi, B., & Dayani, E.: The Nurse Entrepreneur. Reston, VA, Reston Publishing Co., 1982.

Shope, J.: The clinical specialist in epilepsy. Nurs Clin North Am 9(4):761–773, 1974.

Spross, J., & Hamric, A. B.: A model for future clinical specialist practice. In Hamric, A. B., and Spross, J. (eds): The Clinical Nurse Specialist in Theory and Practice. New York, Grune and Stratton, 1983, pp. 291–306.

Teberg, A., et al.: Setting up a PNP Clinic. Am J Nurs 80:1485–1487, 1980.

Tennant, F., et al.: A study of the economic viability of low-cost, fee-for-service clinics staffed by nurse practitioners. Public Health Reports 95:321–323, 1980.

Thomstad, B., et al.: Changing the rules of the doctor-nurse game. Nurs Outlook 23:422–427, 1975.

Vander Zwaag, R., et al.: Cost of chronic disease care. J Chron Dis 33:713–720, 1980.

Wahlquist, G. I.: Impact of a nurse-managed clinic in multiple sclerosis. J Neurosurg Nurs 16:193–196, 1984.

Warner, A.: Innovations in Community Health Nursing. St Louis, CV Mosby, 1978.

Weinstein, P., & Demers, J.: Rural nurse practitioner clinic. Am J Nurs 74:2022–2027, 1974.

# The CNS in Private Practice

Chapter

**21**

Patricia Stewart

## INTRODUCTION

Private nursing practice is an emerging entrepreneurial endeavor for more and more nurses. This approach to delivering nursing care may seem novel, but private practice in the form of private duty nursing has been a role within nursing for decades. Fee for service, an important concept of private practice, was a familiar idea to the private duty nurse of the past, when the nurse was employed directly by the person or family requiring nursing services. However, more autonomy, self direction, and expertise are expected of the clinical nurse specialist (CNS) in private practice today than were expected of the private duty nurse of the past.

Through their activities in the 1960s, psychiatric CNSs are considered pioneers in the development of contemporary private specialty practices (Menard, 1987; Hoeffer, 1983). The movement of nurse practitioners (NPs) into private practice in the 1970s brought more attention and focus to this role as a possible option for the specialized nurse (Kinlein, 1977). Only recently have CNSs outside the field of psychiatry and mental health seen private practice as an alternative for providing direct patient care.

The 1984 American Nurses' Association (ANA) survey of CNSs indicated that an increasing number of nurses are providing service through private practice (ANA, 1986b). This move toward independence parallels economic trends in the 1980s which have emphasized entrepreneurialism and a strengthening of the private sector. Albrecht and Zemke stated that the United States has become a service economy in which relationships have become more important than physical products (1985). The service sector, which provides direct interaction with clients rather than tangible or storable goods (Stanback, 1979), has grown steadily from 54 per cent in 1948 to over 65 per cent in the 1980s (Aronson & Cowhey, 1984).

Certain economic trends support development of private practice for CNSs. A look at national service sector expenditures reflects a shift of dollars to health care. For example, health care expenditures in 1986 continued to rise to 10.8 per cent of the gross national product and are estimated to be at 13.9 per cent for 1990 (Standard & Poor's, 1987). At the same time, professional services (other than physicians and dentists) were 3 per cent of total health expenditures in 1986, representing a quadrupling over the previous 10 years; most other categories of health care costs only tripled during the same period. In addition, cost-containment efforts have resulted in a decrease in inpatient hospital care. This has proven to be a boon for less expensive forms of health care, such as outpatient treatment and free-standing facilities. Areas showing growth include long-term care for the elderly and specialty facilities such as mental health, rehabilitation, child development, elder care, and home health care (Standard & Poor's, 1987).

Consumers who are better informed and more conscious of health, diet, and physical fitness expect quality health care from a variety of health professionals, including CNSs. CNSs are recognizing these economic and social trends and are identifying specific skills that can be marketed to meet the needs of health care consumers (Powell, 1984). With 18 per cent of respondents to the 1984 ANA survey of CNSs indicating that they were in private practice (ANA, 1986b), it seems that CNSs are more actively exploring possibilities available to them in meeting patient needs in the private practice arena.

## WHAT IS PRIVATE PRACTICE?

Private practice has been defined as the practice of nursing within a business framework that is partially or wholly owned and operated by the nurse providing the service (Keller, 1975). For purposes of this chapter, the definition of private practice is limited to those CNSs providing direct care. An assumption of this definition is that the CNS provides a service and is remunerated for that service as an independent contractor rather than as an employee of an agency or of another practice which does not belong in part or whole to that CNS. CNSs in private practice perform the range of subroles identified in Chapter 1. The proportion of time spent in direct care may be higher than that of CNSs employed by institutions.

CNSs who have created successful private practices serve a variety of clientele. The literature describes private practices established by nurses in such specialty areas as mental health and psychiatry (Hoeffer, 1983), care of oncology patients (Holmes, 1985), care of patients who are on home dialysis programs (Norris, 1982), rehabilitation of neuro-logically impaired persons (Wiener, 1983), pediatric health care (Gorke-Felice, 1984), and family health care providers (Dickerson & Nash, 1985).

## WHY PRIVATE PRACTICE?

Peters and Waterman (1982) reflected that vision pulls and pain pushes each of us into various activities. Some CNSs establish private nursing practices as a result of what may be perceived as "negative" forces pushing the individual, i.e., the grant ran out, the CNS lost a previous job, or the CNS perceived a lack of freedom in determining work schedule in response to patient need. Others are drawn into the quest for a way to practice nursing which will allow them to act affirmatively on closely held beliefs about quality care for patients and to achieve the potential satisfaction in seeing ideas and concepts suc-cessfully working to the benefit of those served (Kerfoot, 1982; Jacox & Norris, 1977).

Reasons for choosing private practice are as varied and individual as CNSs themselves. Some CNSs believe that they can generate more income in private practice than in a salaried position (Jacox & Norris, 1977). For others it is a move taken in reaction to frustration experi-enced with bureaucratic policies and a perceived lack of autonomy when operationalizing the CNS role within the institutional setting. The attraction of being one's own boss in the delivery of nursing services is enough to motivate some CNSs to make the move (Riccardi, 1982). Many believe that autonomy, often regarded as the hallmark of a profession, will be more effectively achieved in the private practice arena (Kinlein, 1977). This last idea was borne out by respondents to the 1984 ANA survey of CNSs in which those in private practice (along with those in both private clinical consultation and extended care facilities) reported high professional autonomy in their setting com-pared with CNSs in other settings (ANA, 1986b).

For another group, the need to try something new, to experience a different way of sharing one's expertise rather than accepting a lateral transfer to a similar CNS position in another facility, is the motivation for exploring the possibilities of private practice. Some specialists express awareness of an internal drive that simply says the time is right, given expertise, experience, resources, personal desires, and community needs, to try this new framework of practice. Some also know that not to try is likely to invite a sense of regret at a later time.

Rarely is there only one factor motivating the CNS to go into private practice. Rather, some CNSs sense the decision is based on a combination of values, beliefs, needs, and wishes. The CNS with an interest in private practice must be willing to consider not only potential benefits but also potential risks involved in such an undertaking.

## RISKS OF PRIVATE PRACTICE

There are risks involved in almost any career move and certainly in opening a private practice. Generally, these risks fall into two main categories: professional and financial.

One's professional nursing career is at some degree of risk with entry into private practice. CNSs who have been active in professional organizations and who have been recognized for their contributions to the practice of nursing as salaried employees of an established organization may find that the demands of private practice reduce the time commitments they can make to continuing these activities. The fear that they will "drop out of sight" of professional peers and colleagues and be forgotten as professional associates makes them wonder what will happen if the business fails or if the private practice cannot sustain itself.

Usually the CNS in private practice, especially a solo practice, tends to experience less interaction with professional colleagues. There is less routine contact with non-nurse professionals and sometimes even with people in general. The CNS is alone in decision-making relative to the practice and patient care. This can lead to a great sense of isolation and loneliness, the source of which must be directly confronted and constructively changed (Gorke-Felice, 1984). Establishing a support network is vital to this process, and time should be made for this.

Financial risks are inherent in establishing and conducting a private practice. Since a salary is received only if there is income to the business, there is the decided potential for decreased financial security. Less tangible risks lie in the area of salary continuance during time away for vacations, periods of illness, attendance at continuing education activities, and writing for professional publication. Such absences from income-producing activities mean that salary received during these periods had to have been generated at an earlier time.

Careful consideration and planning of resources must also be given to overhead costs, the expense of operating the actual business of private practice. Overhead costs may create a major drain on financial resources. Yet another major financial issue with which the CNS in private practice must deal is that of retirement planning. Income must be generated for the future as well as for the present.

Although attitudes are changing, conducting a business is often viewed as nonfeminine and especially inappropriate for nurses, since nursing is identified by the public as a service profession. While some peers may view the CNS going into private practice as one who is courageous, is able to take risks, is self-confident, and has a strong belief in one's ability to provide a high level of nursing care, others may criticize the nurse for having become "corrupted" by business concerns and thus being less true to nursing (Powell, 1984). As more CNSs establish and maintain private practices, this attitude on the part of both the public and other professionals will gradually change.

## PRACTICAL STRATEGIES FOR ESTABLISHING A PRIVATE PRACTICE

Paving the way for opening private practice often proves to be as important as the practice itself in achieving success. Advance planning provides a framework for determining the philosophy, goals, and expected outcomes of the practice. Careful planning can greatly contribute to the success of the practice, whereas inadequate planning can jeopardize that success (Holmes, 1985). Potential problems inherent in such a venture can be anticipated, addressed, and constructively solved before launching the practice. CNSs who are considering opening a private practice should undertake a sequence of steps, including self-assessment, market analysis, establishing a business plan, and building a network of consultants, such as lawyers, accountants, bankers, fellow entrepreneurs, and nursing executives. If the CNS decides to proceed, the data collected and resources identified can be used to accelerate implementation of the actual practice.

### Self-Assessment

Although CNSs possess qualifications and clinical skills essential to establishing a private practice, these are not sufficient. Stepping into the enterprise of private practice requires a careful blending of personal and professional talents as well as clinical and managerial skills. To best determine one's entrepreneurial talents, many self-assessment techniques are available.

The values grid (Simon, et al., 1972), or valuing process, can help clarify the personal motivating forces of the nurse. With the prospect of making such a major decision, Simon and his colleagues pose some very insightful questions. Taylor (1982) developed a table of entrepreneurial personality characteristics and role requirements which can be used as a check list for self-assessment. Vogel and Doleysh (1988) outline a process of entrepreneurial self-discovery and self-assessment, including an inventory of the CNS's business and management skills. Scott (1984) also developed a six-step career planning model that suggests a systematic review of one's personal and professional profile as a background for possible career decisions. It can be helpful to complete this process with the assistance of a colleague or consultant or to attend a seminar especially focused on career shifts.

General questions that can be helpful in exploring and identifying areas of personal nursing expertise and interests are identified in Table 21–1. The answers to these questions can serve to focus one's thoughts about potential services to be offered in a private practice. The nurse should determine *why* entry into private practice is desired. An examination of motive might yield interesting results. The wish to escape from an unsatisfying or frustrating work situation might mean simply that obtaining another job is in order (Graham, 1987). High motivation and determination are essential for riding out the rough period of establishing the practice (Graham, 1987).

A careful analysis of past achievements should be done to help assess one's aptitude toward managing a successful private practice. In 1984 Max completed a study that examined the characteristics of self-employed nurses (not necessarily CNSs). Results showed that of the 237 participants, most had completed their education at the master's or doctoral levels and belonged to their professional organization, the American Nurses' Association. They expressed altruistic motives for setting up their practices or businesses and had assumed much responsibility for the practice or business.

Additional characteristics that experience has shown to be of importance include effective communication and interpersonal skills, the ability to be self-directed and work well under stress, the ability to negotiate, ego strength (the phone will ring again!), flexibility, and a willingness to take risks. Specific skills such as typing or basic bookkeep-

**TABLE 21–1. Self-Assessment: Areas of Interest and Clinical Expertise**

- What nursing activities give me satisfaction?
- What nursing activities give me the least satisfaction and should therefore be avoided?
- What do I do well as a nursing expert?
- How well known am I in the health care community where I am interested in opening a private practice?
- Have my teaching and publication activities lent credibility to my professed expertise in the area in which I wish to offer nursing services?
- Would private practice in this specialty help me to achieve my long-range nursing career goals?
- What community health care needs am I interested in satisfying through services offered by my practice?

ing are useful but not absolutely necessary since one can contract for these services.

An analysis of personal resources such as time and energy should also be undertaken. The question of part-time versus full-time involvement in the initial development of the practice might best be answered by considering these as well as other personal resources, such as financial capabilities and degree of commitment to the idea of private practice. Other self-posed questions regarding these issues can be found in Table 21–2. These questions should be asked before opening a private practice. It can be very discouraging to find that such resources are not available once the practice is opened.

Whatever the method or process used for self-evaluation prior to undertaking private practice, it must be tempered with the knowledge that only the individual can fully appreciate and understand the ramifications of the questions and issues. Once this process of self-assessment is completed and internal and/or individual capabilities and characteristics have been examined, the next step is to look at external or market forces that will promote successful practice.

## Identifying the Market

A market assessment to identify potential consumers, their needs, and their ability to pay for the services should be undertaken. Such an analysis can be contracted out or performed by the CNS.

Usually, completion of a very comprehensive and readily applicable market analysis demands the services of a marketing expert. However, the costs of hiring such a professional are expensive and must be considered. Many CNSs will not have the necessary capital initially; instead, utilizing a marketing specialist as a periodic consultant will generally cost less and will possibly provide the CNS with valuable suggestions on how to proceed. In addition, a marketing consultant can provide suggestions for developing a business image, contacting the media regarding the new practice, and maintaining public relations once the practice is established. Local banks or other financial institu-

**TABLE 21–2. Self-Assessment: Personal Resources**

- Would it be appropriate to begin the practice on a part-time basis while maintaining a salary and other benefits of having part-time employment elsewhere?
- Is enough money available to meet personal obligations, i.e., living expenses, until the practice becomes self-supporting?
- Is there a support system among family and friends which will allow me to expend the necessary time and energy required in the practice while possibly reducing the time and energy I can give to these important people?

tions as well as major hospitals can usually recommend marketing specialists for the CNS to contact.

Other sources of information can be obtained from the local city planning office and/or the chamber of commerce. Government librarians or the business research bureau of a local university could assist the CNS in using United States census and other government data. The Small Business Administration can provide information on the practical business use of government statistics (Brannen, 1981). Many books and publications are available to assist the small business newcomer in assessing a particular market potential.

A market analysis not only should yield demographic data about the population of an area but also should reveal the local attitudes toward health care and which services the community will utilize (Simms, 1982). Income levels among the population to be served by the practice must be identified along with potential sources of reimbursement. These data help the CNS to determine if the client base in the community is adequate enough to support the practice (Dalton, 1985).

Prospective clients and potential referral sources should be interviewed to assist in identifying what services are already being provided in the community or potential market. If it is determined that the services that the CNS wants to offer are already provided in sufficient quantity or are simply not needed, perhaps the services can be provided with a different focus, to a different population, or in a different locale. Exploring these options may diminish the chance of duplication and may reduce the potential for competition with other CNSs, NPs, and professionals in the area.

If the market analysis provides data that lead the CNS to decide against going into private practice at the time of inquiry, a later assessment may lead to a different conclusion. Once the market analysis yields positive results, the next step is to obtain legal consultation.

## Legal Consultation

CNSs, whether in private practice, in a hospital, or in other agencies, are usually acutely aware of the fact that their practice must fall within the scope of their particular state's nurse practice act with its rules and regulations governing practice. In private practice, questions are likely to arise which the nurse practice act will not directly answer. The CNS who wants to establish a private practice needs an attorney who is knowledgeable about the state's laws, rules, and regulations that govern both nursing practice (Holmes, 1985) and business structure (Moskowitz & Griffith, 1984). Few attorneys will have the required expertise in both areas of legal practice; therefore, the CNS may need to consult with more than one. The CNS would be well advised to seek such counsel before forming the practice.

Selecting an attorney should be carefully done and can be accomplished in several ways. Contacting the state board of nursing may yield recommendations of several attorneys who have provided legal counsel to that agency and are recognized for their knowledge of the state's statutes governing nursing practice. Other nurses who have formed successful private practices might also know attorneys to recommend. Schools of nursing are often aware of local attorneys who can provide the counsel needed. Physicians have long dealt with the question of corporate versus other forms of business organization for their private practices. Seeking recommendations from a trusted physician colleague could prove beneficial. Local banks and accountants who provide services to private professional practice entities are frequently aware of attorneys whose practices are focused on business rather than other specialty areas. Finally, conducting interviews with several of the recommended attorneys, usually at no cost to the CNS, will help the CNS determine which one to choose for legal assistance.

One of the first tasks for the attorney is to review the written purpose of the practice to determine consistency with scope of practice within the state. A responsible attorney will then instruct the CNS in the various forms of organization or business structure available and will provide assistance in determining what is best for the private practice. Tax and liability issues are major factors utilized in deciding what form the business will take. The four most common business forms available to nurses in private practice are the sole proprietorship, the partnership, the corporation, and the Subchapter S corporation (Gardner, Gardner, and Moore, 1984). The Tax Reform Act of 1986 directly changed the tax liabilities and fiscal concerns of each form of business, but careful review of the advantages, disadvantages, and legal consequences of each entity balanced against the CNS's resources and expectations of the private practice enterprise should clarify the direction needed. An accountant with expertise in professional businesses and tax planning can be very helpful to both the CNS and the attorney at this juncture in the planning process.

## Financial Consultation

Consulting with a certified public accountant during the formative stages of private practice is well worth the investment of time and money. The accountant can provide sound objective guidance in the areas of tax planning and business structure, as well as bookkeeping responsibilities and necessary communication with local, state, and federal agencies. The investment capital required to get the business started and an approximation of the amount of cash flow required for steady operation of the business should be discussed with the accountant.

CNSs wanting to establish a private practice often must overcome the disadvantage of having inadequate business knowledge (Powell, 1984; Diehl, 1986). Basic bookkeeping, accounting practices, billing procedures, completing complex insurance forms, negotiating contracts, establishing fees, obtaining business credit, or signing an office lease agreement may sound threatening initially. The business concerns of running an office are indeed different from the professional concerns to which the CNS is accustomed; however, resources are available for increasing one's knowledge and skill in these areas. It is highly recommended that the CNS seek out an accountant who is willing to work with and instruct the CNS in day-to-day tasks required by the business end of the operation, rather than an accountant who wishes to simply do the bookkeeping (Keller, 1975). This can save a great deal of money over time and will allow the CNS to have an ongoing appreciation of the costs involved in maintaining the practice.

Many accountants work closely with their client's attorney in an effort to provide a coordinated service that gives the mutual client a more efficiently run business. Again, some of the same suggestions offered for finding an attorney hold true for finding an accountant. It may be helpful to ask for recommendations for accountants when interviewing each attorney. The advantage would be that the accountant and attorney usually know each other already and have developed a working relationship.

Other resources are available to CNSs who want to develop a better understanding of business thinking and structure. Contacting the local Small Business Administration and/or community colleges should yield a list of courses or workshops in basic business skills. The Small Business Administration also offers free brochures on many subjects pertaining to establishing and maintaining a business. In some communities, an active Service Corps of Retired Executives (SCORE) provides consultants in office management and other areas of expertise who will assist in setting up the business and designing office systems (Diehl, 1986). Daily operation of the private practice can be guided by an overall business plan, and these resources can be very helpful in developing this document.

### The Business Plan

In the entrepreneurial game, Taylor believed that planning is the key to winning (1982). Realistic, concrete planning is the next step for the CNS to take, developing the ideas and thoughts about the business of the private practice in writing. Vogel and Doleysh (1988) offer practical, detailed worksheets to assist the CNS in generating this written document, called the business plan. It is an important step in that it allows the CNS to test the concept of the practice and plan effectively for its introduction (Newman, 1987).

The business plan for the practice is a statement of information about the business and its long-range future. Initially, the plan should cover at least three to five years of operation with evaluation of the business scheduled regularly. Professional as well as financial goals, both short- and long-range, are stated in the plan, with time lines established for measuring progress (Taylor, 1982). Goals keep the CNS focused and reduce the likelihood of becoming disorganized (Newman, 1987). CNSs are familiar with this phase of planning, although admittedly not as familiar with certain portions of the content that need to be considered.

The business plan requires a realistic and practical look at the business of the private practice. It includes an itemization of capital needed for start-up costs and a projection of profits and/or losses anticipated (Dickerson & Nash, 1985). An assessment of available resources is made, including potential funding sources and a personal financial statement. Business strategies, including marketing plans for promotion of the practice, are also usually outlined. A well-designed business plan can provide the information needed to secure loans for financing the private practice endeavor (Dickerson & Nash, 1985).

In the beginning, the process of developing the business plan may be a rather painful experience for the CNS, since it requires reflective thinking and more self-analysis (Taylor, 1982). An accountant or a business consultant can provide assistance in developing the actual plan, since such professionals are generally more aware of overall business needs and can ask questions to stimulate the CNS's thinking about the different variables. A good business plan, while perhaps difficult in the construction phase, can form a solid base from which the practice routinely operates, thereby allowing the CNS's energy to be concentrated on the crises that will inevitably arise and greatly improving the chances for the practice to succeed (Newman, 1987).

Four areas of the business plan deserve particular consideration, as they form the basis for day-to-day financial operation of the practice and allow the CNS to realize profit. These four areas are: anticipating overhead, establishing fees, identifying reimbursement sources, and devising a budget.

*Anticipating Overhead*

Overhead is the expense of setting up and maintaining the office. Capital is needed in the early stages to cover these expenses, as well as provide for salaries, until a profit can be realized from the business. Depending on the amount of overhead experienced and the amount of income generated, it has been estimated that it can take at least a year (and probably longer) for the business to stabilize and show a profit.

Overhead includes routine costs sustained by the office, such as rent, utilities, telephone charges, postage, and supplies, as well as depreciation on equipment, furniture, a vehicle, or other large purchases. Repayment of a loan acquired to meet initial expenses of starting the business might be a part ot the monthly calculated overhead. Also included are the expenses incurred in utilizing other professionals, such as an attorney, an accountant, a management consultant, or a marketing firm. CNSs who work out of home and who see clients in their homes might find that the most significant start-up costs are incurred in the purchase of business cards and stationery or in the operation of a vehicle for home visits.

Consideration must be given to the potential need for office support personnel such as an office manager, bookkeeper, secretary, or receptionist. This will depend mainly on the anticipated size of the practice. Providing salaries and fringe benefits for office personnel can represent a substantial expense, and the cost of hiring such personnel may not be feasible or necessary initially. While potential clients must know they can reach the CNS quickly and easily, utilizing a local telephone answering service or simply a telephone answering machine may be sufficient during the CNS's absence from the office.

Another financial concern is insurance coverage: health, disability, dental, life, and malpractice. It is a well known fact that costs for these benefits can rise significantly when purchased outside group membership policies. Also, as noted in *The American Nurse* in 1986, malpractice insurance rates for self-employed nurses tend to be somewhat higher than for the nurse who is a salaried employee (ANA, 1986a). Another type of insurance to be considered in overall costs is insurance for the business, covering the business property and legal liability secondary to bodily injury, property damage, or personal injury incurred by someone on the business premises.

An underestimation of working capital requirements can result in failure of the practice. Therefore, anticipated overhead must be carefully assessed and pro-rated into the fee structure along with other considerations (Pearson, 1984).

*Establishing Fees*

Establishing fees for service can be an emotional hurdle for some CNSs to overcome. It is one thing to negotiate within the limits of an identified salary range for a particular position in a hospital or other agency; it is quite another to decide how much will be charged for services rendered as an independent contractor. There is a tendency among CNSs to undervalue the services they can and do provide (Vogel & Doleysh, 1988). What has become somewhat routine and appears relatively simple to the expert practitioner can seem to be of little importance when considering its monetary value as a service offered for a fee. A change of attitude may be needed before the CNS can indicate to a prospective client, clearly and without hesitation, what the established fees are. Certainly, this becomes easier the first time fees are charged and received.

Many different factors must be considered in establishing fees, not the least of which is time. In the business world, the axiom that "time is money" holds true. It indeed takes time to render any service. When the CNS sees patients in an office situation, fees may be established on a per visit basis or may be based on the anticipated time involved in performing various functions, e.g., an initial visit involving a complete physical examination versus a return visit for follow-up of a minor problem. The cost for supplies involved in a particular activity, such as obtaining a Pap smear, might be added to the basic visit fee. Patients seeking direct care from the CNS are usually familiar with this type of fee schedule because it is commonly used by other professional health care providers. Generally when such services are being provided within a particular community, it is helpful to determine the recognized "going rate" in that community for the services being offered (Woodward, 1984)—information obtained as an outcome of the market analysis. As more CNSs develop and maintain financially successful private practices, they can become a valuable resource for other nurses new to this task.

For some services, e.g., consultation provided to a home health agency to set up a nursing care plan for a particular patient, fees may be charged on an hourly basis or the CNS might contract with the agency on a retainer basis when frequent use of services is anticipated. The fee for an educational program to be given at a particular facility may be established on a project basis, including the anticipated time involved in preparation and charges incurred in photocopying hand-outs, rental of films, or other materials and travel expenses involved.

The CNS who provides consultation as an expert witness in legal situations will usually charge for services on an hourly basis, including time spent in medical records review, patient evaluation, report completion, conferences with the attorney, and/or other appropriate activities, plus reimbursement of expenses incurred. Since it is difficult for the attorney to schedule courtroom and deposition testimony dates far in advance, a contract to be available for testifying might require that the CNS maintain a flexible calendar and be able to testify on relatively short notice. Therefore, it is generally considered appropriate to charge more for time spent in these testifying activities. Reimbursement for services should never be allowed on a contingency basis, based on the outcome of the legal suit, since this can present a conflict of interest issue for the CNS.

Determining appropriate charges for selected activities, whether as a direct caregiver or a consultant, is but one facet of establishing the fee structure. Consideration must also be given to the potential sources of reimbursement.

### Reimbursement Issues

Organizational entities, such as hospitals, nursing care agencies, and educational institutions, who utilize the CNS as a consultant may have predetermined fixed rates they will pay for those services, and the specialist may have little latitude for negotiating anything different. Then it becomes necessary for the specialist to decide whether or not the service can be offered profitably within that rate structure.

In direct patient care practices, reimbursement for nursing services rendered becomes a major issue and has been identified as the single most limiting factor to establishing more private nursing practices (Holmes, 1985; Felder, 1983). Consumers have occasionally been required to pay out-of-pocket for health care services, and certainly some private nursing practices have survived under this form of payment (Dickerson & Nash, 1985). However, health care in the United States is more typically paid for through the third-party reimbursement system. The consumer in the third-party reimbursement system participates in a prepaid health insurance or government assistance program. When a provider renders a service to the consumer covered by such a program, the program pays the provider what is usually a predetermined amount for that particular service. In most states, laws governing health insurance do not include provisions for nurses to receive payment for their services through the third-party reimbursement system (LaBar, 1986). State statutes relevant to the community in which the CNS wishes to establish private practice should be carefully consulted when one is establishing fees and determining the potential for third-party reimbursement. The state's board of nursing and nursing organizations can be contacted for the latest developments relevant to that particular state.

However, in some situations, without benefit of state laws supporting third-party reimbursement, nurses have negotiated directly with insurance carriers and have received payment for their services. Other nurses have suggested that their clients submit statements to the insurance carrier for reimbursement even when they know it will be denied, thereby at the very least letting third-party payers know that direct nursing services are being utilized by the public (Dickerson & Nash, 1985).

Federal legislation has done little to improve the general reimbursement picture for nurses, even though mandates for third-party payment have been legislated through certain government sponsored programs, such as in the care of Medicaid and Medicare recipients (LaBar, 1986). The United States Department of Defense provides a medical benefits program called the Civilian Health and Medical Program of the Uniformed Services (CHAMPUS), which directly pays fees for services to three groups of nurses: certified nurse midwives, certified nurse practitioners, and certified psychiatric nurses (LaBar, 1986). For many certified psychiatric and mental health CNSs, benefits to those insured by CHAMPUS have made a significant difference in the specialists' financial ability to provide services through a private practice. This further demonstrates the need for direct third-party reimbursement from privately sponsored programs.

The question of third-party reimbursement is likely to be an issue for years to come, given the number and variety of parties interested in the outcome. The ability to negotiate for direct payment, coupled with creativity and flexibility in payment expectations, is currently the best tool the CNS has for dealing with the question of reimbursement on a regular basis.

### Devising a Budget

In developing a business plan, the final step, and one of the most significant, is devising the budget. Budgeting focuses on the tactical element of the business (Porter-O'Grady, 1979) and addresses the detailed allocation of financial resources in daily operation of the enterprise over a certain period of time, usually one year (Mark & Smith, 1987). According to Mark and Smith, the planning that has occurred to this point would be called strategic planning and includes developing the mission of the private practice, outlining the goals and objectives, and assessing the resources. Allocation of these resources represents a budget based on management priorities, designed to reflect and support the strategic planning component.

Operating and cash flow budgets are very detailed and form a basis for decision-making regarding expenditures. Maintaining adequate cash flow—the timing of cash coming into the business balanced with cash being paid out—is a necessity if the business is to survive; and budgeting identifies how this is to occur. If budgeting is unsuccessful, Mark and Smith emphasize that the achievement of long-range plans is dubious.

A reasonable and realistic budget—one that allows the CNS to also realize profit—should be designed. Profit, that portion of the income received in excess of expenses paid, is both a reward and an incentive for continuing the business of a private practice. It compensates the CNS for the risks taken in establishing the practice and for relying upon expertise and skill in generating and maintaining clients (Pearson, 1984).

## Choosing Suitable Facilities

Depending upon the clientele and practice specialty, the need for space and/or office facilities is determined. For the solo practitioner, a small single office space may be sufficient; for CNSs in a group practice, possibly several examining rooms would be required. CNSs who see patients in group therapy and/or patient teaching groups should consider a setting that allows several patients to be present simultaneously. Local laws in some communities require offices, as well as restrooms and parking, to be wheelchair-accessible. The CNS who plans to see patients with disabilities might also wish to utilize examination tables that could be raised for ease of the CNS examiner and lowered for wheelchair transfers. Providing a waiting room for clients will add extra space requirements. The need for workspace for other office personnel, such as a secretary or a receptionist, must also be considered.

A realistic assessment of space requirements includes decisions on furniture and office machinery to be used (Wright, 1981). Desks and chairs, waiting room seating, examination tables, computers and printers, data retrieval systems, file cabinets for record storage, photocopy and dictation equipment, typewriters, and the need for storage of supplies will affect the amount and kind of space required.

In anticipation that the practice will expand over time, consideration must also be given to furture space needs (Dalton, 1985). Other CNSs might possibly be invited to join the practice. Record storage will likely increase as the practice grows. A typewriter may be sufficient in the beginning of the practice, but word processing capabilities may be required as the practice expands or changes.

Office location must be given consideration. Factors influencing location include expense, locale, age of the building, and whether to buy or lease space. Also to be considered is proximity to patients' homes and places of business, access to public transportation routes, and desired proximity to other support services such as a pharmacy (Dalton, 1985). Closeness to other health care providers, such as physicians, NPs, physical therapists, or other health care agencies, may be helpful in increasing the potential for referrals and may possibly allow for greater ease of mutual consultation.

## Promoting the Practice

Identifying potential clients for the practice was a key issue in completing the market analysis earlier; the next step is letting clients know what services the CNS offers, how they can be obtained, when and where they will be provided, and how much they will cost. Serious attention must be given to the issue of attracting clients. Durham and Hardin (1983) believe that promoting the private nursing practice is essential to success in today's competitive market.

Consumers have an ever-increasing number of health care resources with whom they can directly negotiate for services. Competition is keen for the health care dollar, and one potentially serious drawback for CNSs setting up private practice is the public's image of nursing and an overall confusion about nursing qualifications, responsibilities, and roles. When informed that a CNS is about to open private practice, a public lacking accurate information about CNSs' capabilities might very well question what a nurse has to offer in a private practice separate from a hospital or a physician and even if it is legal to operate such a practice. Questions such as these would not engender trust or foster the likelihood of seeking out the CNS's services; both are a necessity if the practice is to succeed. Thus, education of the public is an important thread running through all efforts to promote the practice.

There is another element of concern which must be addressed by some CNSs in the promotion of their practice. These are the nurses who are uncomfortable with the idea of advertising an offered service, seeing this as somewhat unprofessional and self-promoting (Durham & Hardin, 1983). This places the CNS in a bind: how to inform the public while not appearing self-serving. The CNS must overcome this self-defeating attitude. One way to change such an attitude is to think of the services offered as being separate from one's self, or in other words, placing value on the service offered rather than on the person offering it. True, the CNS is the "service" of the business in that it is the CNS's expertise that is the essence of what is being offered. And it is the service that is promoted, not the person. It is important for the CNS to also believe that what is being offered is worthwhile and is making a useful contribution to society (Wilson, 1972). For the CNS to then receive remuneration for the provided service results in a reciprocally beneficial relationship for both parties, an important principle of marketing (Durham & Hardin, 1983).

Promoting the practice can be accomplished in many ways. It is well recognized that satisfied consumers will always be the best form of advertising (Woodward, 1984) and an important source of referrals. However, information about the practice can also be generated and shared with the public more formally while possibly reaching many more potential clients. One method is to inform the media (i.e., newspapers, television, radio) of what the CNS is planning. The media can be very helpful in promoting the practice. Local newspapers usually have columns discussing businesses that are starting up in the community, and they are always looking for new and different ventures to highlight. Sending out a press release has led some CNSs to be invited guests on local television and radio talk shows at which they were interviewed about the role of nursing in society, the laws that allowed them to open a private practice, what their practice entails, what problems or concerns might lead the public to seek their services, and other particulars such as hours of availability.

The CNS might consider attracting clientele through public offerings. Writing a newspaper article or holding a public workshop on some aspect of health care relevant to the CNS's practice can draw much attention to the services offered. For example, the CNS might give a workshop on the premenstrual tension syndrome and follow up with the offer of a free counseling session for any woman who attended the workshop, thereby providing a public service and attracting clientele at the same time. Or the CNS establishing a practice focused on counseling adolescents might contact career counselors at local high schools, explain their services to the counselors, and volunteer to discuss nursing career opportunities with students at a class seminar or on a "career day," again offering a public service and becoming visible to potential clients.

Almost anything and everything the CNS does professionally represents the practice and has the potential for enlarging the professional support network and attracting referrals. Presentations at professional workshops and conferences, as well as publishing in the professional literature, speak to the level of expertise and keep the CNS's name in mind. Making appointments to meet with other professionals in the local area to inform them of the CNS's practice and to discuss the differences in services offered by each can serve to decrease feelings of threat and potential competition while leading to the possibility of referrals. Reciprocal referrals to these same professionals will further enhance the visibility of the CNS and potentially lead to new business.

Printed information that can be distributed at appropriate places and times are helpful reminders of the practice. Information that presents a professional image, qualifications, services, and other such information can be printed in the form of a brochure or flyer and distributed appropriately. Business cards exchanged at professional meetings, given to colleagues, and/or enclosed with mailed brochures or flyers become a reference in the future for those who wish to contact the CNS or refer others to the practice.

## Expanding the Professional Support Network

As was noted in the discussion about the risks involved in establishing a private practice, a reduction in interaction with professional colleagues usually occurs and carries with it the potential for developing a sense of isolation and loneliness. Gorke-Felice (1984) emphasized peer support and involvement as being critical to dealing with this problem. An expanded network can help the CNS maintain perspective during the ups and downs of the practice as well as provide the new private practitioner with resources for problem-solving and decision-making.

Persons and Wieck (1985) viewed networking as a power strategy in relation to its impact on career goals. In this light, activities that establish contact with other professionals, even if social in nature, can become tools for increasing one's power base in private practice.

How does the CNS proceed in attempting to expand the professional support network? Participating in peer review activities, as described by Winch (see Chapter 14), provides support and validation. Many of the activities identified earlier in promoting the practice will lead quite naturally to establishing greater contact with colleagues and peers. Often the individual must then actively seek out further contact and development of the relationship. Following up new contacts with telephone calls, exchange of business cards, and/or planning for a future meeting can be initiated.

The CNS should attempt to find other CNSs who have formed successful private practices and plan for discussion with them regularly, if only by telephone. Forming a group with other CNSs who are starting or who are already in private practice can prove especially helpful to the beginner in allowing for collegial sharing time. Meeting frequently for purposes of sharing business pressures and/or difficulties provides an opportunity to express frustrations and obtain suggestions for problem-solving. Sharing of successes and gaining approval of peers reinforces the CNS's ego strength and helps one to persevere during the rougher periods.

## SUMMARY

Entering the adventure of private practice requires effort well worth the risks involved. CNSs are succeeding in this entrepreneurial endeavor in many states and in various clinical fields. Others have failed, usually for a number of reasons addressed directly and indirectly throughout this chapter. Experience has shown that a fundamental requirement of a successful practice is balancing creative initiative with self-discipline. Success is measured in many ways. While income may remain comparable with the income of CNSs in other employment settings, as reported in the 1984 ANA survey, CNSs in private practice also tend to report high job satisfaction (ANA, 1986b). This is one of the payoffs for devoting the extraordinary time, effort, and energy required to develop the practice.

With success comes new challenges. Maintaining a successful private practice is a demanding, exciting, and dynamic process; the practice must constantly change and evolve to meet new challenges.

*References*

Albrecht, K., & Zemke, R.: Service America! Doing Business in the New Economy. Homewood, IL, Dow Jones-Irwin, 1985.
American Nurses' Association: ANA Contracts for New RN Liability Insurance Programs. Kansas City, American Nurses' Association, 1986a.
American Nurses' Association: Clinical Nurse Specialists—Distribution and Utilization. Kansas City, American Nurses' Association, 1986b.
American Nurses' Association: Nursing—A Social Policy Statement. Kansas City, American Nurses' Association, 1980.
Aronson, J. D., & Cowhey, P. F.: Trade in Services—A Case for Open Markets. Washington, DC, American Enterprise Institute for Public Policy Research, 1984.
Brannen, W. H.: Practical Marketing for Your Small Retail Business. Englewood Cliffs, NJ, Prentice-Hall, 1981.
Dalton, J. B.: Guide to private practice office planning. Nurs Pract 10(5):43–56, 1985.
Dickerson, P. S., & Nash, B. A.: The business of nursing: Development of a private practice. Nurs Health Care 6(6):326–329, 1985.
Diehl, D. H.: Private practice—out on a limb and loving it. Am J Nurs 86(8):907–909, 1986.
Durham, J. D., & Hardin, S. B.: Promoting private practice in a competitive market. Nurs Econ 1(4):24–28, 1983.
Felder, L. A.: Direct patient care and independent practice. In Hamric, A. B., & Spross, J. (eds): The Clinical Nurse Specialist in Theory and Practice. New York, Grune and Stratton, 1983, pp. 59–71.
Gardner, J. C., Gardner, K. L., and Moore, V. M.: Tax factors and choice of business forms for nurses. Nurs Econ 2(4):250–257, 1984.
Gorke-Felice, M. B.: Practitioner/proprietor. Pediatr Nurs 10(1):67–69, 1984.
Graham, J.: Pre-entrepreneuring. Sylvia Porter's Personal Finance 5(2):57–62, 1987.

Hoeffer, B.: The private practice model: An ethical perspective. J Psychosocial Nurs Mental Health Serv *21*(7):31–37, 1983.

Holmes, B. C.: Private practice in oncology nursing. Oncol Nurs Forum *21*(3):65–67, 1985.

Jacox, A. K., & Norris, C. M.: Organizing for Independent Nursing Practice. New York, Appleton-Century-Crofts, 1977.

Keller, N. S.: The why's and what's of private practice. J Nurs Admin *5*(3):12–15, 1975.

Kerfoot, K.: Hanging out a shingle: The joys and sorrows of private practice. *In* Lynch, M. L. (ed): On Your Own: Professional Growth Through Independent Nursing Practice. Monterey, CA, Wadsworth Health Sciences Division, 1982, pp. 116–125.

Kinlein, M. L.: Independent Nursing Practice with Clients. Philadelphia, J. B. Lippincott Company, 1977.

LaBar, C.: Third party reimbursement for services of nurses. *In* Mezey, D. M., and McGivern, D. O. (eds): Nurses, Nurse Practitioners—The Evolution of Primary Care. Boston, Little, Brown and Company, 1986, pp. 450–470.

Mark, B. A., & Smith, H. L.: Essentials of Finance in Nursing. Rockville, MD, Aspen Publishers, 1987.

Max, S.: Personal communication, February 1984.

Menard, S. W.: Possibilities and predictions. *In* Menard, S. W. (ed): The Clinical Nurse Specialist—Perspectives on Practice. New York, John Wiley & Sons, 1987.

Moskowitz, L. D., & Griffith, S.: To incorporate or not to incorporate. Nurs Econ *2*(4):246–249, 1984.

Newman, J.: Risk-taking—the entrepreneur's handbook. Bostonia *61*(4):40–41, 1987.

Norris, M. K.: Other options: Super opportunities outside the hospital—in independent practice. Nurs Life *2*(3):45–49, 1982.

Pearson, L. E.: Self-employment income: Professional fees and tax considerations. Nurs Econ *2*(1):52–56, 1984.

Persons, C. B., & Wieck, L.: Networking: A power strategy. Nurs Econ *3*(1):53–57, 1985.

Peters, T. J., & Waterman, R. H.: In Search of Excellence. New York, Warner Books, 1982.

Porter-O'Grady, T.: Financial planning: Budgeting for nursing, part I. Supervisor Nurs *10*(8):35–38, 1979.

Powell, D. J.: Nurses—"high touch" entrepreneurs. Nurs Econ *2*(1):33–36, 1984.

Riccardi, B. R.: You: The nurse entrepreneur. *In* Riccardi, B. R., and Dayani, E. C. (eds): The Nurse Entrepreneur. Reston, VA, Reston, 1982, pp. 5–8.

Scott, P. P.: Executive career planning. Nurs Econ *2*(1):58–63, 1984.

Simon, S. B., Howe, L. W., and Kirschenbaum, H.: Values Clarification. New York, Hart, 1972.

Simms, E.: How to start a private practice. *In* Lynch, M. L. (ed): On Your Own: Professional Growth Through Independent Nursing Practice. Monterey, CA, Wadsworth Health Sciences Division, 1982, pp. 2–28.

Stanback, T. M.: Understanding the Service Economy—Employment, Productivity, Location. Baltimore, The Johns Hopkins University Press, 1979.

Standard & Poor's: Industry Surveys. April 16, 1987 (Section 4).

Taylor, C.: The business ownership game. *In* Riccardi, B. R., and Dayani, E. C. (eds): The Nurse Entrepreneur. Reston, VA, Reston, 1982, pp. 17–29.

Vogel, G., and Doleysh, N.: Entrepreneuring—A Nurse's Guide to Starting a Business. New York, National League for Nursing, 1988.

Wiener, S. M.: Rehabilitation nursing in the private sector. Rehabil Nurs *8*(2):31–32, 1983.

Wilson, A.: The Marketing of Professional Services. London, McGraw-Hill, 1972.

Woodward, J. A.: The private practice nurse practitioner. J Obstet Gynecol Neonatal Nurs (Supplement) *13*(2):97s–100s, 1984.

Wright, B. L.: An independent practice setting. Can Nurs *77*(2):34–36, 1981.

# INDEX

Note: Page numbers in *italics* refer to illustrations; page numbers followed by (t) indicate tables.